CONTENTS

Encyclopedia of Birth Control

Marian Rengel

Oryx Press
2000

The rare Arabian Oryx is believed to have inspired the myth of the unicorn. This desert antelope became virtually extinct in the early 1960s. At that time, several groups of international conservationists arranged to have nine animals sent to the Phoenix Zoo to be the nucleus of a captive breeding herd. Today, the Oryx population is over 1,000, and over 500 have been returned to the Middle East.

Published by The Oryx Press
4041 North Central at Indian School Road
Phoenix, Arizona 85012-3397
www.oryxpress.com

Published simultaneously in Canada
Printed and bound in the United States of America

∞ The paper used in this publication meets the minimum requirements of American National Standard for Information Science—Permanence of Paper for Printed Library Materials, ANSI Z39.48, 1984.

Library of Congress Cataloging-in-Publication Data

Rengel, Marian.
Encyclopedia of birth control / Marian Rengel.
p. cm.
ISBN 1-57356-255-6 (alk. paper)
1. Birth control—Dictionaries I. Title.
HQ766.R442 2000
363.9'6'03—dc21

00-009598
CIP

PREFACE

Birth control: The phrase is a common one in modern society. To many it means preventing pregnancy. To others it means preventing birth. Virtually everyone in the world has heard the phrase, and has at least a vague understanding of its meaning. In economically and medically advanced societies people generally regard the ability to choose when to allow sexual intercourse to lead to pregnancy as a natural part of adulthood. In less economically developed countries, people see "birth control" as a possible choice they may or may not have, or they may see birth control as contrary to the expectations of adulthood. Despite such common familiarity with the phrase "birth control," reproductive health professionals, social scientists, demographers, and non-professionals alike find that individuals have inadequate understandings of the complexities of the biology, chemistry, sociology, politics, culture, and law that surround the role of birth control, contraception, and even abortion in their lives. Personal, cultural, and medical beliefs and expectations intertwine to make birth control a complex and intimate part of a person's reproductive life.

The *Encyclopedia of Birth Control* brings together in more than 200 entries, arranged in A-to-Z format, a portrait of the complex modern issue that birth control has become with advances in medicine and biochemistry of the twentieth century. Specifically, this book will help people gain a preliminary understanding of many of the issues surrounding birth control as they prepare to do more in-depth research on a specific topic. It will serve well students beginning their work on either the science or sociology of family planning, but will also serve well people seeking answers to questions of the medicine of contraception and to questions of the role of birth control in many societies. The book is aimed at both the student and the consumer of birth control.

The book presents entries on basic reproductive biology, information which summarizes the human physiology of reproduction. The material here was drawn primarily from recent physiology texts which offer people clear explanations of how their bodies function as biological processes. Among those texts are the sixth edition of John Hole's *Human Anatomy and Physiology* (1993), the fifth edition of *Anatomy and Physiology* by Rod Seeley, Trent Stephens, and Philip Tate (2000), and the fourth edition of *Anatomy and Physiology* by Gary Thibodeau and Kevin Patton (2000). Also of value as further reading are home medical guides such as the *Merck Manual of Medical Information.*

From the basics of physiology, the book moves on to present entries on the methods of preventing or interrupting a pregnancy, from the ancient act of withdrawal to the ubiquitous birth control pill and the non-chemical fertility awareness methods of contraception. Entries also examine the future of birth control methods and the choices users of birth control may expect into the twenty-first century.

Biographical entries tell the stories of the inventors of major forms of contraception and those people who struggled to make birth control acceptable to the public. While many people worked during the nineteenth and twentieth centuries to bring the topics of pregnancy, population, and birth into the realm of public discussion, some, such as Margaret Sanger, an American nurse, and Aletta Jacobs, a Dutch doctor, struggled more publicly and became leaders of a social movement that would change attitudes toward family planning around the world. In a similar way, some inventors, such as John Rock and Etienne-Emile Baulieu, played more public roles in securing public access to their family planning methods than did other inventors. The prominent roles these people played in the story of birth control qualified them to be part of this *Encyclopedia*.

The prominent laws and legal cases that surrounded the birth control movement, primarily U.S. laws, also earned attention in this *Encyclopedia* and serve as examples of the legal struggles that many other nations experienced as the birth control movement traveled around the globe.

Entries on a sampling of countries and regions explore how individual nations and their people and governments experienced the increasing world demand for family planning methods. Those chosen for entries here represent nations where contraception has become an expected part of adult life, for example, the nations of western Europe, and nations where birth control is a matter of strong social and governmental concern, particularly the nations of China and India. Every nation has a birth control story to tell, but the nations included in this *Encyclopedia* have stories for which readers will readily find additional research to further their learning.

All entries except a few on the basic biology conclude with "Further reading" listings, which guide readers to selected books, journal articles, Web sites, and other research materials on each topic. Cross-references in each entry point to further discussion of the topic elsewhere in the book.

Illustrations, photographs, and charts help readers capture at a glance the nature of birth control devices and methods, and to understand in visual forms some of the complex issues surrounding a person's choice of birth control, or a nation's efforts to bring modern birth control methods to their people. The charts included in the *Encyclopedia* illustrate birth control use statistics and fertility patterns for a variety of nations and a variety of devices. The data used to form these charts came primarily from databases provided to the public by the U. S. Census Bureau and the Alan Guttmacher Institute. The author compiled the charts from this data, as well as from data included in Census Bureau reports.

A bibliography and a subject index follow the *Encyclopedia*. In addition, a list of topics covered is provided in the front of the book to enable the user to quickly access areas of interest.

Family planning is a rapidly changing aspect of adult life, with inventions, product development, and scientific discoveries occurring almost daily. In fact, as the book was in print organizations around the world were making decisions on contraceptive availability, emergency contraception policy, and the safety of new products seeking a place in markets around the world. Organizations and people were leading efforts to bring greater reproductive freedom to more people and to ensure prevent sexual intercourse from leading to pregnancy came to be of such common social awareness. The history of birth control, covering mainly the twentieth century, though dipping further back in time when the need for making connections arises, illuminates how birth control became, around the world, an important aspect of a person's reproductive life.

This *Encyclopedia* brings together in one convenient source many, though by no means all, of the aspects surrounding the issue of birth control in contemporary adult life. It explores the personal choices and personal methods of preventing pregnancy and the social significance and social value of providing women and men with the right to determine when and if they have children and with the means to fulfill that choice.

INTRODUCTION

A woman and a man unite during sexual intercourse. Their reasons for coupling can be as varied as the people involved, from love to violence, from the urges of the moment to the fulfillment of the plans of a lifetime. In some acts of intercourse both man and woman feel free to express their sexual emotions, their basic physical desires. Some acts occur as the result of coercion, force, manipulation. Some are a matter of choice on the part of both partners. Some are not. Virtually all such acts between women and men of reproductive age, from about age 12 or 13 to the early 50s for women and well into old age for men, have the potential of leading to reproduction, the conception of a child, a pregnancy.

For many of the more than 6 billion people living on the earth as the calendar turned from 1999 to 2000, separating the expression of sexual desires from child-bearing had become an almost automatic aspect of adult life. Conscious, planned action which these adults took—birth control—eliminated the chance of pregnancy associated with sexual intimacy. For many, but far from all, adults, science, technology, and social progress had granted them the ability to do what humans for eons had tried to do: have sex without having children.

From the earliest days of the understanding of the cause and effect relationship between sexual intercourse and pregnancy, people have sought to disconnect that connection. First they relied upon abstinence, then upon the man withdrawing his penis from the woman's vagina before he released his male seed, or sperm, his half of the biology needed to begin human life. Eventually people turned to natural products to free themselves from the consequence of pregnancy when they engaged in sexual intercourse. They turned, so historians have discovered, to animal skins to use as condoms, to ends of lemons to serve as vaginal barriers. Many tried herbal concoctions taken before and after intercourse to induce menstruation and prevent pregnancy.

When those measures failed, women, who bear the consequences of pregnancy, turned to abortion to end pregnancies they would not or could not continue. Abortion, a highly controversial act and moral issue in the late twentieth and early twenty-first centuries, has long served women and men as an alternative to bearing children they do not want. History also records physical and chemical means of interfering with a pregnancy and records societies' reactions to the act of stopping a pregnancy once it has begun. That reaction has varied from acceptance to abhorrence.

Fertility rates had begun to decline in western Europe and the United States as early as the late 1700s, though scientific understanding of reproduction was slight and contraceptives still primitive. Somehow, historians argue and attempt to explain, families were able to begin to limit the number of children they had without modern contraceptive measures. Families found they could preserve resources and provide a higher quality of life for their children if they had fewer children than their parents had. Some historians point out, as did the activists of the late nineteenth and early twentieth centuries in Europe and the United States, that those declines in the number of children women could expect to have in their lifetimes were not spread equitably across society. Poor women were deprived access to the medical information that wealthy women could afford. Those least able to care for large families had the least access to information to help them prevent pregnancy. The unwillingness of society, even medical doctors, to discuss with women methods for blocking the path of sperm on its way to an egg prevented information from spreading. Doctors, either through ignorance of their own or through an unwillingness to discuss sex with their patients, would often tell women to simply not share a bed with their husbands. In blunt terms, doctors told women not to have sexual intercourse. The options were therefore few for most women: sex or no sex. However, in the human quest for love and emotional nurturance, sex most often prevailed.

With the advent of modern technology as a social force, and with the inventions of the late industrial revolution, humankind began to achieve the long sought-after goal of sexual intercourse without risk of unwanted pregnancy. The innovations that led scientists, businesspeople, and societies to adopt the machine as the means to achieving their goals, the arrival of tools of the machine age, medical answers to the plagues of life, and modern inventiveness brought with them, slowly, the application of modern scientific understanding toward helping to fulfill the desire to separate sexual intercourse from reproduction. The advent of highly effective means to separate this particular cause from this biological effect finally allowed choice concerning when sexual intercourse would result in adding a member to a family.

In the late 1800s and early 1900s, the birth control revolution began.

More than 100 years later, the struggle to bring reproductive choice to all people continued to be a concern for all nations and a significant public issue around the world. In 1994, at the International Conference on Population and Development, in Cairo, Egypt, 179 members of the United Nations reached a consensus that firmly established family planning and reproductive health as basic human rights. What began as a social movement scattered across Europe and North America in the late 1800s became, by the turn of the twenty-first century, a right to which all adults were entitled. The agreement arrived at during the Cairo convention made clear that nations and societies had the obligation to provide individuals with the means to exercise that right. Preventing pregnancy had moved from a personal desire to a fundamental, morally valuable choice that many nations now uphold as essential to being human.

The battle to bring social acceptance and access to modern, highly effective methods of preventing pregnancy began in the late 1800s in western Europe. Many scholars credit Aletta Jacobs (1854–1929), the first female Dutch physician, with creating public awareness of women's need for access to the means to prevent unwanted pregnancy. Others credit the battle for women's rights, particularly the right to vote, as the driving force that would lead to the acceptance of women in medical schools, which in turn would lead to a greater understanding of reproductive health needs. By the early 1900s, women fighting for the rights of their gender engaged directly in the battle to bring the right to choose when to become pregnant to all women. In England, Dr. Marie Stopes, a botanist, and in the United States, Margaret Sanger, a nurse, led the fight to make pregnancy prevention a part of every woman's life—to bring to poor women (who were bringing many unwanted children into their lives of inadequate housing, food, and shelter) what people perceived as the privilege of the wealthy: to bear fewer children, and to bear them when wanted.

The early days of the fight involved far more than providing women with the meager means then available for blocking the path of sperm—an early diaphragm, spermicides, and a rubber condom. It involved fighting with society to make sex, reproduction, and pregnancy acceptable topics for public discussion. The struggle to bring pregnancy prevention into the public domain (focused in Western Europe and North America during the early 1900s) coincided with the struggle for women's rights and the social changes that followed World War I. Although discussing sex, advocating for sexuality education, and even considering the selling of contraceptives was illegal in most industrialized, economically advanced societies, attitudes were changing. War had brought out the real danger of venereal diseases among civilian forces and soldiers. With the U.S. Army distributing condoms to soldiers, many people in society had to admit that the discussion of sex, disease, and pregnancy prevention had moved from the bedroom to the public forum. Historians credit the success of European and American women, fighting in the late 1800s and early 1900s, as the driving force that would lead society to a revolution that in turn would separate sexuality from pregnancy, that would require highly effective, almost certain means of preventing unplanned pregnancies.

The term "birth control" entered the public discussion in 1914 when friends and associates of Margaret Sanger gathered to create an expression that would capture the essence of their objectives—to give women control over pregnancy—without threatening society, as did such phrases as "voluntary motherhood," then popular in the United States and Europe. "Birth control," they felt, would separate in people's minds the act of sexual intercourse from the act of raising children. They sought a term that would separate sex from birth. Controlling the timing of conception gave a woman authority over her body, yet did not threaten her potential or current role as mother. Many advocates of the early birth control movement, however, abhorred abortion. Once conception had occurred, they argued, at least publicly, a woman had a moral obligation to carry the pregnancy to term. Birth control, as they used the phrase, meant controlling birth before conception, not after conception, though the phrase itself does not preclude that option.

In the mid-1900s, as the public became more aware of the availability of reliable pregnancy prevention methods, leaders of the social movement and medical and scientific researchers worked to understand the biology of reproduction in the hopes of devising methods for more effective control of conception. In the early 1930s, scientists began to isolate the steps in the female reproductive system. They discovered the follicles on the ovaries that contained mature eggs. They discovered newly fertilized eggs in uteruses removed during hysterectomies. They discovered hormonal control of the menstrual cycle. Changes in society, with women moving rapidly into the workforce, freed people to discuss sex, to ask questions about preventing pregnancy. The combined forces of people seeking the gratification of sexual expression without risk of pregnancy and of women moving from their nearly exclusive roles as mothers and wives, fueled the scientific research that ultimately lead to what social scientists and historians refer to as the first revolution in birth control.

The development of synthetic imitations of the hormones that control the female reproductive cycle led in 1960 to the development, manufacture, and sale of the hormonal contraceptive pill. "The Pill": women turned to it eagerly, quickly. Throughout the United States and Europe, women sought the new birth control pill to help them achieve their family goals. Sex, for these women, no longer held the great risk of pregnancy. By the mid-1970s, spurred by the success of the pill, biochemists and pharmaceutical companies had developed alternate ways to move the contraceptive hormones into the woman's body. Doctors could either inject the hormones or implant small rods under the woman's skin. Hormonal contraceptives, like no physical barrier had before them, has separated sex from pregnancy. A woman could take a pill every morning and be 99 percent sure, if she accurately followed directions, that sex she may have later in the day would not result in a sperm uniting with an egg.

The birth control revolution brought about by the pill did not universally free women, and men, from unwanted pregnancy. As in earlier days, access to the new highly effective means of birth control became available first in the wealthy nations of the world. In Europe, Canada, and the United States women turned quickly to the new contraceptives. By the 1990s, almost all adults in Sweden, France, Norway, Italy, and Spain had access to modern birth control and effectively used it. In the United States and Canada more than 90 percent of sexually active women used modern birth control methods, particularly hormonal contraceptives and modern surgical sterilization, to limit the number of children to which they gave birth.

By the 1990s, many of the nations of western Africa still had not benefited from easy and convenient access to modern birth control. In Chad, a central African nation, women and men had little if any access to condoms, oral contraceptives, intrauterine devices, female sterilization, or vasectomy. Indeed, people in that nation had had slightly better access to this pool of modern contraceptives in 1982 than they had in 1994. In some nations of Asia—Laos, Cambodia—and South America—Argentina—where access to birth control had spread rapidly in the 1970s and 1980s, people still had very poor access to any modern forms of contraception. As tracked by Population Action International, only 11 nations had excellent access to contraceptives in 1996 and all of them were among the wealthier, economically developed nations of the world. No developed nations, which include the former republics of the Soviet Union, had poor access. In contrast, no developing nations had excellent access to modern contraceptives and 12 nations had very poor access.

An international humanitarian concern with the world's rapidly growing population began to take root in the 1950s. Nonprofit charitable organizations began forming that would set as their goals helping nations achieve access to means of birth control and family planning to slow what were then considered skyrocketing population increases. Developed nations would begin sending money and technical aid to nations to help them create plans for offering birth control to families.

Modern technology and modern medicine had improved the quality of life worldwide, eliminated diseases, prevented infant deaths, and extended the life expectancy of almost all people. Recognizing that declining death rates if not accompanied by declining birth rates could overwhelm a society's ability to care for its people, nations from China and South Korea to Brazil and Mexico developed national programs and often national political policies to support and encourage family planning. Many nations of the developing world turned to the nations of the developed world for money and resources to provide access to modern birth control methods. With the evolution of the 1994 U.N. agreement that access to family planning was a human right, these nations also increased efforts, and in some nations began efforts, to improve the education of women. With education, women often choose for themselves smaller families, not only out of the self-interest of recognizing in themselves the ability to fulfill roles in society other than wife and mother, but also in the interest of improving the quality of life for their children.

From the basic sexual urges of individual human beings to the international global concern with a rapidly growing world population, birth control evolved through the course of the twentieth century from a social movement to a human right. Its name changed—voluntary motherhood, birth control, population control, family planning, reproductive freedom. Its scope changed, from a concern of the individual to the concern of the society to the concern of the planet. In the beginning of the twenty-first century, adults still demand that science and society provide them with the means to plan their families and that demand motivates societies, including those of the developed world, to improve access to contraceptive options.

Recognizing that a woman or couple's successful use of birth control depends upon that woman's personal and emotional needs and on her preference for one method over another, scientists, drug companies, and public health workers are struggling to create the next contraceptive revolution. They are working to find methods of biological contraception as effective as or more effective than injectable or implantable contraceptives, which have success rates of 99.9 percent, but which have fewer side effects and are even easier and more convenient to use than current methods. Researchers are also struggling to discover methods of contraception that allow men to participate more fully in planning families, in controlling the impact of their sperm on the women with whom they have sexual relations.

Throughout the development of contraceptives, gender imbalances in the discovery of methods and the use of those methods have made birth control a woman's issue. While the condom is an increasingly popular form of contraception and disease prevention and its use is rising rapidly around the world, women often find a dependence on men to use condoms to be an ineffective way to protect themselves from pregnancy. Women prefer, according to survey results from many nations and many cultures, methods they can control or male methods that make the man temporarily infertile, as the pill makes women. Such male contraceptives, which would incapacitate sperm but not men, are under study around the world by such organizations as the World Health Organization and the United Nations Fund for Population Activities.

Societies around the globe still wrestle with the moral and ethical aspects of birth control and family planning. Though virtually every adult alive at the turn of the calendar from 1999 to 2000 had at least heard of birth control, widespread disagreement, fueled mainly by the Roman Catholic Church, but also by religious conservatives of Islam, Judaism, and by most Hindus, over the need for family planning, the need for reducing the world population, and the right of women and men to prevent an act of God or nature, stirred emotions and limited the access to birth control for people who did not share these beliefs. In Ireland and the Philippines, the Catholic Church exercised significant influence over government and limited access even to condoms. Disagreement over the teachings of the Qur'an in the Moslem faith separates people of that faith; nations such as Indonesia, a Moslem nation, turn aggressively to family planning policies, whereas nations of northern Africa develop more limiting policies. Within all societies, people worry that access to birth control will lead teens to promiscuous, unhealthy sexual lives, that birth control will lead women to reject motherhood altogether, and that birth control deprives one or the other partner in a relationship from exercising his or her right and responsibility to conceive children.

The shift in attention by public health, population, medical, and social professionals and activists in the 1990s from considering birth control as a means of limiting birth to a human right is beginning to shift people's attitudes across societies. If family planning is a human right, as asserted in the U.N. agreement signed in Cairo in 1994, then each individual born into this world of more than 6 billion deserves access to that right. Advocates for the full implementation of the Cairo agreement argue that it will be the responsibility of all people, all nations, to bring those rights to each other. It will also be the responsibility of each adult, they argue, to learn of and understand those rights so that she or he can fully exercise them, so that he or she can teach their children of those rights and how to fulfill them. Not all parties to the U.N. agreement, or all people in the world, agree to that stand. International human rights and reproductive rights communities still must work to present the family planning and reproductive health as human rights. The revolution is not yet over.

Sexual education, or lack of it, many advocates believe, is one of the greatest hindrances to achieving the goal of universal reproductive rights. Too few adults, even in the United States and Western Europe, where the modern contraceptive revolution began, fully understand their own bodies, human fertility, and human reproduction. Without understanding the personal aspects of their ability to reproduce, people will not be able to make the choices that reproductive rights activists seek to secure for them. The *Encyclopedia of Birth Control* will teach readers about their biology, about the science of birth control, and about the social struggle that separates sexual intercourse from childbearing. Through the entries in this book, people will learn that, though ubiquitous, birth control is a still developing, still growing aspect of a modern adult human being's life.

GUIDE TO SELECTED TOPICS

Birth Control Advocates and Inventors
Baulieu, Etienne-Emile
Dennett, Mary Ware
Guttmacher, Alan F.
McCormick, Katharine Dexter
Pincus, Gregory Goodwin
Rock, John Charles
Sanger, Margaret Higgins
Stopes, Marie C.

Cases and Legal Issues
Comstock, Anthony
Comstock Laws
Dennett, Mary Ware
Eisenstadt v. Baird
Griswold v. Connecticut
Obscenity
Privacy Laws
Roe vs. Wade
Sanger, Margaret Higgins

Contraceptive Methods
Abortifacient
Abstinence
Barrier Contraceptives
Basal Body Temperature Method
Billings Method
Biological Methods of Contraception
Breastfeeding
Cervical Cap
Combined Oral Contraceptives
Condom—Female
Condom—Male
Contraception
Contraceptive
Dalkon Shield
Depo-Provera
Diaphragm
Douching
Effectiveness (of Contraceptives)
Emergency Contraception
Endometrial Ablation
Failure Rates
Fertility Awareness
Future Methods of Contraception
Hormonal Contraceptives
Hysterectomy
Implants
Injectable Contraceptives
Intrauterine Device
Lea Contraceptive
Long-Term Contraceptives
Male Contraceptives
Menstrual Regulation
Mifepristone
Modern Contraceptive Methods
Monthly Contraceptives
Non-hormonal Pill
Norplant
Oral Contraceptives
Patch (Contraceptive)
Pessary
PREVEN
Progestin-Only Contraceptives
Rhythm Method
Spermicides
Sterilization

A

Abortifacient

Abortifacients, whether chemicals or objects, cause abortions, the termination of a pregnancy. However, because the definition of pregnancy varies, opinions vary greatly over just which contraceptive or fertility control methods involve abortifacients.

For example, procedures such as vacuum aspiration, which are performed during the first 12 weeks of pregnancy after a test has confirmed that an egg has been fertilized and after the egg has been implanted, are clearly seen as abortifacient techniques. However, oral contraceptives and intrauterine devices, which most often prevent fertilization, but which may disrupt implantation should fertilization occur, are considered by people who see fertilization as the beginning of life as abortion-inducing chemicals and objects, and are considered methods for preventing conception by people who do not see fertilization as the beginning of life.

Chemicals, whether modern pharmacological substances or traditional mixtures of herbs and liquids, are referred to as either menstrual regulators, because they force menstruation to begin, or as abortifacients, because they would force an embryo, should one exist, to be washed out with the menstrual blood. Postcoital or emergency contraception uses heavy doses of oral contraceptives to force the onset of menstruation. Women who use this protection against unwanted pregnancy soon after having unprotected intercourse or if a barrier device fails, do not know before taking the drugs if a sperm had fertilized an egg. However, because that chance exists, some people see postcoital contraceptives as abortifacients.

Discussions over when life begins and when pregnancy begins, at fertilization of an egg by sperm or implantation of a fertilized egg days later in the uterus, lead to differences in definition of whether a birth control device is a contraceptive or an abortifacient. *See also* CONCEPTION; CONTRACEPTIVE; EMERGENCY CONTRACEPTION; FERTILIZATION; IMPLANTATION (OF EGG); LIFE (BEGINNING OF); MIFEPRISTONE; ORAL CONTRACEPTIVES

Further reading: Knight, James W., and Joan C. Callahan. *Preventing Birth: Contemporary Methods and Related Moral Controversies.* Ethics in a Changing World 3. Salt Lake City: University of Utah Press, 1989.

Abortion

Whether legal or illegal, natural or induced, performed safely or unsafely, an abortion stops a pregnancy and forces the prebirth removal of the embryo or fetus and its placenta. Abortion, when used as a form of fertility control to limit the number of children born to a woman or a society, is not considered a form of contraception, which seeks to prevent the union of a female egg with a male sperm. Neither do most scholars consider abortion a form of birth control, a phrase which from its invention in the early 1900s did not include advocacy of abortion.

The medical processes of abortion are clearly known and widely practiced around the world. However, moral, ethical, and legal issues surrounding the "abortion issue" vary greatly from country to country and within countries. Even the relationship between contraception and abortion provides opportunity for disagreement and debate.

Nature alone stops approximately 50 percent of all pregnancies. Most of these spontaneous abortions occur within two weeks of ovulation and one week of implantation. In fact, most women never realize conception occurred; their periods arrive on schedule as the uterus sheds the lining and the unaccepted egg. Spontaneous abortions are less common after the first two weeks of embryo development. Of the pregnancies that are evident by a missed period, approximately 15 percent end in miscarriage.

People can also halt pregnancies, with or without medical assistance. These abortions may be legal or illegal, depending on the laws of a specific country, and either performed safely under approved medical supervision or unsafely in unsanitary and dangerous conditions. Medically safe, legal abortions are performed in clinics that specialize in the procedure, in doctors' offices, and in hospitals. Under a doctor's care, with specialized instruments and sanitary conditions, the abortion procedure is medically twice as safe as a tonsillectomy. Unsafe, illegal abortions, often performed by the women themselves by inserting objects through the vagina and into the uterus or by less trained people in unsanitary conditions, often lead to the serious medical complications of a septic abortion, a procedure that usually requires medical attention and which often results in death.

Vacuum aspiration (also known as suction curettage) is the most commonly used procedure for aborting pregnancies in the early stages. Medical professionals agree that it is the safest, simplest, and most effective way of performing an abortion. Medical professionals perform vacuum aspirations during the first 12 to 14 weeks of pregnancy. While many clinics require women to be at least five or six weeks pregnant, as measured from the first day of their last period, the procedure is becoming safer during the earliest stages of pregnancy. Recently developed tests that detect the body's chemical and hormone changes can determine an existing pregnancy earlier than older tests allowed, thus allowing medical professionals to perform abortions earlier in the fetal development process.

During a vacuum abortion, while the woman is under local anesthetic, doctors insert small rods into the cervix until that opening has stretched wide enough for the insertion of a suction tube or cannula, which is attached to a small pump. When turned on, the pump vacuums out the contents of the uterus. The process takes between five and 15 minutes and is done on an out-patient basis.

Some doctors perform similar procedures within four to five weeks of the beginning of a pregnancy, using a large hand-held syringe to extract the uterine lining and its contents. Known as manual vacuum aspiration, MVA is used more frequently in developing countries, where it provides medically safe abortions. In Bangladesh, Indonesia, and several other Asian nations where abortions are illegal, this early procedure is allowed soon after a missed menstrual period if a pregnancy is not confirmed.

After the twelfth or fourteenth week of confirmed pregnancy, medical professionals use the dilation and evacuation (D&E) for abortions. The D&E procedure takes longer to open the cervix than does vacuum aspiration, but uses the same method for removing the contents of the uterus. Small match-stick sized laminaria, made of sterile seaweed, are inserted into the woman's cervix. The farther along the pregnancy, the more laminaria are needed to open the cervix. Usually, these rods, which soak up fluid and expand, are inserted the day before the evacuation takes place. On that second visit, the woman again receives a local anesthetic while the cannula is inserted and the vacuum pump activated. When the laminaria are inserted, many doctors also inject chemicals into the uterus to stop the fetal heartbeat and to stop development of the fetus.

Chemical means have also been developed for medical abortions. In the early 1970s, French chemists searched for an "antiprogestin," a chemical that takes the place of progesterone, a hormone that helps maintain the uterine lining during pregnancy. In 1980, biochemists at Roussel Uclaf, now part of Aventis Pharma, created RU-486, now known as *mifepristone*. This antiprogestin takes the place of the natural hormone in the uterine lining and prevents the lining from receiving the signal necessary for continued development from the progesterone. Without that natural signal, the lining begins to shed. Now the primary chemical means of inducing medical abortions, mifepristone is used under a doctor's medical supervision to ensure that pregnancy has not implanted in the fallopian tubes during an ectopic or tubal pregnancy. Mifepristone does not work in this situation and such a pregnancy can be very dangerous to the woman. The drug also causes severe cramping, extended days of menstrual bleeding, and nausea.

Another form of chemical abortion involves *methotrexate*, which has been used in the United States since 1954 to treat cancer and arthritis. Methotrexate blocks the action of folic acid, and stops the development of the fetus. While poisonous in larger doses, a small amount of methotrexate is not harmful to the woman. Several days after taking methotrexate, the woman also takes another chemical, misoprostol, which forces cramping and contraction of the uterus.

Researchers continue looking for other forms of chemical abortions that would have less severe side effects than mifepristone and be less complicated to use than methotrexate.

Worldwide in 1995, approximately 26 million women underwent legal abortions and 20 million women underwent illegal abortions. The legal abortions were performed in the 69 countries where procedures to stop a pregnancy are permitted by law, though some are accounted for in Mexico, Brazil, and Sudan, where abortions are only permitted to save the woman's life. The illegal abortions occurred in the 33 countries where

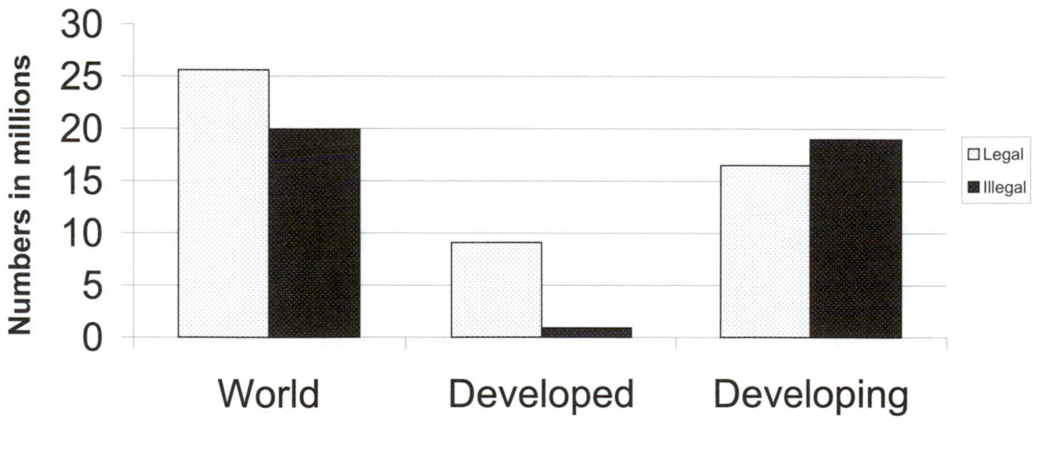

Abortions: 1995

Source: Alan Guttmacher Institute

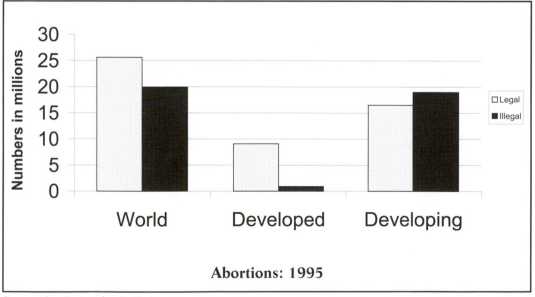

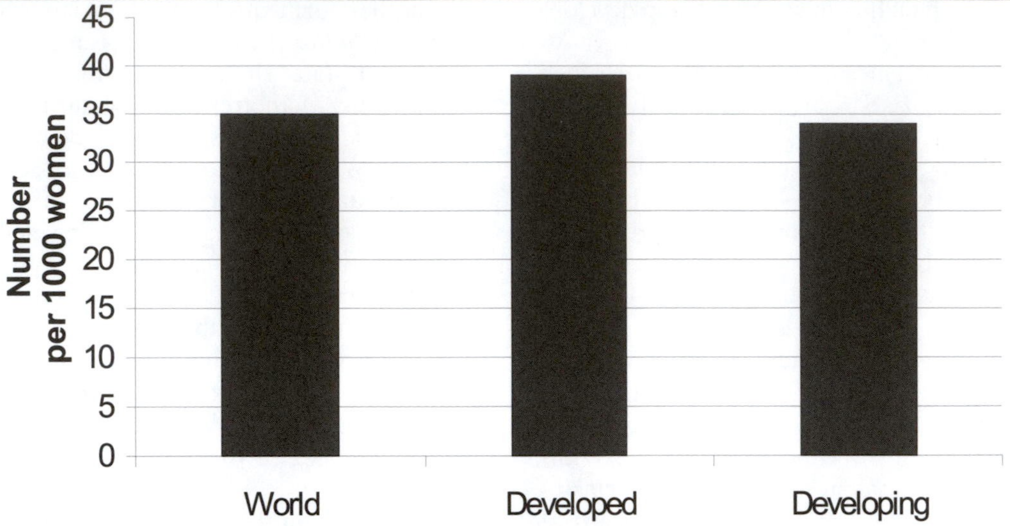

Abortion Rate 1995

Source: Alan Guttmacher Institute

abortion is illegal and in countries where the legal procedure is limited and difficult to obtain. Illegal abortions are commonly performed in dangerous situations where women attempt to induce their own abortions or seek the help of people who are underqualified and unregulated and who work in unhealthy conditions.

Complications from illegal abortions kill between 60,000 and 120,000 women every year, according to the World Health Organization. Most of these deaths occur in south Asia, sub-Saharan Africa, and rural Latin America. Even in countries where abortions are legal, insufficient provision of medical abortions lead 4 to 5 million women to seek illegal abortions each year. The rate of injury from illegal abortions is also high, resulting in infection, damage to the uterus and vagina, and infertility.

In the United States, where abortion is legal but where opposition to the procedure on religious and moral grounds is high, the abortion rate is falling. From 1992 to 1996, the abortion rate decreased from 26 to 23 abortions for every 1,000 women aged 15 to 44. The number of abortions decreased from 1,529,000 in 1992 to 1,366,000 in 1996. Seventy percent of those abortions were performed in clinics, and only 7 percent were performed in hospitals. The remainder were performed in physicians' offices. As of 1998, the number of women choosing chemical means of abortion were too small to be measured and factored into the national statistics. More people using contraceptives, more people using them better, and the development of more effective contraceptives, as well as declining sexual activity by teens accounts for most of this decline. The rate at which women facing an unplanned pregnancy choose to keep the child has also increased.

Moral and ethical resistance to abortion centers around the debate of when life begins and of concern for the well-being of the woman and the "conceptus," a term ethicists use to refer to the cells that grow from the joining of a fertile egg with a fertile sperm. One argument, put forth most notably by the religious leadership of the Roman Catholic Church, posits that life begins with conception, when the egg and sperm combine. Other arguments state that life begins sometime later in pregnancy, most likely when a conceptus, if born, would be able to survive on its own and be cared for by someone other than the woman in whose body it grew. Medical technology has since the 1970s been pushing this point closer to conception; ever younger fetuses are surviving spontaneous abortions and this is in turn fueling the debate over when life begins.

Those who believe that life begins at conception view any means of interfering with the ensuing biological process as an abortion. They see devices that interfere with implantation, even if that interference is only a part of its function, such as intrauterine devices and hormonal contraceptives, as abortifacients. Many people with these beliefs seek to prevent the use of and even outlaw such devices. Others see a difference of morals and ethics in the primary function of the device itself and may accept hormonal contraceptives and IUDs as acceptable means of preventing pregnancies, not stopping them.

People making the opposing argument state that, though a conceptus has the potential to become a person, as a seed has the potential to become a tree, that conceptus is not a person in the same sense that an infant is a person. Having life, they hold, does not equal personhood and the level of rights bestowed upon human beings after birth. This distinction between personhood and life influences the debate over abortion, which in turn influences the availability of abortion procedures around the world.

Contraceptives, research shows, reduce the need for abortions. In the United States, women using contraceptives are far less likely to have an abortion than women who use no contraception. Fifteen percent of contraceptive users seek abortions compared to 85 percent of women who use no contraceptives. The Netherlands, where contraceptives are easily and widely available and abortion legal, has the lowest abortion rate in the developed world.

Because no contraceptive is 100 percent effective—the best modern method, Norplant, prevents pregnancies 99.91 percent of the time—and women and men often fail to use or misuse the contraceptives they do choose, some people believe there will always be a demand for abortion. *See also* ABORTIFACIENT; CONCEPTION; CONTRACEPTIVE; ISLAM; JUDAISM; LIFE (BEGINNING OF); MIFEPRISTONE; PROTESTANTISM; ROMAN CATHOLIC CHURCH.

Further reading: Alan Guttmacher Institute. *Sharing Responsibility: Women, Society, and Abortion Worldwide*. New York: Alan Guttmacher Institute, 1999. Henshaw, Stanley K., Susheela Singh, and Taylor Haas. "The Incidence of Abortion Worldwide." *International Family Planning Perspectives* 25 (1999): Supplement S30–S38. Kaufman, K. *The Abortion Resource Handbook*. New York: Fireside—Simon and Schuster, 1997. Kulczycki, Andrzej, Malcolm Potts, and Allan Rosenfield. "Abortion and Fertility Regulation." *Public Health* 347 (1996): 1663–1886.

Abstinence

Abstinence, defined as refraining from sexual intercourse that leads to a man ejaculating his sperm in a woman's vagina, is the only certain way to avoid pregnancy. Abstaining from all intimate sexual contact with another person is also the only certain way to prevent contracting sexually transmitted diseases. As a means of preventing diseases and preventing unwanted childbirth, abstinence became an increasingly used option in the late 1990s.

Primary abstinence, or virginity, involves people who have never engaged in complete sexual intercourse. Secondary abstinence involves people choosing abstinence for a period of time after having sexual intercourse at least once. People choose this option for a variety of reasons, from not being involved in a relationship to valuing a celibate lifestyle. Couples may choose together to refrain from intercourse and explore a variety of alternative intimate forms of communication and expression.

Abstinence grew in popularity among U.S. teenagers in the 1990s. From 1991 to 1997, the rate of sexually active teens fell 11 percent. In 1997, 48.4 percent of students in ninth through twelfth grades were sexually active, compared with 54.1 in 1991. High school boys were as likely to remain virgins as high school girls. White students were more likely to choose abstinence than black students, of whom 73 percent were sexually active, and Hispanic students, of whom 52 percent were sexually active.

Education programs that emphasize abstinence, greater involvement by parents in their children's education, and disease prevention programs greatly influenced this increase in sexual abstinence. Throughout the 1990s, education programs in sexual abstinence grew across the United States, with organizations pushing for Congressional support of abstinence-only sex education programs. However, opposition groups expressed concern that abstinence-only programs that did not mention birth control and sexually transmitted diseases jeopardized the health and well-being of teenagers.

Adults might choose abstinence as an important option for protecting themselves from sexually transmitted diseases and from unwanted pregnancy. About 17 percent of the women surveyed in the 1995 *U.S. National Survey of Family Growth* reported that they had not had sexual intercourse by choice in the three months prior to the survey.

The main drawback of abstinence for healthy adults is the denial of the expression of emotion through sexual encounters. Researchers have shown that emotional denial has adverse effects on relationships just as can unwanted intercourse. In an effort to balance protection from unwanted pregnancy and disease with a full range of emotional expression, health professionals and counselors encourage people to explore a wider range of sexual communication and contact that do not include penile-vaginal intercourse.

Celibacy, a long-term, lifestyle choice, involves refraining from sexual encounters for the purpose of exploring other means of emotional expression and personal fulfillment. As a full expression of abstinence, celibacy represents a different goal than the physical prevention of pregnancy and sexually transmitted diseases. *See also* CONTRACEPTION; INTERCOURSE

Further reading: Carlson, Margaret. "A Girl's Best Friends: Alma Powell and Elayne Bennett, One Pro-choice, the Other Pro-life, Find Common Ground on Teens and Sex." *Time,* 22 January 1996, 32. Kowal, Deborah. "Abstinence and the Range of Sexual Expression." In *Contraceptive Technology,* 17th rev. ed., edited by Robert Hatcher, James Trussel, Felicia Stewart, and others. New York: Ardent Media, 1998. Stryker, Jeff. "Abstinence or Else! The Just-Say-No Approach in Sex Ed Lacks One Detail: Evidence that it Works." *The Nation,* 16 June 1997, 19–21.

Access (to Contraceptives)

Women and men around the world gaining control of their reproductive health was a goal established by the international community in the 1990s. Improving access to modern contraceptives is a means to that goal.

By 1999, 51 percent of the world's married women used some form of modern contraceptive to limit the number of children to which they gave birth. In the developed world, more than 90 percent of the sexually active women used contraceptives, from simple barriers to surgical sterilization and including hormonal contraceptives. Rates in the developed world ranged from 70 percent in Brazil to less than 5 percent in Nigeria to virtually none in several central African countries.

In certain parts of the world, people's access to modern contraceptives rose sharply in the 1980s and early 1990s. In Bolivia, approximately 2 percent of women used contraceptives in 1982. By 1994 more than 50 percent did so. In Iran during the same time period, the rate rose from near 10 percent to more than 60 percent. Despite similar increases in access and use around the world, population analysts expect that the demand for modern birth control methods will increase by 20 percent in those countries that currently report high use and convenient access and by 110 percent in nations, such as the Congo and Chad in central Africa, where contraceptives were virtually unavailable in the mid-1990s.

With the world population continuing to grow, at least into the middle of the twenty-first century, according to projections from the United Nations, more and more women each year will be demanding easy access to contraceptives. The world's population of people between the ages of 15 and 24 years stood at 1 billion at the beginning of 2000. The number of people in that age group is likely to increase into the 2020s, and that increase in people will increase the demand for contraceptives. Governments, health care providers, manufacturers, and volunteer family planning organizations will face challenges to providing the contraceptives that people will demand. Limited access to, as well as supply of, contraceptives may create difficulties for people seeking contraceptives if government and nongovernment organizations, many of which subsidize the cost of contraceptives in poorer nations, cannot afford to keep up with demand.

Many factors may limit a woman's or man's access to contraceptives. Geography presents difficulty when people need to travel for several hours to receive the medical attention often necessary to receive contraceptives. Women in many African villages must walk from their villages to the nearest clinic, which can be hours away. Women in the island nations of the Philippines or Indonesia experience gaps in the supply of contraceptives due to the isolation of the island on which they live.

The monetary costs of contraception can also limit people's access. Trade agreements can raise the price of contraceptives in some parts of the world to more than 200 times the prices that same item might be elsewhere. In 1994, 100 condoms cost between US$2 and $3 in Tunisia, China, and Egypt. That same amount cost more than $70 in Brazil, Burundi, and Venezuela. In the United States, a lack of insurance coverage for contraceptives deprives people of as easy access to contraceptives as they have to the medicines that treat illness.

Government regulations also limit people's access to the contraceptives of their choice. Japan's government did not approve the sale of hormonal contraceptive pills until 1999, citing risks to the nation's morals, side effects, and environmental harm as reasons for keeping birth control pills, which had been available in the United States and Europe since the early 1960s, out of Japanese pharmacies.

Social circumstances can also keep people from using contraceptives they might otherwise choose. Sexually active teens, around the world, may not protect themselves from unwanted pregnancy for fear of the reputation they might gain if people find out they use contraceptives. Women may experience social pressure to prove their ability to have children and not use contraceptives when they themselves would choose to do so. Even wives' fears of their husbands' reactions can deprive them of access to contraception. *See also* AFRICA; JAPAN; UNMET NEED (FOR CONTRACEPTION)

Further reading: "Battle of the Bulge: Population." *The Economist,* 3 September 1994, 23–25. Bureau of the Census. Report WP/98. *World Population Profile: 1998.* Washington, DC: U.S. Government Printing Office, 1999. Population Action International. *Contraceptive Choice: Worldwide Access to Family Planning.* Washington, DC: Population Action International, 1997. Online: http://www.populationaction.org/programs/rc97.htm, 11 October 1999.

Acquired Immunodeficiency Syndrome (AIDS)

Sexual intercourse brings with it for women and men the risk of contracting sexually transmitted diseases (STDs) as well as the risk of unwanted pregnancy. With the advent of acquired immunodeficiency syndrome (AIDS), a lethal, currently incurable STD that has reached epidemic proportions around the world, the relationship between contraception and disease protection has received intense study and educational efforts on the parts of public health professionals and disease and reproductive researchers. Very often the people who seek protection from unwanted pregnancy are also people who need protection from sexually transmitted diseases. Public health advocates believe that combining efforts at educating people about both contraception and disease prevention could have a significant impact on reducing both.

As of the end of the twentieth century only latex male condoms proved highly effective at preventing the spread of the human immunodeficiency virus (HIV). The male synthetic condom and the new female condom, both made of polyurethane, were undergoing studies for their effectiveness at blocking sexually transmitted diseases. Preliminary tests suggested both were as effective as latex male condoms but confirmation of that effectiveness awaited further testing. Current spermicides, notably nonoxynol-9, the leading spermicide used in the United States, showed success in the laboratory at incapacitating HIV, though evidence had not clearly shown that spermicides protected against HIV/AIDS during intercourse. Reproductive health research by pharmaceutical companies focused in the 1980s and 1990s on developing chemicals effective both as spermicides and as microbicides. Hormonal contraceptives appear to have no effect in preventing sexually transmitted diseases. Since they are highly popular contraceptives, however, experts urged clinicians and physicians to specifically discuss AIDS prevention as they counseled women in contraceptive choice.

Condom use has risen steadily worldwide since AIDS became a public health crisis in the 1980s. In Ethiopia, for example, condom sales rose from 4 million in 1991 to 21 million in 1996. In Brazil, the sales numbers rose from 3 million in 1991 to 27 million in 1996. By 1996, marketing campaigns were underway in 60 nations. They focused on use by unmarried people with several sex partners as well as monogamous married couples. The AIDS epidemic has actually made condoms more acceptable as a contraceptive than they had been before the rise of AIDS.

Despite these significant increases in condom use, many groups of people at risk from HIV/AIDS and other sexually transmitted diseases still do not use condoms regularly. In the United States between 1988 and 1995, condom use accounted for most of the increase in the overall use of contraceptives by women between the ages of 15 and 44. Condom use rose faster among African-American and Hispanic women than among white women. Condom use by unmarried women also increased significantly. Despite those increases, only between 15 and 20 percent of the women in those categories used condoms regularly during intercourse.

In the late 1990s, social and health scientists around the world were advocating combining efforts to reduce the number of unwanted pregnancies with decreasing people's risk from AIDS. Research had revealed that women who chose long-term contraceptives, such as implants and injectable hormonal contraceptives, often quit using condoms. This behavior decreased their risk from unwanted pregnancy, but increased their risk from AIDS and other sexually transmitted diseases. Women who had been counseled while choosing those contraceptives to continue using condoms were more likely to have maintained their use of condoms than were women who received no such advice.

By 1999, more than 33 million people worldwide lived with HIV/AIDS. The number of women infected was rising rapidly. During 1998, HIV-associated illnesses killed approximately 2.5 million people, including 900,000 women. More than 95 percent of HIV-infected people live in developing countries where access to contraceptives and treatment for AIDS and related illnesses are still significantly less than in developed countries. Combining efforts to bring protection from AIDS to the people of the developing world could bring with it the added effect of increasing contraceptive use and effectiveness. *See also* BARRIER CONTRACEPTIVES; CONDOM—FEMALE; CONDOM—MALE; SAFE SEX; SEXUALLY TRANSMITTED DISEASES

Further reading: Cushman, Linda F., et al. "Condom Use Among Women Choosing Long-Term Hormonal Contraception." *Family Planning Perspectives* 30 (1998): 240–243. Hines, Alice M., and Karen L. Graves. "AIDS Protection and Contraception among African American, Hispanic, and White Women." *Health and Social Work* 23 (1998): 186–194.

Adolescents

As they work their way through the second decade of life, through puberty and the onset of the functioning of their reproductive systems, adolescents face special challenges in understanding and learning to deal with their sexuality. People between the ages of 10 and 19 made up one-sixth of the world's population, 1.1 billion, as of the end of the twentieth century. Almost 90 percent, 913 million, lived in developing nations, and 160 million lived in developed countries. With most of them entering sexual maturity between the ages of 12 and 15 and with changing attitudes worldwide concerning adolescent sexuality and pregnancy, the medical, health, and social communities began recognizing the need to pay special attention to adolescents and their reproductive health needs.

Attitudes toward adolescence as a life phase vary around the world, and those societies' perceptions of teen pregnancy and teen sexual activity also vary. In many developing countries, girls are expected to marry young, premarital sex by unmarried teens is socially unacceptable, and before they are 18, married girls are expected to start having children. In more developed countries, most women marry after their twentieth birthdays, frequently engage in premarital sex, and often delay pregnancy. In some countries, such as the United States, people view teen pregnancy as a problem. In others, such as Nigeria, society sees more of a problem in teenaged married women not having children. In all countries attitudes toward adolescents is changing toward allowing teens time to mature as they progress through puberty before they have children. Adolescent marriages are declining worldwide, with the greatest decrease in southeast Asia and the slowest decrease in sub-Saharan Africa.

Overall, young women experience greater health and social consequences of teen sexual behavior, specifically sexual intercourse, than do teen boys. Girls risk becoming pregnant, contracting difficult-to-diagnose sexually transmitted or reproductive tract diseases, undergoing abortions, and enduring social stigmatism for their experimentation in sexual intercourse. In some societies, men may share some of the social risks, but they do not share the biological risks of teen pregnancy. Many societies still encourage boys to begin having sexual activity as teens, though they do not tolerate girls engaging in sex before, or outside of, marriage. The preponderance of negative consequences to teen girls as they develop sexually and begin to explore and express that sexuality has focused adult attention on understanding and helping girls decrease these risks in their lives and in helping boys recognize and share in preventing the risks that girls face.

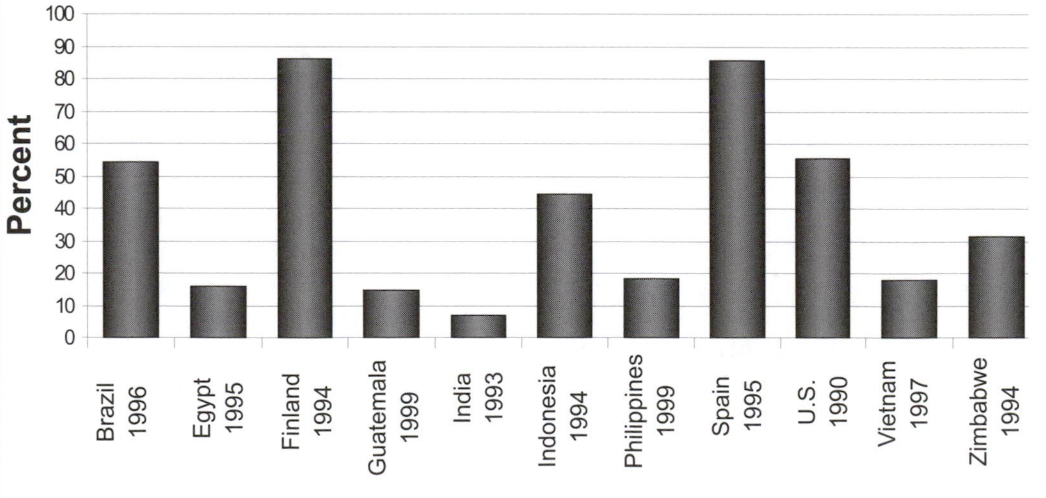

Prevalence of Contraceptive Use by Women Ages 15–19

Source: U.S. Census Bureau International Data Base

Girls experienced the onset of menstruation, known as menarche, much earlier at the end of the twentieth century than they did 150, or even 100, years earlier. Presently in Western developed countries, menstruation typically begins at 12.5 years old. In poorer developing countries menarche occurs around age 15. That age had been declining approximately three months for every decade since the 1850s, when menstruation is known to have begun at age 16 or 17 in those Western countries. Historians attribute this shift to improvements in the quality and the quantity of people's diets and in the meeting of nutritional needs. This lowering of the age of menarche means a woman experiences more years of fertility and faces greater risk of pregnancy before reaching physical and emotional maturity.

Girls in the 1990s experienced first sexual intercourse earlier in their lives than did girls in the mid-1900s. In the United States in the 1950s, 27 percent of adolescent girls had their first experience with sexual intercourse by age 18. In the 1990s that figure had risen to 50 percent. In the United States in the 1990s the typical age of first sexual intercourse for girls was 17 and for boys was 16. In sub-Saharan Africa sexual activity for teens commonly starts before 18, while in Asia, Latin America, and the Caribbean the average age of first intercourse was 20 years.

Worldwide in 1995, 15 million adolescent girls gave birth, accounting for 10 percent of the world's births. That percentage had been steadily falling through the last half of the twentieth century. Fewer women aged 20 to 24 in 1995 had given birth before age 20 than had women ages 40 to 44. In the Sudan, for example, 61 percent of women in the older group reported having had their first children before age 20, whereas 26 percent of women 20 to 24 had done so. In the United States, where the birth rate among teens was declining in the 1990s, 11 percent of girls ages 15 to 19 became pregnant in 1998.

Most of those teen pregnancies, especially in developed countries, were unplanned, either unwanted or mistimed. In the United States during 1998, 73 percent of teen pregnancies were unplanned, giving the United States the highest teen pregnancy and unplanned teen pregnancy rate in the developed world. The rate of unplanned teen pregnancies varies in developing countries but is generally higher than 20 percent.

Younger teens in the United States are more likely than older teens to seek abortions to end unplanned pregnancies; overall 31 percent of teen pregnancies were terminated in abortion in 1994. Declines in the teen birth rate in the mid-1990s was mirrored by a decline in the abortion rate. Worldwide, teens face the same risks from illegal abortions as adult women, but teens are more likely to use traditional, or nonmedical, means of ending an unwanted pregnancy.

Teen girls face a much higher risk from pregnancy than do adult women. Though a teenage girl begins ovulating soon after menarche, the rest of her body takes longer to reach its full ability to healthily bear children. Adolescent girls have a heightened risk of experiencing premature labor, miscarriage, and stillbirth. They are four times as likely as adult women to die from pregnancy-related causes. These risks are greater where medical services are inadequate or unavailable. Girls who receive good prenatal care during pregnancy have far less risk of complications than do girls who do not have easy access to medical care. Social stigma, family and friend disapproval, or denial of a pregnancy, however, often lead teens to avoid seeking medical care early in a pregnancy, and that avoidance increases the risks of complications.

Emotional and social maturity also place teens at greater risk than adults from sexual activity. The common attitudes among teens that they are invulnerable can lead teens to disregard information on the risk of pregnancy and the risk of sexually transmitted diseases with each act of sexual intercourse. With the newness of the emotions of the sexual experience, teens may have a harder time remembering risks and recognizing them when they are involved in the emotional turmoil that precedes intercourse.

Despite this, contraceptive use by teens is rising. In the late 1990s in the United States, 81 percent of sexually active teens report using a modern birth control method. The older the teen, the more likely she will be to use a contraceptive; the rate was 84 percent for girls 18 to 19 and 71 percent for girls 15 to 17. Teens in the 1990s were far more likely to use a contraceptive on first intercourse than women were in the 1970s. Worldwide, the number of teenage women not using contraception is slowly decreasing, yet more than 11 percent of sexually active teens who do not want to become pregnant are not using a method of birth control.

The issues surrounding teenage sexuality, pregnancy, and marriage are complex and highly influenced by cultural differences around the world. As societies work to provide women, including teens, with reproductive rights, including the right to choose when to marry and the right to choose when to have children, teen advocates and reproductive health experts see a trend of fewer teen pregnancies developing around the world. To achieve that goal, experts recommend changes in societies and cultures that encourage health care providers, counselors, and teen educators to provide parents with information to support and guide their teens, increase efforts to provide educational opportunities for teens, especially girls and young women, and to help young people understand the physical, emotional, and social consequences of sexual relationships. *See also* OLDER REPRODUCTIVE-AGE WOMEN

Further reading: Alan Guttmacher Institute. *Into a New World: Young Women's Sexual and Reproductive Lives*. New York: Alan Guttmacher Institute, 1998. *Studies in Family Planning* 29.2 (1998). Entire issue focuses on adolescents. Zabin, Laurie Schwab, and Sarah C. Hayward. *Adolescent Sexual Behavior and Childbearing.* Developmental Clinical Psychology and Psychiatry 26. Newbury Park, CA: Sage, 1993.

Adoption

While not a form of fertility or birth control, adoption becomes an issue in the discussions concerning the moral and ethical aspects of preventing birth, especially forms of birth prevention that occur after a female's egg has been fertilized by a male's sperm. Critics of abortion argue that a human life begins upon fertilization and that the human life started at that moment has all the rights society gives to human life after birth. These critics maintain that adoption gives the child a chance at life denied by abortion, and provides a more humane solution to an unwanted pregnancy for the child and the birth mother than abortion.

Other people argue that the rules surrounding adoption in most countries make it an extremely time-consuming and needlessly difficult process, so difficult that it will not help ease the dependence on abortion until countries relax those rules. They see the suggestion that adoption in any form can replace a need for abortion as unworkable and as imposing undue burden upon the pregnant women. Still others suggest that to make adoption a workable option to abortion would require far greater social, financial, and emotional support of pregnant women than governments can or should offer. *See also* ABORTION; REPRODUCTIVE RIGHTS; UNPLANNED PREGNANCY

Further reading: Bartholet, Elizabeth. "Adoption Rights and Reproductive Wrongs." In *Power and Decision: The Social Control of Reproduction,* edited by Gita Sen and Rachel C. Snow, 177–203. Boston: Harvard University Press, 1994. Richards, Arlene Kramer, and Irene Willis. *What to Do If You or Someone You Know Is Under 18 and Pregnant.* New York: Lorthrop, Lee & Shepard—William Morrow, 1983. Welton, K. B. *Abortion Is Not a Sin: A New-Age Look at an Age-Old Problem.* Costa Mesa, CA: Pandit Press, 1987.

Africa

In the southern portion of Africa, often referred to as sub-Saharan Africa, children are being born at a faster rate than in any other region of the world. Fewer women there use modern contraceptives than women in any other region in the world. For the people of north Africa, only their neighbors to the south use fewer modern contraceptives and live in countries that are growing faster in population.

As a global region, with high levels of poverty, high levels of sexually transmitted diseases (STDs), including acquired immunodeficiency syndrome (AIDS), and a wide mix of cultures, governments, and traditions, Africa presents challenges for its own people and the world aid community in ways to improve the quality of life for its citizens, including access to and understanding of family planning.

From the middle of the twentieth century to the early 1990s, sub-Saharan Africa's rate of population growth increased steadily from near 2 percent a year in 1950 to 2.75 percent in the late 1980s. After this, the population growth rate began slowing. United Nations projections suggest that by 2020, this region of Africa will once again be increasing its population at less than 2 percent each year.

North Africa experienced a sharper increase in population growth, reaching a high of 3 percent in the early 1980s, but also experienced a rapid decrease in the rate of population growth, and by 1990 was growing at about 2.4 percent a year. Since the early 1990s, the nations of north Africa have slowed their rates of growth at a somewhat faster pace than did the nations of sub-Saharan Africa. Projections from the United Nations and the U.S. Census Bureau suggest that annual population growth rates will continue to decline faster for north Africa than for sub-Saharan Africa.

The rate of modern contraceptive use in sub-Saharan Africa by married women of childbearing age remained well below 20 percent with few exceptions. In the nation of South Africa 52 percent of married women used contraceptives. Contraceptive use in north Africa by the mid-1990s for women of childbearing age was substantially higher with four nations—Tunisia, Egypt, Algeria, and Morocco—approaching 50 percent. More developed nations around the world have prevalence rates over 80 percent.

Use of modern contraceptives has a direct bearing on the number of children a woman can expect to give birth to in her life, a figure known as the total fertility rate. In nations where contraceptive use is low, total fertility rates are high, and population growth is equally high. Sub-Saharan Africa, with such low levels of use of modern birth control methods, has correspondingly high rates of fertility. In Uganda in 1995, for example, women could expect to have seven children in their lives, and less than 5 percent of both men and women used modern contraceptives. In Tunisia that same year, women could expect to have an average of 2.5 children, and more than 50 percent of married women between the ages of 15 and 44 used modern contraceptives.

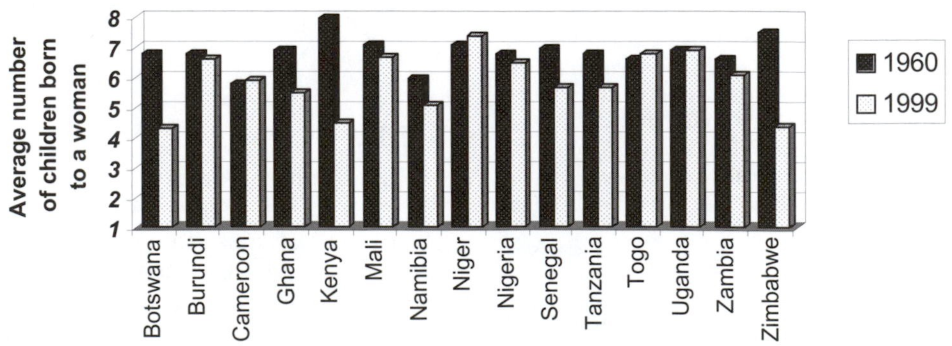

Sub-Saharan Africa: Total Fertility Rates: 1960 v. 1999

Source: Alan Guttmacher Institute (1960); International Planned Parenthood Federation (1999)

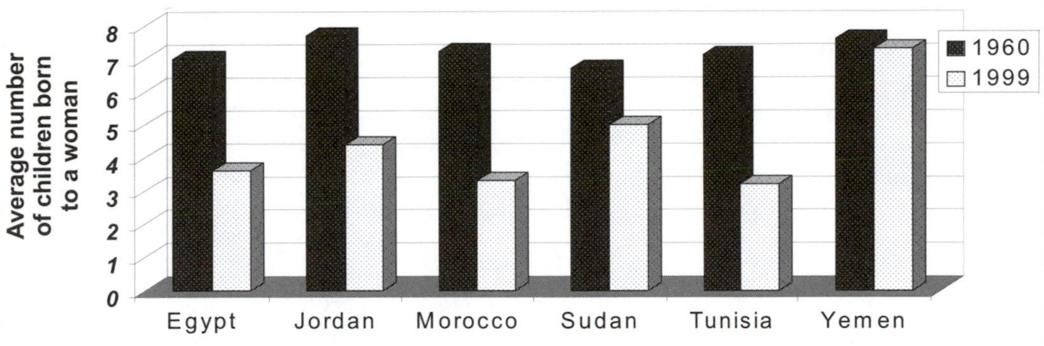

North Africa: Total Fertility Rates: 1960 v. 1999

Source: Alan Guttmacher Institute (1960); International Planned Parenthood Federaton (1999)

While use of modern contraceptives across Africa has generally risen, it has done so erratically and at tremendously varying rates. In the small country of Benin, use of modern contraceptives by married women crept up from near zero in 1982 to barely 5 percent in 1995. Zimbabwe saw a rapid increase in use of contraceptives from just above 10 percent in the late 1970s to almost 40 percent in the mid 1980s; since then increases in contraceptive use in Zimbabwe have risen steadily to its 1995 rate near 50 percent.

Generally, however, African women and men have very low rates of access to modern contraceptives. According to a 1997 study by Population Action International, three nations—Tunisia, Botswana, and Mauritius—provide their citizens with very good access to contraceptives, measured by people needing less than two hours and less than one percent of a month's wages to obtain a month's supply of modern contraceptives. People in those countries could easily obtain condoms, oral contraceptive pills, and intrauterine devices. They also had ready access to permanent sterilization. Thirteen nations had poor access to contraceptives by the same scale, though even for the two countries with the least access—Cote D'Ivorie and Central African Republic—access had improved significantly during the early 1980s.

Many social and health issues influence the value of modern contraceptives to Africans. Questions of cultural differences and issues of development influence the desire of people to use contraceptives. Many people in Africa favor large families and see contraception as a means to give women's bodies the rest from childbearing that will allow them to have more healthy children. The woman's physical well-being more than a desire to give birth to few children often leads sub-Saharan women to consider using contraceptives.

The advancement of the AIDS epidemic will have a significant impact on the lives of people in sub-Saharan Africa through the first decade of the twenty-first century. United Nations estimates suggest that much of this region, due to AIDS, will experience much higher overall death rates and much higher infant mortality rates than other parts of the world. In sub-Saharan Africa, a high percentage of the population, more than 5 percent, have been infected with the human immunodeficiency virus (HIV) that leads to AIDS. In 1998, AIDS had already lowered the life-expectancy rate from 61 years to 40 years in Botswana. The impact of AIDS and other diseases on family life could determine people's willingness to use modern contraceptives, such as condoms and spermicides that contain agents to destroy viruses, to either have more children to ensure the survival of some, or to have fewer children to decrease the risk of each child to disease.

A refocus in international aid attention from trying to force lower population growth rates and higher use of contraceptives to incorporating family planning in the larger scheme of reproductive health of women,

men, and nations, is seen as a culturally tolerant way of helping the people of Africa achieve higher quality of life standards and decrease the strains of rapidly increasing population growth. Helping the people of Africa achieve the levels of economic growth and population size achieved in Latin America and Southeast Asia has become a goal of African governments, non-governmental organizations, and international aid agencies. *See also* ACCESS (TO CONTRACEPTIVES)

Further reading: Bledsoe, Caroline, Fatoumatta Banja, and Allan G. Hill. "Reproductive Mishaps and Western Contraception: An African Challenge to Fertility Theory." *Population and Development Review* 24 (1998): 15–57. Bureau of the Census. Report WP/98. *World Population Profile: 1998.* Washington, DC: U.S. Government Printing Office, 1999. Kirk, Dudley, and Bernard Pillet. "Fertility Levels, Trends, and Differentials in Sub-Saharan Africa in the 1980s and 1990s." *Studies in Family Planning* 29 (1009): 1–22.

African Americans

Birth control and family planning play complex roles in the lives of African Americans. As they struggle to achieve success despite lingering racism, black Americans, who make up 12 percent of the United States population, face social obstacles and challenges to their reproductive health. With more than 26 percent living below the poverty level, black Americans must deal with government programs aimed at assisting people in poverty with meeting their reproductive health needs. As a group, African Americans work to understand and influence high rates of unwanted pregnancies in teens. As they move into the middle class, African Americans also face the challenges of delaying childbirth so that women and men can complete their education and achieve financial success and security before beginning families.

Contraceptive use among all black women ages 15 to 44 in the United States rose steadily from 51.6 percent in 1982 to 62.1 percent in 1995. The number of sexually active women not using contraceptives decreased by almost half from 13.6 percent in 1982 to 7 percent in 1995.

By 1995, black women who used modern contraceptives relied most heavily upon female sterilization, at 40 percent. Second most commonly used were the hormonal pill at 24 percent, and third were the male condom at 20 percent. The rate of male condom use by black women increased by 16 percentage points from 1982 to 1995. Almost all of that increase was among black women ages 15 to 24. Studies suggest that women often used condoms as protection from AIDS as well as from unintended pregnancy.

Black women from an early reproductive age begin choosing female sterilization to prevent pregnancy. Approximately 30 percent of women in their late 20s who used a modern method of birth control had undergone permanent sterilization. The percentages increase steadily through their reproductive lives until 70 percent of black women ages 40 to 44 report having undergone a sterilization procedure. Researchers suggest that greater proportions of black women complete their families early in their reproductive years and choose the highly reliable methods of preventing further pregnancies.

During the mid-1990s, the number of black teens giving birth began a steady decline. By 1999, the teen birth rate had dropped by more than 24 percent over the 1991 rate. More than 84 percent of sexually active black teens between 15 and 19 years old reported using contraceptives in 1995. Contraceptive use for black women of this age changed substantially with the availability of Norplant, an implantable hormonal contraceptive. In 1988, 75 percent of black teens who used birth control relied upon hormonal contraceptive pills. By 1995, that rate had dropped to 32 percent; 19 percent of black teens were using Norplant. A sharp increase in the use of condoms by black teens, from 20 to 30 percent, accounted for part of the shift from pills. The percentages of black teens who become pregnant each year also declined steadily and rapidly in the 1990s. From 1991 to 1996, that rate dropped by 20 percent.

The 1997 total fertility rate for all black women hovered during the mid-1990s at just above 2.0, as did the United States national total fertility rate. That figure shows that on average a black woman is as likely as any woman in the United States to give birth to two children during her lifetime.

Statistics tell only part of the story of family planning in black families in the United States. A three-times greater proportion of African American families live in poverty than do white families. Access to contraceptives for poor black women may be limited by the governmental programs and the welfare services that help pay for reproductive care for families in poverty. Reports of coercive measures against poor black women by government and legal agencies to encourage them to use the new injectable contraceptives led to charges in the early 1990s of racism and inequality of access to contraceptives by black families. Critics charged that many black women experienced family planning as a way for the government to control their fertility rather than as a way for women to control their own fertility.

As the number of African Americans achieving economic and social success increased, more black women and men put off having children until their 30s. This change in the timing of childbirth also accounted for increases in contraceptive use, decreased fertility rate, and increased problems with infertility among black families.

Further reading: Horner, Louise L., ed. *Black Americans: A Statistical Sourcebook*. 1998 ed. Palo Alto, CA: Information Publications, 1998. Roberts, Dorothy. *Killing the Black Body: Race, Reproduction, and the Meaning of Liberty*. New York: Pantheon, 1997. Taylor, Robert Joseph, James S. Jackson, and Linda M. Chatters, eds. *Family Life in Black America*. Thousand Oaks, CA: Sage, 1997.

Alan Guttmacher Institute

Staff at the Alan Guttmacher Institute (AGI), a U.S. not-for-profit organization, conduct extensive research into reproductive health issues, including contraceptive use, abortion, and unwanted pregnancies. Employees also analyze governmental policies and public education efforts that influence reproductive health and provide policy makers with the statistical information they need to make decisions on reproductive health issues.

Through careful, detailed data collection, AGI compiles information on national, state, and even county levels and presents that information through a wide variety of publications, including those for the general public and specialists. The staff, with more than 60 members working from offices in New York and Washington, DC, gathers the often scattered evidence needed to support reproductive rights and individual's efforts to control their reproductive health. While in its early years, AGI staff focused on the United States, in the 1980s and 1990s, this organization expanded its research work to gather information internationally. While its primary focus remains on the United States, the institute works with a growing network of scientists and opinion leaders around the world.

In 1968, the Planned Parenthood Federation of America (PPFA) founded the Center for Family Planning Program Development to offer policy expertise and data collection resources that might assist discussions by the people and government of the United States as issues of reproductive health gained public acceptance and began gaining public attention. Dr. Alan F. Guttmacher, obstetrician and gynecologist and then president of PPFA and himself an experienced statistical researcher, oversaw and nurtured the organization. In his honor after his death in 1974, the organization changed its name to the Alan Guttmacher Institute. In 1977, AGI became an independent corporation, though it remains a special affiliate of PPFA.

AGI has as its corporate mission to protect reproductive choice for women and men, nationally and internationally. Its goals, to achieve that mission, include supporting efforts to develop sexual and reproductive health rights, promote the prevention of unintended pregnancy, guarantee women the freedom to terminate pregnancies, help women have healthy pregnancies and births, encourage social support for parents and parenting, and promote gender equality.

To achieve those goals, AGI has gathered and maintained reproductive health information on all of the states and counties in the United States. It documented a 16 percent drop in the level of unplanned pregnancies in the United States between 1987 and 1994, focused research attention on the role of private insurance and managed care organizations to providing people with access to contraceptives, issued materials that demonstrate the relationship between contraception and abortion, examined the publicly provided reproductive health services provided by all U.S. counties, and gathered statistics on the rights of minors and the threats to their reproductive health.

Dedicated to sharing its information with a wide audience, the Alan Guttmacher Institute publishes *Family Planning Perspective*, begun in 1968, and *International Family Planning Perspectives,* begun in 1974, both peer-reviewed scholarly journals. In regular reports, AGI releases statistical information on topics from abortion and unwanted pregnancy to the differences in age between young women and their sexual partners and the influence of that age difference on the woman's reproductive well-being. The institute also publishes book-length reports, including *Hopes and Realities: Closing the Gap Between Women's Aspirations and Their Reproductive Experiences* (1995) and *Sharing Responsibility: Women, Society and Abortion Worldwide* (1999).

Funding for AGI comes from a diverse mix of sources including revenue from its publications and private donations. Little of its revenue comes from government agencies or pharmaceutical businesses. Its budget in 1997 included $10 million in assets. *See also* GUTTMACHER, ALAN F.; PLANNED PARENTHOOD FEDERATION OF AMERICA

Further reading: Alan Guttmacher Institute Web site. http://www.agi.usa.org. Goldsmith, Marsha F. "Researchers Amass Abortion Data." *Journal of the America Medical Association* 262 (1989): 1431–1432.

Androgens

Androgens are sex hormones that create masculine traits. Testosterone, the primary androgen, forms primarily and dominantly in the testicles. It controls the development of the male reproductive system during puberty and the development of sperm throughout adulthood. The adrenal glands, in men and women, located just above the kidneys, also produce testosterone as do a woman's ovaries.

Researchers have synthesized several artificial forms of testosterone. In efforts to develop male hormonal contraceptives that influence the male reproductive cycle, scientists focus on testosterone cypionate and testosterone enanthate, both of which are given through injections into large muscles. The synthetic hormone elevates testosterone levels, which suppresses the pituitary gland's secretion of luteinizing hormone (LH) and follicle-stimulating hormone (FSH), both of which the testicles require to trigger the production of sperm. While tests show synthetic hormones suppress sperm development to the point of being effective contraceptives, the shots must be given weekly and cause unwanted side effects such as weight gain and acne. Testing continues, however, to develop synthetic forms of testosterone to use as contraceptives without these drawbacks.

Synthetic progestins in oral contraceptives, derived from testosterone, suppress a woman's production of testosterone, a result known as an antiandrogenic process. The progestins actually reduce the effects of the testosterone produced naturally by a woman's adrenal glands and ovaries. Progestins have been shown to reduce unwanted hair growth, oily skin, and acne. However, some women do experience minor androgenic side effects of progestins. Progestins may also cause unacceptable weight gain, changes in cholesterol levels, and decreased libido. Balancing the androgenic effects of oral contraceptives with the woman's personal biology and the contraceptive effects of the estrogens and progestins in oral contraceptives becomes an important element in a woman and her health care provider finding the right hormonal contraceptive to meet her needs with few side effects. *See also* HORMONES—SYNTHETIC; TESTOSTERONE

Further reading: Thorneycroft, Ian H. "Update on Androgenicity." *American Journal of Obstetrics and Gynecology* 180, pt. 2 (1999): S288–S294. World Health Organization Task Force on Methods for the Regulation of Male Fertility. "Contraceptive Efficacy of Testosterone-Induced Azoospermia and Oligozoospermia in Normal Men." *Fertility and Sterility* 65 (1996): 821–829.

Andrology

The rather young medical specialty of andrology, which literally means "study of men," involves the scientific study of male physiology and the diseases of men with a focus on the reproductive organs. The field draws on specialists from other areas of scientific study, most notably urology (the study of the urinary tract), endocrinology, gynecology, cell biology, and clinical practitioners.

Most of the work of the International Society of Andrology, founded in 1981, concentrates on sperm production and function, fertility, and contraception. Scientific research by the society includes work on hormonal secretions that could inhibit the production of sperm and lead to the development of an effective, convenient male contraceptive similar to the hormonal contraceptives available to women.

As an area of medical and scientific emphasis, andrology is growing as its own specialty. Thirty-six nations worldwide belong to the International Society, which has more than 8,000 members. Many of those nations had formed societies of andrologists before the International Society took form. The British Andrology Society, for example, was formed in 1977. *See also* HORMONAL CONTRACEPTIVES; HORMONES—SYNTHETIC; MALE CONTRACEPTIVES

Further reading: Davis, W. Marvin. "Andrology: Pharmacotherapies for Man Only." *Drug Topics* 141 (1997): 86–95.

Asia

Asia is home to the world's two most populated nations: China and India. It is also home to a nation, Japan, where very few children are being born and where the number of elderly retired people could soon equal the number of workers. Faced both with nations that, according to their own views, are growing too quickly and nations that have successfully stopped population growth, Asian social, environmental, and political activists see the challenge of population within its nations as a dominant quality-of-life concern that needs constant and careful attention and effective solutions.

With the exception of Japan, the nations of Asia established family planning policies in the middle of the twentieth century in an attempt to limit population growth. Improvements in health conditions and medical resources in the early part of the century led in Asia, as it did throughout the world, to rapidly decreasing death rates for infants and elderly, and steadily increasing birth rates. Weak economies and low levels of industrial development prevented the Asian nations from improving living conditions and employment opportunities, two conditions that allowed the nations of North American and western Europe to experience a slow transition from high birth rates to low birth rates. Family planning programs in the 1960s and 1970s, where governments provided access to contraceptives, subsidized the cost of birth control, and actively persuaded citizens to limit family size, helped many nations throughout Asia achieve rapid transition to strong, industry-based economies.

By 1965, South Korea, Taiwan, Thailand, and Indonesia had established aggressive family planning programs that dramatically increased access to modern, effective contraceptives. These nations also established education programs for girls, created opportunities for women to enter the work force, and encouraged late marriage among its citizens. All of these factors contributed to rapid decreases in national fertility rates. In the 1950s and early 1960s women in these nations could expect to give birth to between four and six children in their lifetimes. By the mid-1990s, total fertility rates in South Korea, Taiwan, Thailand, Singapore, and Hong

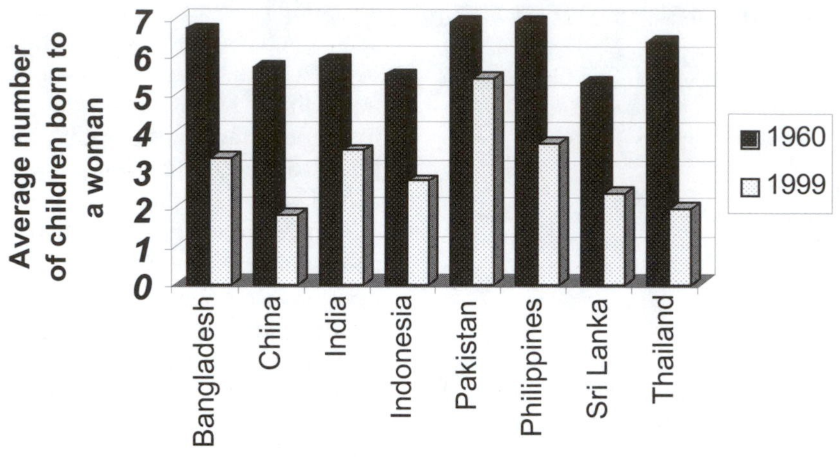

Asia: Total Fertility Rates: 1960 v. 1999

Source: Alan Guttmacher Institute (1960); International Planned Parenthood Federation (1999)

Kong had fallen to an average of fewer than two children for every woman, a level lower than the birth rate in the United States, and equal to many nations in Europe. In Indonesia and Malaysia fertility rates had fallen rapidly to near three children for every woman by the mid-1990s.

With now low fertility rates and increasing economic and industrial activities, Indonesia, Malaysia, and Thailand are expected to follow the pattern of the older Asian economies and greatly increase opportunity for their people as they further decrease the rate of population growth.

Governments that invested in family planning programs over long periods of time benefited from the cost savings in educating ever smaller groups of school-age children. They benefited when families could put more of the family income into savings accounts and spend less of it on feeding greater numbers of children. Providing women with opportunities in addition to motherhood increased the labor pool and decreased the number of children women were willing to have. Decreasing the size of the overall work force meant that more jobs were available to women. This force also contributed to greater opportunity for women.

The availability of contraceptives alone could not have brought about Asia's fertility change. However, without easy and convenient access to contraceptives, people would not have had effective means to bring about the social change of delayed childbearing and women would have been delayed from entering careers by pregnancies and family care.

The government of the Democratic Republic of Vietnam established in 1963 the first family planning program in southeast Asia. India had established unsuccessful programs in the late 1950s and struggled with changing attitudes and approaches to addressing its rapidly growing population. Singapore began its program in 1965, Indonesia in 1968, and the Philippines in 1970. Before the mid-1960s, only the people of Japan had successfully limited population growth and they did that without access to modern contraceptive except condoms. After the mid-1960s, the other nations of Asia turned aggressively to modern contraceptives to help limit population growth. China in 1978 began its "one-child" policy that encouraged couples to support a below replacement birth rate.

The development of the hormonal contraceptive pill in the 1950s lead quickly to worldwide marketing and by 1970, a contraceptive revolution had swept much of the world, except sub-Saharan Africa. In Asia, modern contraceptives, particularly the pill and intrauterine devices, became very popular in government programs and to individuals for their long-term effectiveness.

Permanent contraceptive sterilization also became increasingly common in many nations. Women of older reproductive age turned increasingly toward sterilization, and with 23 percent of women across the entire region having undergone surgery, tubal sterilization is the mostly frequently used form of birth control throughout Asia. India and China have both turned aggressively to sterilization, on occasion against the woman's wishes, in attempts to dramatically influence population. Male sterilization accounts for approximately 6 percent of the contracepting sexually active people of Asia and that percentage is rising. China's development in 1974 of the no-scalpel method for vasectomies, male surgical sterilization, spread rapidly through southeast Asia. The no-scalpel method takes far less time to perform than a traditional vasectomy which cuts the skin, and causes fewer complications and side effects.

The role of abortion varies greatly across Asia. It is available upon request in Vietnam, Singapore, North Korea, Mongolia, China, and Cambodia. It is easily available to protect the health of the woman, and for economic and social reasons, in India, Japan, and Taiwan. In other nations, abortion is highly restricted. The legal status of abortion, however, is only one measure of abortion's availability. Where it is not legal, women still find doctors who will perform abortions or turn to traditional methods. Of the 26.8 million abortions performed in Asia in 1995, 37 percent were illegal. That represents one-quarter of all Asia's pregnancies. Approximately 290 women die as a result of illegal procedures for every 100,000 abortions performed in Asia; in developed countries the death rate is between 0.2 and 1.2 for every 100,000 abortions. With high maternal death rates and higher rates of complications from illegal pregnancies, those nations that have greatly restricted abortion spend a significant percentage of their medical resources treating women who did not have easy access to contraceptives.

Family attitudes have changed considerably in much of Asia and are changing quickly in others. As they faced the pressures of large populations and the inability caused by those numbers to improve standards of living and economic opportunity, nations adopted policies that encouraged late marriage, by making later the legal age of marriage, and encouraged education of women. They also have shifted to preferring small families, as in Japan, and have even made remaining single socially acceptable for women and men. Within this effort, most nations of Asia remain committed to improving people's access to reliable, safe, and effective means of birth control, while maintaining their cultural uniqueness. *See also* CHINA; INDIA; INDONESIA; JAPAN; PHILIPPINES; VIETNAM

Further reading: Eberstadt, Nicholas. "Asian Population Change: What It Means for Policy." *Current* 409 (1999): 33–39. Jones, Gavin W. "Population and the Family in Southeast Asia." *Journal of Southeast Asian Studies* 26 (1995): 184–195. Singh, Susheela, Deirdre Wulf, and Heidi Jones. "Health Professionals' Perceptions about Induced Abortion in South Central and Southeast Asia." *International Family Planning Perspectives* 23 (1997): 50–67.

B

Barrier Contraceptives

Barrier contraceptives block the path of the male sperm into the uterus and thus prevent the fertilization of a female egg. They are among the oldest known contraceptives and if used properly, barriers provide adequate protection from pregnancy.

Some barrier contraceptives provide physical barriers to the sperm in the form of a plastic or latex device placed either over the penis or in the vagina. Others provide chemical barriers that kill most of the sperm before it enters the uterus. Many barrier contraceptive methods combine physical devices with chemicals to increase their effectiveness.

The methods of making barriers available to couples who wish to use them differ from country to country. In the United States, contraceptive barriers, such as male and female condoms and sponges, are easily available in drug stores, at pharmacies, in clinics, or through the mail without a prescription. Others, such as the diaphragm and cervical cap, which are inserted into the vagina, require that a woman have a prescription before purchasing these devices. Generally as of 1997, developed nations had easy access to several barriers, most commonly the male condom. As of 1997, access to barriers in developing countries ranged from easy access in Singapore and South Korea to no access at all in Laos and the Congo.

Barriers provide less protection against pregnancy than hormonal contraceptives or intrauterine devices. Barriers expose people to the risks associated with that particular device only when the barrier is in place. The diaphragm, cap, and sponge carry slight risks of developing toxic shock syndrome, but only when the device is in the vagina.

The success rates of barrier contraceptives (when people follow directions for their use precisely) range from 20 percent for a vaginal sponge to 3 percent for the male condom. (The percentage represents the number of women who are likely to become pregnant during the first year of use.) As opposed to "perfect use," the typical use of barrier contraceptives range from 36 percent for the sponge to 12 percent for the condom. The huge difference is primarily the result of people not accurately following package directions for the barrier's use, or through the less frequent occurrence of the device breaking or developing holes during use.

Barriers provide protection for only a few hours and need to be applied shortly before or during intercourse, and they are most often chosen by people who have intercourse infrequently, who do not feel a need for the constant protection of hormonal contraceptives. People often carry their devices with them. Many people, however, find such planning unsettling and inconsistent with the spontaneous nature of sexual intercourse. The need to plan ahead for sex is an important characteristic of choosing to use a barrier contraceptive. Also barrier contraceptives require that the user touch his or her genitals to put the device in place, and some people find doing so uncomfortable.

Researchers are currently working to develop new forms of barrier contraceptives to provide more people with more choice in meeting their contraceptive needs. *See also* CERVICAL CAP; CONDOM—FEMALE; CONDOM—MALE; DIAPHRAGM; EFFECTIVENESS (OF CONTRACEPTIVES); FAILURE RATES; FERTILITY AWARENESS; VAGINAL SPONGE

Further reading: Chez, Ronald A., and Daniel R. Mishell, Jr. "Control of Human Reproduction: Contraception, Sterilization, and Pregnancy Termination." Chap. 34 in *Danforth's Obstetrics and Gynecology*. 7th ed. Philadelphia: J. B. Lippincott, 1994. Speroff, Leon, and Philip Carney. *A Clinical Guide for Contraception.* Baltimore: Williams and Wilkins, 1992.

Basal Body Temperature Method

The basal body temperature method of the fertility awareness approach to family planning measures a woman's body heat in an attempt to predict when she has ovulated. This method of what is also called natural family planning is based upon the scientific discovery that many women's lowest daily body temperature rises slightly but constantly after a mature egg emerges from an ovary. Women use this procedure to either avoid conceiving a child by avoiding intercourse close to ovulation or to try to conceive a child by having sexual intercourse before or closely after ovulation.

Each morning, immediately upon waking and before getting out of bed, a woman takes her temperature and records the result on a temperature/date graph. The activity of the day raises a person's body temperature so it is an important feature of this method that a woman take her temperature after she has been asleep for at least three hours. The method requires a special basal thermometer which shows readings between 90 and 100 degrees Fahrenheit marked every 0.1 degrees. The woman may take her temperature either orally, rectally, or vaginally but must use the same location each day.

This signal of ovulation is triggered by the increases in progesterone levels that follow the eruption of a mature egg from the ovary. Once a mature egg has been expelled from an ovary, the surrounding follicle transforms into the *corpus luteum*. The circular form releases progesterone during the last 14 days of the menstrual cycle, and the progesterone raises the body temperature.

For most women, the temperature reading for the days of her cycle preceding ovulation will be a noticeable 0.5 to 1.0 degrees cooler than for the days immediately following ovulation. Some women's base temperature drops then rises sharply 12 to 24 hours after ovulation. The sharp drop signals ovulation. After ovulation, the higher temperature caused by increased progesterone levels persists until her menstrual flow begins. However, since an egg is only able to be fertilized by a sperm within 24 or 48 hours of ovulation, the woman becomes infertile again about two days after her temperature rises until her menstrual period begins.

Not all women show this temperature variation. As many as one in every five women do not register a different body temperature even though they do ovulate. Many women who do show the persistent temperature increase after ovulation will not show the downward spike in temperature that indicates ovulation.

The success rate of the basal body temperature method of natural family planning varies. It is most commonly used in conjunction with other methods of fertility awareness such as charting the consistency of cervical mucus. *See also* BILLINGS METHOD; BIOLOGICAL METHODS OF CONTRACEPTION; FERTILITY AWARENESS; OVULATION; REPRODUCTIVE SYSTEM—FEMALE; ROMAN CATHOLIC CHURCH

Further reading: Pasquale, Samuel A., and Jennifer Cadoff. *The Birth Control Book: A Complete Guide to Your Contraceptive Options*. New York: Ballantine, 1996. Weschler, Toni. *Taking Charge of Your Fertility: The Definitive Guide to Natural Birth Control and Pregnancy Achievement.* New York: HarperCollins, 1995.

Baulieu, Etienne-Emile (1926–)

French biochemist Etienne-Emile Baulieu led the teams of researchers working for a French pharmaceutical company and for France's national health and medical research institute that developed in the early 1980s mifepristone, also known as the "abortion pill," a synthetic molecule that interferes with the functioning of progesterone in a pregnant woman and interrupts that pregnancy.

Baulieu was born Etienne-Emile Blum 12 December 1926, in Strasbourg. After the death of his physician father when Baulieu was age four, Baulieu's mother moved the family to Paris. When the Germans invaded France in World War II, the Blum's fled to Grenoble. As a young man, Baulieu sympathized with communist philosophies and activists, a circumstance that brought him to the attention of the Gestapo, the secret police of Nazi Germany. In 1942, he obtained false identification papers under the name Baulieu. In the last years of the war he served in the French Army and worked with the French underground. Baulieu chose to keep that name and used it in his adult life.

In 1945, Baulieu studied medicine in Paris and after earning his medical degree continued on to earn a doctorate in science. In 1956, he joined the biochemistry department at the Faculty of Medicine in Paris. While working both as a physician and a researcher,

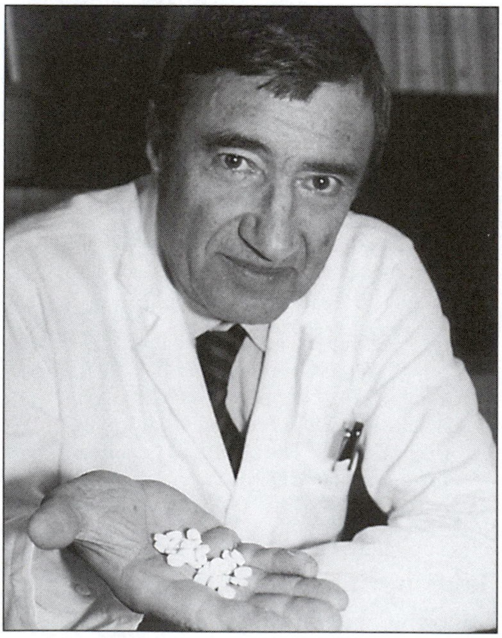

French biochemist Etienne-Emile Baulieu led the team that developed RU–486. *AP/Wideworld Photos*

Baulieu discovered dehydroepiandrosterone sulfate, a water-soluble hormone produced by the adrenal gland. That discovery brought him professional attention that eventually led in 1961 to his spending a year as a visiting lecturer at Columbia University in New York. While in the United States, Baulieu met Gregory Pincus, who with John Rock, had developed the hormonal contraceptive pill, which reached the U.S. market in 1960. His meeting with Pincus inspired Baulieu to devote his talents and skills as a researcher to work on contraceptives. With the advent of molecular biology in the mid-1960s, Baulieu was able to combine his work with steroids with a new interest in reproduction.

In 1963, Baulieu became director of a research unit in France's national institute of health and medical research. He also accepted a consulting position with Roussel Uclaf, one of the country's largest pharmaceutical companies. Developments in the understanding of cell function and the role of hormones in triggering that function led to the discovery of chemicals that could combine with a cell in the same position that a hormone would. These chemicals, known as antihormones, would then block the action of that hormone. When a Roussel-Uclaf researcher developed a molecule that disrupted the function of cortisone, Baulieu realized the role that molecule could also play as an antiprogesterone, a drug that interferes with the function of the sex hormone progesterone. Baulieu exerted his expertise and influence to persuade Roussel Uclaf not to discard the molecule, known as RU–38486, when it failed at its designed purpose.

Baulieu began tests on animals and soon was able to demonstrate the power of RU–486—Roussel Uclaf had shortened its designation and given it the name mifepristone—which effectively blocked the ability of progesterone to bind with cells in the uterine lining. By disrupting that union, mifepristone proved 80 percent effective at disrupting a pregnancy either by preventing a fertilized egg from implanting in the uterine lining or causing the uterus to shed its lining shortly after implantation. Baulieu later discovered that mifepristone used with misoprostol, a chemical that helped the uterus shed its lining, led to a 95 percent effectiveness rate in halting pregnancies less than nine weeks from conception. France approved sale and use of mifepristone as a chemical abortifacient in 1988.

Baulieu had become in the mid-1960s a member of a World Health Organization panel of experts dealing with problems of overpopulation, reproduction, and the high number of women who died as the result of illegal abortions. After France approved sales of mifepristone, Baulieu campaigned around the world for governmental approval of mifepristone. In 1990, he published an autobiographical and scientific account of the development of that drug: *The "Abortion Pill:" RU–486, A Woman's Choice.*

Baulieu is a tireless researcher who believes that scientists need to personalize science to help people understand its achievement and limitations. In the 1990s, Baulieu focused his research attention on steroid hormones produced in the brain. *See also* MIFEPRISTONE

Further reading: Baulieu, Etienne-Emile. *The "Abortion Pill:" RU–486, A Woman's Choice.* New York: Simon and Schuster, 1991. "Baulieu Etienne-Emile." *Current Biography–1995.* New York: H. W. Wilson, 1995.

Billings Method

In the 1950s, Dr. John Billings and Dr. Evelyn Billings began the scientific study that would lead to the development of the ovulation method, also known as the Billings method, of using cervical mucus to anticipate a woman's fertile period.

Based upon cultural and medical anecdotes that reported the flow of a slippery, stringy, lubricated mucus that comes from women's vaginas, John Billings in 1953 began a careful, planned study of this consistent, predictable biological event. By the 1970s, scientific understanding of ovulation and research around the world, including the 1978 study by the World Health Organization, established that learning and understanding the changes in her cervical mucus could help a woman estimate when she would be fertile or not fertile.

To use the method, a woman learns to recognize differing consistencies in her cervical mucus. Before ovulation, a thick mucus plugs her cervix; this substances is known to block the path of sperm and to inhibit sperm function. As an egg matures on a woman's ovaries, its follicle gives off increasing amounts of estrogen, which alters the cervical mucus to allow sperm to pass through. Because a woman is only fertile for approximately 24 hours after a mature egg erupts from her ovary during ovulation, she can learn to use these changes in her cervical mucus to help predict when she could safely have unprotected intercourse.

From the beginning of menstruation until several days before ovulation, most women have dry days when no mucus discharges from the vagina. Then, several days before ovulation most women will feel and see that the mucus is becoming thinner and more elastic. When the moist mucus is present in the cervix, sperm can live for up to three days in the lining of the cervix. The last day that wet, slippery mucus appears is the peak of her fertility, at or very close to ovulation. The sperm swim through the mucus, which has also been nourishing the sperm and now provides channels to speed the sperms' journey.

To avoid pregnancy, a woman must abstain from sexual intercourse from the day she first notices a change in her mucus until three days after the peak day. This phase of her cycle lasts approximately 10 days, though this figure varies depending on the overall length of a woman's specific menstrual cycle.

Most often, women learn this method from women teachers trained in the method. Offices of Natural Family Planning provide information and teachers. As she learns, the woman keeps charts of the mucus she observes with each trip to the bathroom. By wiping near her vagina with toilet paper or her fingers before she urinates, a woman samples the mucus and describes, for herself, its texture and moisture content. At the end each day she writes the changes on the chart. The woman also notes on her chart when she has intercourse. After one lesson and one month's chart, 90 percent of women are able to accurately recognize changes in their mucus. Generally, it takes women three months to effectively chart and interpret the changes in cervical mucus.

During the lessons, teachers help women learn not to mistake for cervical mucus the lubricating substance her body makes during arousal or to mistake the man's semen which is also discharged. She also learns not to confuse cervical mucus with spermicides used with barrier contraceptives.

The Billings method provides greatest success when the woman and the man are very conscientious about abstaining from intercourse or using a barrier method of contraception during the fertile period. Under perfect use, the Billings method is 97 percent effective at preventing pregnancy. However, like other methods of fertility awareness, typical use results in an 80 percent effectiveness rate. Should a couple have unprotected intercourse on or just before the peak day of mucus discharge, they have an 85 percent chance of conceiving, the same chance of pregnancy as a couple that takes no action to prevent pregnancy.

The advantages of the Billings method make it a valuable choice for many people. It requires no special devices, requires cooperation by both partners, and can support religious convictions against the use of other contraceptives. *See also* BASAL BODY TEMPERATURE METHOD; BIOLOGICAL METHODS OF CONTRACEPTION; FERTILITY AWARENESS; OVULATION; REPRODUCTIVE SYSTEM—FEMALE

Further reading: Billings, Evelyn, and Ann Westmore. *The Billings Method: Controlling Fertility without Drugs or Devices.* New York: Random House, 1980. Weschler, Toni. *Taking Charge of Your Fertility: The Definitive Guide to Natural Birth Control and Pregnancy Achievement.* New York: HarperCollins, 1995. Winstein, Merryl. *Your Fertility Signals: Using Them to Achieve or Avoid Pregnancy Naturally.* Saint Louis: Smooth Stone Press, 1994.

Biological Methods of Contraception

Biological methods of birth control (sometimes referred to as "natural" methods) work without women or men needing to insert drugs, chemicals, or objects into their bodies or cover their reproductive organs with devices to block the path of sperm.

The earliest forms of preventing pregnancy involved only knowledge of human reproduction and included two essential biological methods, withdrawal and abstinence, which, historians conclude, have been used since humankind discovered that pregnancy was the result of sexual intercourse. People who did not have intercourse, who remained virgins, or who chose abstinence after experiencing sex, never conceived children. Men who withdrew their penises during intercourse immediately before ejaculation, a procedure known formally by the Latin phrase *coitus interruptus*, were frequently successful at not fathering children. Both of these biological methods are still commonly practiced around the world, quite successfully by some people, even as science and technology devise modern artificial forms of contraception.

Abstinence is known as the only 100 percent certain way to prevent pregnancy. In the narrowest definition, abstinence means refraining from the man inserting his penis into the woman's vagina. Broader definitions include no sexual contact at all. People often choose varying degrees of abstinence as a temporary pregnancy prevention measure or as a lifestyle.

Withdrawal involves a man removing his penis from the woman's vagina moments before he feels he is about to ejaculate. The semen then erupts from his penis outside of the woman's body. This method depends greatly upon the man's willingness and ability to remove his penis.

Fertility awareness methods of birth control also rely upon an understanding of human biology to be successful at preventing pregnancy. In the 1950s, researchers discovered that the mucus that blocks a woman's cervix changes during her menstrual cycle, from dry and sticky in the early days as eggs mature on the ovaries and in the later days as the endometrium sheds in menstruation, to wet, sticky, and slimy during the middle days immediately before and after ovulation. Scientists also discovered in the 1950s that the resting body temperature for many, though not all, women, rose sharply from 0.5 to 1 degree at ovulation and remained high during the remainder of her cycle until menstruation. These two science-based biological methods of birth control, known as the basal body temperature method and the Billings method, require that couples abstain from intercourse when physical conditions indicate ovulation is about to or has occurred. Both methods have success rates comparable to most barrier methods, such as the diaphragm and the condom, when both people are dedicated to fertility awareness methods and use them accurately.

The calendar method of fertility, sometimes still referred to as the "rhythm" method, is the least reliable because it depends upon a woman keeping track of the length of her cycles and then counting back 14 days from the typical cycle length as the way of anticipating when ovulation has occurred. While ovulation is known to consistently occur 14 days before menstruation, the length of a woman's cycle before ovulation varies significantly from month to month and from woman to woman. Modern uses of the calendar are based upon an accurate understanding of the timing of ovulation. Before the mid-1900s, however, people did not understand that ovulation occurred in midcycle and proponents of the "rhythm" method, recommend intercourse at midcycle to prevent pregnancy. This misunderstanding lead to significant failure of this method and to its low reputation today, though that error has been corrected in modern training.

Breastfeeding women may also take advantage of biological circumstances to help prevent pregnancy. The lactational amenorrhea method (LAM) of contraception depends on the fact that a child sucking at a woman's breast which is producing milk suppresses ovulation and creates a natural form of infertility. Very specific criteria for the amount of nutrition a mother must provide through direct breastfeeding make this approach highly successful when a woman follows those criteria.

Research and study have provided people with biological options to drugs and devices, but all biological methods, to be highly successful at preventing pregnancy, require cooperation from both partners and a dedication to the method. That dedication and the communication it requires challenge many couples who choose biological methods. The challenge of that dedication often leads to typical success rates less than 80 percent, where one in every five women will become pregnant during the first year of use. Perfect use of fertility awareness methods would give success rates ranging from 91 percent for the calendar method to 98 percent for the basal temperature and cervical mucus method. The lactational amenorrhea method can offer women success rates as high as 99.5 percent when used correctly. *See also* ABSTINENCE; BASAL BODY TEMPERATURE METHOD; BILLINGS METHOD; BREASTFEEDING; FERTILITY AWARENESS; TRADITIONAL METHODS OF CONTRACEPTION; WITHDRAWAL

Further reading: Hatcher, Robert, James Trussel, Felina Stewart, and others. *Contraceptive Technology.* 17th rev. ed. New York: Ardent Media, 1998.

Birth Control

The meaning of the phrase "birth control" has evolved and expanded since the phrase was first publicly coined in 1914 by women's advocate Margaret Sanger (1879–1966). Sanger gives credit to Otto Bobsein, a young friend, for putting the words together as more publicly appealing way to refer to the cause that had become important in her life, helping women learn of ways to limit the number of pregnancies they had without sacrificing their sexuality. It replaced such terms as "family limitation" or "voluntary motherhood" that in Europe and the United States had been used by social advocates to describe the plight of the poor in remaining ignorant about contraception.

The phrase soon caught on and became part of the title of several groups that worked toward increasing knowledge and public awareness of contraception and the plight of poor women who often bore more children then they could afford and than was healthy for them. In 1915, women advocates formed The National Birth Control League, led by Mary Ware Dennett (1872–1947), to lobby against laws that restricted the sale of contraception and the dissemination of information on contraceptives. That year, Sanger herself formed the New York Birth Control League, which published the *Birth Control Review.*

The original intent of the people who used the term publicly was to provide women with information on preventing pregnancy, but the use of the word "control" carried with it connotations of coercion from outside forces and as a title for organizations it fell out of popularity, to be replaced by terms such as "family planning" and "planned parenthood."

Birth control had become a popular term to describe the influence people had over their ability to reproduce, and with the invention of the "birth control pill" in the 1950s and its arrival on the U.S. market in 1960, the term had become publicly accepted and widely used. By the end of the twentieth century, "birth control" generally referred to the means women and men could use to prevent unwanted pregnancies before fertilization or viability. This included such means as withdrawal, which had been used since ancient times to avoid pregnancy; condoms, invented in the 1800s; diaphragms; intrauterine devices; and hormonal contraceptives. By the late 1970s, birth control also referred to processes known as fertility awareness and periodic abstinence, which uses the biological indicators of body temperature and cervical mucus discharge to determine when ovulation was likely to have occurred. Based upon these indicators, a couple refrains from intercourse for a period of days, often two weeks, around the expected day of ovulation. Before these signs had been carefully studied, people used the "rhythm" method, a highly unreliable and often incorrectly understood method of avoiding a woman's most fertile time that early advocates of birth control rejected as too unsuccessful. Fertility awareness, however, has become a highly regarded and accepted form of birth control and the only modern method approved of by the Catholic Church.

Occasionally, scholars use the term birth control to refer only to modern, artificial means. In this regard, birth control is synonymous with contraception, methods that do not require abstinence but that prevent the ejaculated sperm from reaching the mature egg in the woman's body. According to varying religions, cultures, and moral beliefs, birth control and contraception may also refer to products that prevent a fertilized egg from implanting in the uterine wall, such as progestin-only contraceptives, and chemicals that would induce menstruation, regardless of whether fertilization or implantation had occurred. Some people believe that products that work after fertilization are abortifacients and not contraceptive or birth control devices.

Though commonly considered birth control because it prevents the live birth of a child, induced abortion is seen by many scholars, researchers, health care workers, and feminists not as a form of birth control but as a form of fertility control. Abortion provides women with an option, whether it is legal or not, when birth control devices fail.

Family planning, contraception, fertility control, and birth control often refer interchangeably to processes that allow adults to choose when and if they want to bear children. Fertility control may refer to traditional methods of preventing pregnancy or stimulating menstruation long used by people who believed in their effectiveness but which may or may not have scientific proof of that effectiveness. This term may also refer to abortion methods, whether modern or traditional. Contraception refers most specifically to modern methods of preventing pregnancy, not including abortion. Family planning and birth control refer most often to the aspect of choice in the function of products that prevent unwanted pregnancies.

In common practice and most publications, people make little, if any, distinction between the terms birth control, contraception, family planning, and fertility control. This lack of distinction in turn leads to confusion and often disagreement over the moral and social acceptability of any method of purposely disrupting the reproductive process. *See also* CONTRACEPTION; FAMILY PLANNING; SANGER, MARGARET HIGGINS

Further reading: Back, Kurt W. *Family Planning and Population Control: The Challenges of a Successful Movement.* Boston: Twayne, 1989. Harper, Michael J. K. *Birth Control Technologies: Prospects by the Year 2000.* Austin: University of Texas Press, 1983. Kennedy, David M. *Birth Control in America: The Career of Margaret Sanger*. New Haven, CT: Yale University Press, 1970.

Brazil

Brazil, the world's fifth largest country in total population size (172 million in 1999), experienced a dramatic decline in its total fertility from the early 1960s through the late 1990s, and showed strong indications of continued decline into the 2000s. While rapid social changes appear to have greatly influenced the decrease in the number of children women were having, initiatives by women themselves led directly to that decline. Recent involvement by government planners to support further declines in population growth and involvement in improving women's and children's health is seen as an important path to continued population decline.

In 1965, women throughout Brazil could expect to give birth to 6 children in their lifetimes. By 1995, that total fertility rate had decreased to 2.5. While much of that decreased interest among women in having children took place in the nation's cities, which grew rapidly in those decades, the more rural, poorer states in Brazil's northeast region experienced a similar decline in the number of children women were bearing. In 1965, in the northeast region, women typically could expect to give birth to 7.44 children. By 1995, that figure had dropped to 2.5 children.

That dramatic decrease in the total fertility rate led to an equally dramatic slowing of the growth of Brazil's population. However, the population was large enough from past growth to more than quadruple in size from the 1940s to the 1990s. In 1940, 41 million people lived in Brazil; by 1999, its population had reached 162.1 million. In the late 1950s, the number of people living in Brazil was increasing at a rate of 2.9 percent each year. By the mid-1990s, growth had slowed to 1.4 percent each year. With falling birth rates, Brazil should see steadily decreasing numbers of children under the age of 15, a category that demographers expect to drop by 16 percent between 1995 and 2020.

The grassroots decisions by women to use abortion and contraception accounted for most of that fertility decline. Women frequently turn to abortion, which is illegal in Brazil except in the cases of rape or to save a mother's life. Some estimates suggest that nearly 50 women out of every 1,000 between the ages of 15 and 44 have abortions each year. Other studies report that for every 1,000 births each year there are between 266 and 444 abortions, suggesting that between 20 and 33 percent of pregnancies end in abor-

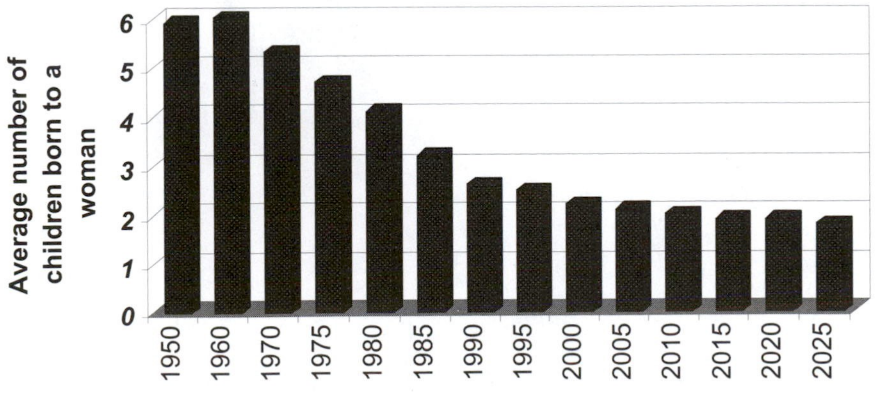

Brazil: Total Fertility Rate: Actual and Projected

Source: U.S. Census Bureau International Data Base

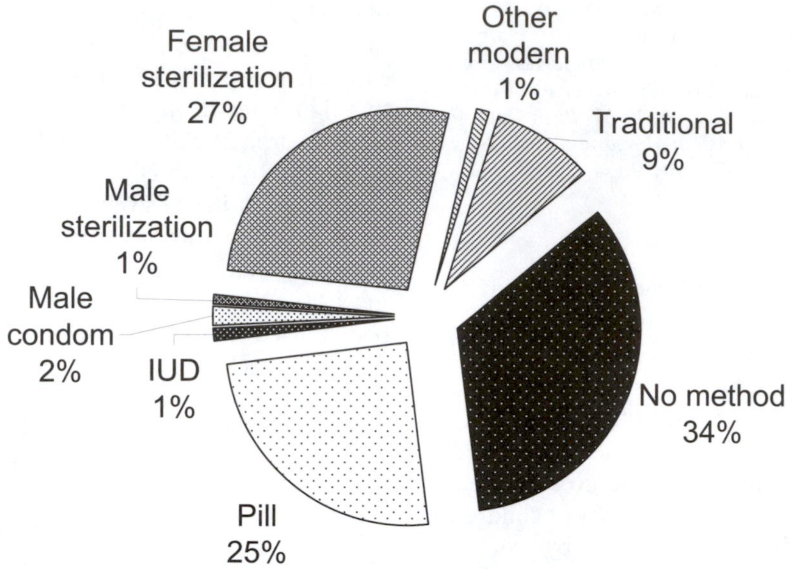

Brazil: 1986 Contraceptive Use by Married Women Ages 15–49

Source: U.S. Census Bureau, *World Population Profile 1998*

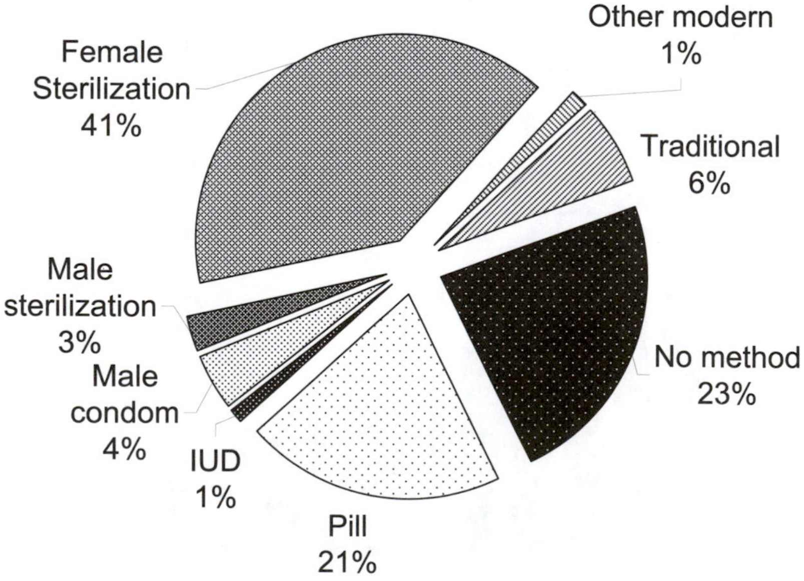

Brazil: 1996 Contraceptive Use by Married Women Ages 15–49

Source: U.S. Census Bureau, *World Population Profile 1998*

tion. Many of those abortions are self-induced where women use commonly known chemical and traditional methods of stopping a pregnancy. Abortions account for 12 percent of women in Brazil who die from pregnancy-related causes.

Sterilization and hormonal contraceptive pills account for a very high use of modern birth control methods in Brazil. More than 70 percent of women in Brazil use modern contraceptive methods to prevent pregnancy. Sterilization, researchers have found, is often performed after cesarean section deliveries, and Brazil has one of the highest rates of cesarean sections in the world. In 1996, 40 percent of the women using contraceptives had been sterilized. Estimates suggest that 75 percent of those sterilizations were performed after the cesarean section delivery.

In contrast, 20 percent of women using modern contraceptives relied upon the birth control pill to prevent pregnancy and to space births, and 78 percent of women of reproductive age had ever used the pill. Women in Brazil have easy access to contraceptive pills, which are available without a prescription in pharmacies.

Other contraceptive methods were used more rarely by Brazil's women. Condom use rose from 1.7 percent in 1986 to 4.4 percent in 1996, due in part to people seeking protection against acquired immunodeficiency syndrome (AIDS), which increased rapidly in the 1990s. AIDS was expected to decrease Brazil's life expectancy average by four years by the early 2000s. Intrauterine devices and injectable contraceptives accounted for a little more than 1 percent of modern contraceptive users and only 2.6 percent of the women had partners who had undergone vasectomies.

Demand by women for contraceptive methods led directly to Brazil's fertility decline. The social forces that caused that demand varied, but among the strongest was rapidly increasing rates of education, particularly of women. Literacy, a prime measure of education, rose as rapidly as fertility declined among Brazil's population, mostly among women, from less than 50 percent in 1950 to more than 83 percent in the late 1990s. The gap between men and women's literacy rates closed completely from 11 percent in the 1950s. In fact, Brazilian women under the age of 30 have a higher literacy rate than men of the same age.

Unlike many other developing countries, Brazil developed no specific governmental population program until late in the 1980s. Actions taken by the governments to solve other Brazilian problems, however, created circumstances that encouraged families to have fewer children. Many social and economic changes, brought about first by a military government in power from 1965 to 1985, then by efforts to democratize Brazil's government and economy, created social policies that had strong if unplanned influences on child bearing and family size. Efforts to transform Brazil into a consumer nation and to provide credit for poorer people, increased the cost to a family of having more children. The more children they had the fewer consumer goods people could afford. Maternal and child health care eventually became a social issue with the increase of the number of medical professionals in Brazil and the government policy of supporting private medicine. Providing immunizations for children and paying for insurance coverage for childbirth also increased the cost to a family of having a child and led to a decline in the fertility rate.

More than the government, however, scholars credit women themselves and the rise of the Brazilian women's movement for bringing about this and further fertility decreases. Women originally fought against the military rule in Brazil and when the government became democratic, women shifted their attention to fighting for women's rights, including reproductive rights.

Further declines in the fertility rate, compounded by Brazil's rapidly increasing rate of deaths from the AIDS epidemic, will work in the twenty-first century to further slow that nation's rate of population growth. *See also* ACCESS (TO CONTRACEPTIVES)

Further reading: "Brazil 1996: Results from the Demographic and Health Survey." *Studies in Family Planning* 29 (1998): 88–92. Bureau of the Census. *Population Trends: Brazil*. Washington,

DC: U.S. Department of Commerce, Economics and Statistics Administration, Bureau of the Census, 1993. Martine, George. "Brazil's Fertility Decline, 1965–1995: A Fresh Look at Key Factors." *Population and Development Review* 22 (1996): 47–75.

Breastfeeding

Women who rely on breastfeeding to nourish their newborn children have a highly effective natural means of contraception to turn to. Known formally as the lactational amenorrhea method (LAM) of contraception, women throughout history have often relied upon breastfeeding to help them space the births of their children. Now scientific research has firmly established that exclusive breastfeeding delays the return of menstruation and offers contraceptive benefits to mothers for the months after the birth of a child.

Research in northern Italy in the late 1980s established that women who fully or nearly fully breastfeed and do not have their monthly menstrual periods return have a less than 2 percent risk of becoming pregnant during the first six months after delivery. An infant's sucking seems to suppress the production of gonadotropin releasing hormone (GnRH) in the mother. The lack of this hormone, produced in the hypothalamus, would prevent the pituitary gland from making and building up luteinizing hormone (LH), which is released in a sudden surge about mid-menstrual cycle. Without sudden burst of LH, the follicles on a woman's ovary never release mature eggs during ovulation.

While this delay of menstruation and ovulation offers women a natural, and traditional, method of preventing the conception of another child while she is suckling one baby, to be effective, LAM requires exclusive breastfeeding, frequent and long feeds day and night, and dedication. To expect the 98 percent success rate when using LAM, a woman must follow a strict set of requirements. She must begin breastfeeding as soon as possible after delivery. Her child must feed directly from her breast; pumping breast milk for feeding from a bottle does not have the same contraceptive effect. The woman's monthly period must not have resumed, and the breastfeeding child must be less than six months old. The mother would need to feed the child on demand, not on a schedule, with no long intervals between feedings and without giving the child food supplements.

The longer a woman breastfeeds, the more likely she is to begin menstruating while breastfeeding, for the contraceptive effectiveness of breastfeeding diminishes over time. When a woman's menstrual period returns within six months of delivery, it generally does so without ovulation having taken place first. Beyond six months, the likelihood that ovulation has occurred before the return of a woman's period increases significantly, from a 33 percent chance at six months that ovulation preceded the return of menses to an 87 to 100 percent chance at 12 months after birth that ovulation preceded the return of menses. After six months, a woman can expect a steadily decreasing success rate, or a steadily increasing failure rate, using the LAM method of contraception.

Studies in Pakistan and the Philippines suggest that breastfeeding is tolerant of some error on the woman's part, showing little or no difference in the success rate of women who used LAM correctly or almost correctly. The studies also show that LAM can be as effective as non-medicated intrauterine devices, barrier methods, and spermicides, though not as effective as hormonal contraceptives such as the pill and implants.

In developing countries, breastfeeding plays a major role in providing a natural form of contraception. In sub-Saharan Africa, for example, mothers breastfeed their babies, on average, for 21 months. However, the rate at which mothers feed their babies exclusively through the child sucking at the breast varies widely across the region. By adding other feeding methods to the child's diet, the mother reduces the contraceptive effectiveness of breastfeeding and increases her risk of becoming pregnant. Thus lactational amenorrhea as a contraceptive has varying success. In the Philippines, researchers found LAM to be highly effective for women who had never used modern contraceptives. For these women, the naturalness of breastfeeding allowed them preliminary access to family planning methods. They were then more likely to choose a modern method after weaning the child.

Breastfeeding, while growing in popularity in the United States, is still chosen by less than half of new mothers. Those who do choose breastfeeding usually continue it for only 13 weeks. Some researchers believe more women would choose breastfeeding if they were more aware of its contraceptive benefits immediately after childbirth. *See also* BIOLOGICAL METHODS OF CONTRACEPTION

Further reading: Ramos, Rebecca, Kathy I. Kennedy, and Cynthia M. Visness. "Effectiveness of Lactational Amenorrhoea in Prevention of Pregnancy in Manila, the Philippines: Non-comparative Prospective Trial." *British Medical Journal* 313 (1996): 909–912. Van Look, Paul F. A. "Lactational Amenorrhoea Method for Family Planning Provides High Protection from Pregnancy for the First Six Months after Delivery." *British Medical Journal* 313 (1996): 893–894.

C

Canada

Canada, the largest and northernmost country in North America, shares in the low fertility and low population growth common in the industrialized nations of the late twentieth century. Within its borders, which reach from the Great Lakes to the Arctic Ocean, and from the Atlantic to Pacific oceans live just more than 30 million people who experience a wide variety of access to modern contraceptives and to modern medical services.

Canada's women could expect to give birth to an average of 1.6 children in their lifetimes as of 1998. That rate had fallen from 2.66 in 1961 and 1.98 in 1981. With a total fertility rate below the level needed to simply replace the current population, which demographers calculate at 2.08 children for every woman, Canada's population was growing at only 0.5 percent each year and much of that was due to immigration. Demographers estimate that by 2020, Canada's population growth will end with about 40 million people living in its 10 provinces and two territories. After 2020, Canada is likely to experience more deaths than births within its population, a situation that is likely to be common throughout western Europe.

Ninety percent of the sexually active women in Canada use modern contraceptives. In the major metropolitan areas, people have easy access to all modern birth control methods. People living in the more remote areas of British Columbia and the Northwest Territories, however, have minimal access to reproductive health care services and methods to prevent pregnancy. As a result, women in the Northwest Territories have the highest regional total fertility rate in Canada at 2.69 children. The eastern province of Newfoundland has the lowest total fertility rate at 1.4 children. Provincial governments have responsibility for providing family planning to their residents and the degree to which they meet that responsibility varies also and influences success. Ontario has a strong family planning program and easy access for people, whereas Prince Edward Island has no public family planning clinics.

Canadians turn most often to permanent surgical sterilization in their choice of contraceptive methods. Twenty-nine percent of Canadian women are protected from unwanted pregnancy by sterilization, either male vasectomy or female tubal sterilization. Canada has one of the highest sterilization rates in the world. However, the ratio of men to women who undergo sterilization is much different from other nations. In Canada as of 1997, vasectomies, a simpler procedure performed through the skin of the scrotum, equaled the number of tubal sterilizations, which require surgery through the abdominal wall or during a cesarean section delivery. Worldwide, tubal sterilizations out–number vasectomies two to one. A change in

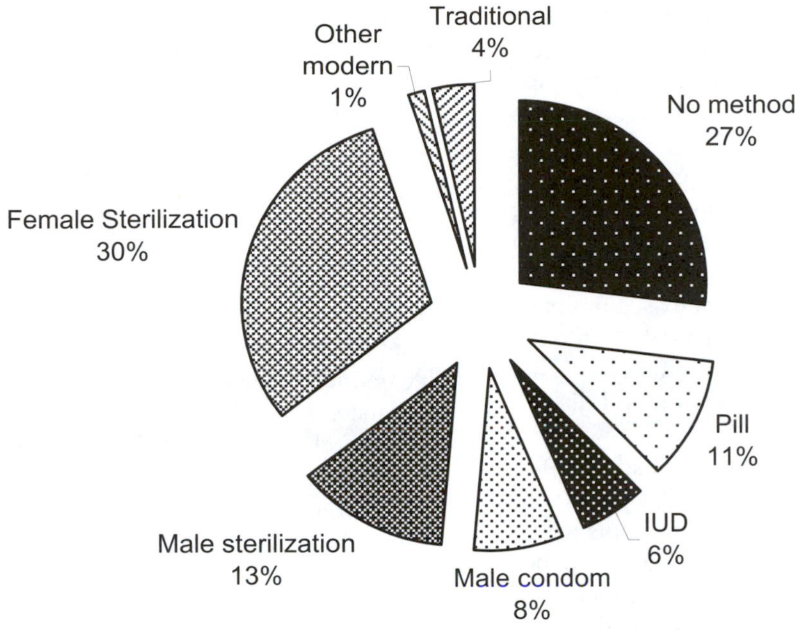

Canada: 1984 Contraceptive Use by Women Ages 15–49

Source: U.S. Census Bureau International Data Base

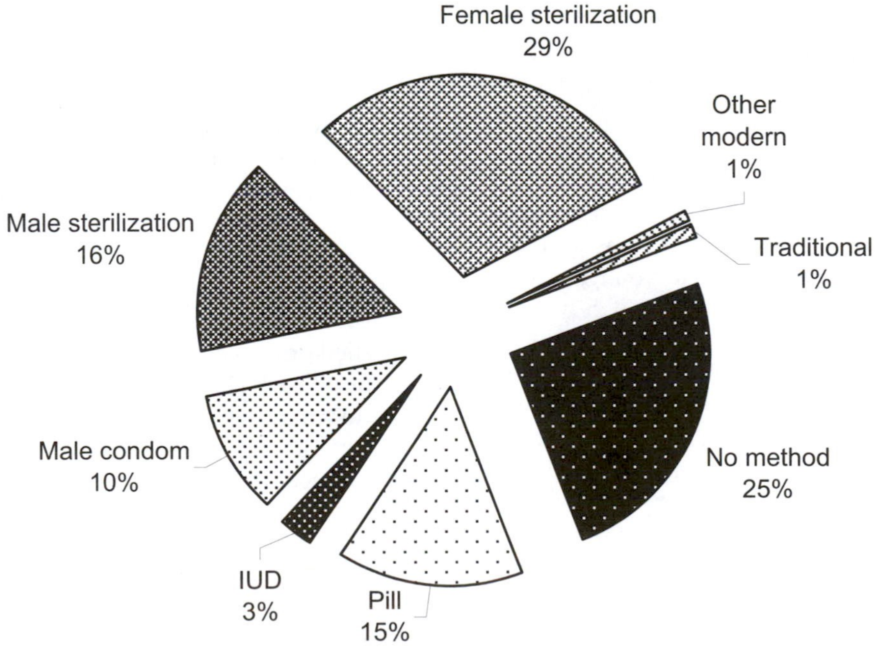

Canada: 1995 Contraceptive Use by Women Ages 15–49

Source: U.S. Census Bureau International Data Base

attitude among the men of Canada accounts for a shift toward greater male responsibility in family planning that began in the early 1980s. By 1986 in the province of Quebec, as many men as women had undergone permanent sterilization. The nation reached that balance by 1993.

Canadians turn next to contraceptive pills, with 27 percent of women using this method, and condoms, at 21 percent use rate. Women report a high degree of satisfaction with hormonal pills. Condom use increased dramatically in Canada from the mid-1980s into the 1990s. Young Canadians turned to this method for both contraception and disease prevention.

Abortion became legal in Canada in 1988 when the Supreme Court of Canada ruled that forcing a woman to carry a fetus to full term was a "profound interference" with her body and an infringement upon her security. Canada, like its neighbor the United States, has faced social unrest as opponents of abortion struggle to overturn that ruling. The number of abortions performed in Canada rose sharply after that decision, from 70,000 in 1987 to 102,000 in 1993. By the late 1990s, 20 out of every 1,000 women had an abortion each year in Canada. Half of Canada's unplanned pregnancies end in abortion, and 40 percent of all pregnancies are unplanned.

Teenagers and their reproductive health represented the largest challenge facing Canada as it began the twenty-first century. At increasing rates, Canada's teens were beginning their sexual lives at younger rates. By 1998, 42 percent of 16-year-olds had begun sexual activity. Use of male condoms on first intercourse increased among teens more dramatically than among the population at large with between 40 and 64 percent reporting that they used condoms at the time of their first sexual intercourse. However 26 percent of women between 15 and 18 years old used no contraceptives. Teen pregnancy rates show the same regional variation as does contraceptive availability. In Quebec, 30 of every 1,000 teens become pregnant each year. In the Northwest Territories, 125 of every 1,000 become pregnant. Decreasing these numbers through improving education and reproductive health services is the goal of Canada's family planning organizations.

Further reading: McLaren, Angus, and Arlene Tigar McLaren. *The Bedroom and the State: The Changing Practices and Politics of Contraception and Abortion in Canada, 1880–1997*. 2nd ed. Toronto: Oxford University Press, 1997.

Cancer

Concerns over a relationship between hormonal contraceptives and cancer and a possible connection between induced abortions and cancer led in the 1990s to much debate and research in the scientific community on both of these issues.

Since they were first marketed in 1960s, hormonal contraceptives have been intensely studied to detect and understand their influence on cancer. Forty years after their development scientists and health experts struggle with continuing questions. Because these contraceptives contain artificial forms of the two reproductive hormones, estrogen and progesterone, and because medical research has indicated that cancers of the female reproductive system depend in part on sex hormones to form and grow, health professionals and cancer experts have carefully studied the influence of the artificial hormones on cancer. The results have been mixed and varied. Combined oral contraceptives (COCs) appear to offer protection for women against some forms of reproductive cancers and at the same time seem to increase women's risk of other reproductive cancers.

Most of the attention has focused on the combined oral contraceptive pill, or the birth control pill, which contains doses of estrogen and progesterone. These pills appear to influence different cancers in varying ways. COCs appear to slightly increase a woman's risk of developing breast cancer, but research has since 1985 presented inconsistent evidence. Debate continued in 1999 after the release of studies that showed that women's risk from breast cancer increased during COC use, then decreased after they stopped taking the pills, until 10 years later when the women showed no more risk of breast cancer than women who had never used COCs. The patterns revealed in this study, which included most of the breast cancer and combined oral contraceptive studies conducted since 1985, also confused experts since they did not match the patterns of other cancer risk factors, such as smoking. Experts are still divided concerning the relationship of COCs to breast cancer.

Women who used contraceptive pills for many years also showed an increased risk from cancer of the cervix, the lower neck of the uterus that fits into the vagina. While studies seemed to indicate that women who use COCs for five years or more were at slightly greater risk of cervical cancer than women who never used COCs, the exact nature of the risk was still unclear almost 40 years after the pill was introduced.

To the contrary, combined oral contraceptives appeared to offer women the positive benefit of decreasing their risk from ovarian and endometrial cancers. Eighteen years of study show a woman's risk from ovarian cancer decreases the longer she uses the pill. Even women who take COCs for only three to six months receive this positive influence. While the cause of COCs' influence on ovarian cancer is unclear, scientists estimate that the pill each year helps 1,700 women in the United States avoid ovarian cancer.

The pattern persists for the reduction of a woman's risk from cancer of the endometrium, the inner lining of the uterus. Studies have shown that women who use COCs for at least one year cut their risk of developing endometrial cancer in half as compared to women who never have taken contraceptive pills.

The relationship between other forms of hormonal contraceptives and cancer were also studied in the 1980s and 1990s, again with mixed results. While implantable contraceptives that contain only a progesterone, such as Norplant, seemed to show no relationship to cancers, depot medroxyprogesterone acetate (DMPA), an injectable progesterone contraceptive was linked to an increased risk of breast cancer. In fact, the U.S. Food and Drug Administration (FDA) for more than 15 years delayed approval of DMPA for use due to results that suggested it too greatly increased a woman's risk of developing breast cancer. However, studies by the World Health Organization and researchers in New Zealand established that DMPA caused no greater risk of breast cancer than combined oral contraceptives. In light of that evidence, the FDA removed its objection to DMPA, marketed as Depo-Provera, and approved its use in 1992.

Controversy also surrounded in the 1990s studies aimed at determining a relationship between induced abortions and breast cancer. While a series of studies seemed to indicate a significant risk from breast cancer for women who had abortions, a study of health databases found no difference in the risk from breast cancer between women who had never had an abortion and women who had.

Barrier contraceptives, such as the diaphragm and the condom offer women some protection from cervical cancer, blocking viruses that appear to lead to this form of cancer. Female surgical sterilization also offers women protection from ovarian cancer. Clinical studies showed that tubal sterilization offered women of all ages a significant protection from ovarian cancer, no matter how many children they had had. Hysterectomy, the removal of a uterus and ovaries, also showed a positive influence in reducing a woman's risk from ovarian cancer.

Douching, which research has firmly established as being ineffective as a contraceptive, disturbs the natural, beneficial organisms in the vagina. This disruption increases a woman's risk from pelvic inflammatory disease and other diseases of the vagina, which can, in turn, increase a woman's risk from cervical cancer. *See also* COMBINED ORAL CONTRACEPTIVES; DEPO-PROVERA; RISK

Further reading: Gammon, Marilie D., Joan E. Bertin, and Mary Beth Terry. "Abortion and the Risk of Breast Cancer: Is There a Believable Association?" *Journal of the American Medical Association* 275 (1996): 321–322. Skegg, David C. G., et al. "Depot Medroxyprogesterone Acetate and Breast Cancer: A Pooled Analysis of the World Health Organization and New Zealand Studies." *The Journal of the American Medical Association* 273 (1995): 799–804. Speroff, Leon, and Carolyn L. Westhoff. "Breast Disease and Hormonal Contraception: Resolution of a Lasting Controversy." *Dialogues in Contraception* 5.3 (1997): 1–4.

Center for Reproductive Law and Policy

From offices in New York City and Washington, DC, the Center for Reproductive Law and Policy, a nonprofit legal organization, studies international laws and the laws in the United States and other countries, advocates and argues for laws that support women's reproductive rights, and trains lawyers in reproductive law.

The center works to protect women's reproductive rights where they exist, including access to legal abortion and contraception, and works to establish reproductive law where it does not exist. Staff lawyers have supported women's rights to abortion, including the rights of adolescent girls, in legal cases in the United States, investigated the arrest and imprisonment in Chile of women who received abortions, and uncovered abuses against women in Peru.

Through its fellowships and education funds, the association helps lawyers learn international law and strategies to improve the legality of reproductive rights. It works to guarantee that low-income women have equal access to contraception and abortion as women of greater financial means and examines legal issues involved in providing universal access to contraceptives and abortion.

The center publishes *Reproductive Freedom News*, a news letter discussing legal issues relating to birth control and abortion worldwide. It also publishes a series of books, videos, and reports, including two in its *Women of the World: Laws and Policies Affecting Their Reproductive Lives* series, the first on Latin America and the Caribbean and the second on anglophone Africa. *See also* REPRODUCTIVE RIGHTS

Further reading: Center for Reproductive Law and Policy Web site. http://www.crlp.org. Wise, Daniel. "ACLU Battles with Ex-Unit Over Breakup." *The National Law Journal,* 29 June 1992, 12.

Cervical Cap

A barrier contraceptive, the cervical cap fits snugly over the cervix and prevents sperm from entering the uterus. The reusable thimble-sized plastic cap, with its upturned brim, is about 1.5 inches in diameter. Women apply a small amount of spermicide inside the cap before inserting it. They may leave the cap in for two days.

First described in 1838 by a German gynecologist, caps made of silver and copper were popular with upper class Victorian women. Cervical caps were in common use in Europe and the United States until the development of the oral contraceptive pill in the United States in the early 1960s.

In 1988, the U.S. Food and Drug Administration (FDA) approved for use the Prentif Cavity-Rim cervical cap.

The clear silicon FemCap, the newest version of the cervical cap, is, as of the end of the twentieth century, under development and testing. Looking like a sailor's cap with a wide brim, FemCap fits securely over the cervix with its brim lodging against the wall of the vagina. This wide brim gives FemCap a tighter fit than that of older cervical caps. When inserted properly, the deep brim of FemCap catches the sperm-filled semen and thus offers an extra barrier to the round dome that fits over the cervix and blocks the path of the sperm. FemCap was designed to be used with a vaginal spermicide foam or gel.

Women visit a doctor or clinician for a vaginal exam, pap test, and fitting and require a prescription to obtain cervical caps. (The flexibility in sizing of FemCap—based on a woman's obstetrical history, if she has never delivered a child, if she has or has not delivered a child vaginally—may allow developers to sell FemCap without a prescription.) A prime candidate for a cap is a woman with a symmetrical cervix that is free of scars and lacerations that prevent the cap from forming a strong bond with her cervix. Once inserted, suction holds the cap in place, so fit is very important to the success rate. Caps are reusable and need careful cleaning with soap and water after use.

With proper use, cervical caps are 85 percent effective at preventing pregnancy in women who have never been pregnant. Women who have been pregnant who choose to use caps generally experience a 64 percent effectiveness rate. Early tests of the new device, FemCap, showed that it had a typical effective rate of 86.5 percent, which is more than for a diaphragm and about the same as the Prentif Cavity Rim Cervical Cap.

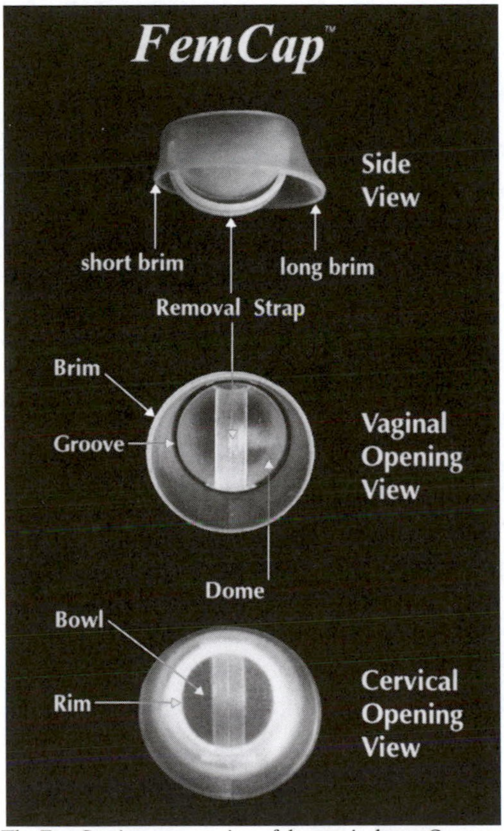

The FemCap is a new version of the cervical cap. *Courtesy of FemCap, Inc., and Alfred Shihata, MD*

As a barrier contraceptive, a cap is easily under the control of the woman who chooses to use it and presents none of the changes to her body as do hormonal contraceptives. Its effective use, however, does depend on the woman remembering to insert the device shortly before she engages in sexual intercourse.

Minor problems with cervical caps include irritation from the spermicide and a very low risk of toxic shock syndrome. *See also* BARRIER CONTRACEPTIVES; DIAPHRAGM; EFFECTIVENESS (OF CONTRACEPTIVES); FAILURE RATES; TOXIC SHOCK SYNDROME

Further reading: Knowles, Jon, and Marcia Ringel. *All About Birth Control: A Personal Guide.* New York: Three Rivers—Crown, 1998. Segal, Marian. *Cervical Cap: Newest Birth Control Choice.* Rockville, MD: U.S. Department of Health and Human Services, 1988.

Cervical Mucus. *See* BILLINGS METHOD

Cervix

The cervix, at the lower portion of the uterus, which is the central organ in the female reproductive system, provides an opening into the upper portions of the uterus and the fallopian tubes. The cervix is also the opening through which a baby leaves the uterus during childbirth.

This neck-shaped canal is lined with glands that secrete various types of mucus needed during different stages in the female reproductive cycle. These glands become capable during ovulation of storing live sperm which can survive there for two or three days and then later move through the uterus and into the fallopian tubes where they can fertilize an egg.

As the opening of the uterus, the cervix provides the entry for male's sperm into the female reproductive organs in which fertilization of an egg can occur. That function also makes the cervix a place where mechanical devices can help keep sperm from reaching the mature eggs. Several devices, such as the cervical cap and diaphragm, cover the cervix and block the route sperm take on their way to the egg.

During most days of a woman's monthly reproductive cycle, a thick plug of mucus blocks this neck of the uterus and prevents sperm from entering. However, during ovulation, the time when a mature egg is ejected from an ovary and travels through a fallopian tube, that mucus becomes very liquid and allows the sperm to pass through and continue towards the descending egg. The mucus flows from a woman's body through the vagina. Careful observation allows a woman to use that mucus as an indicator that ovulation has occurred or is occurring. *See also* BILLINGS METHOD; CERVICAL CAP; DIAPHRAGM; FERTILITY AWARENESS; REPRODUCTIVE SYSTEM—FEMALE; UTERUS

Chemical Contraceptives. *See* BARRIER CONTRACEPTIVES; SPERMICIDES

Child Mortality

The use of contraceptives by women and men is seen as an important way to decrease the rates of infant and child mortality around the world. Estimates show that more than 31,000 children under age five die in the world each day or 11 million each year. The vast majority of these deaths, more than 95 percent, take place in developing countries. There, poverty and lack of access to family planning methods by parents leads to many children being born closely spaced, less than two years after the birth of their next oldest sibling. Providing people with the means to spread farther apart the years and months between their children could help improve the survival rate for children and infants.

The age of the mother, the number of children she has borne, and the years that separate her children all contribute to the risk of death her children face. Of those risk factors, spacing of children has the greatest impact for determining the chances of the child dying before the age of five. While malnutrition is the leading immediate cause of infant deaths in the developing world—half of all infant deaths in developing countries are associated with hunger—inadequate means of family planning and family spacing is one of the major contributors to that lack of food and resources for the child. Improving family planning, vaccinations, improving nutrition, and providing safe water and sanitation working together can further improve a child's chances of surviving and continue the decline in infant mortality that marked the twentieth century.

In the 1970s and 1980s, studies of child spacing conducted in the Europe and the

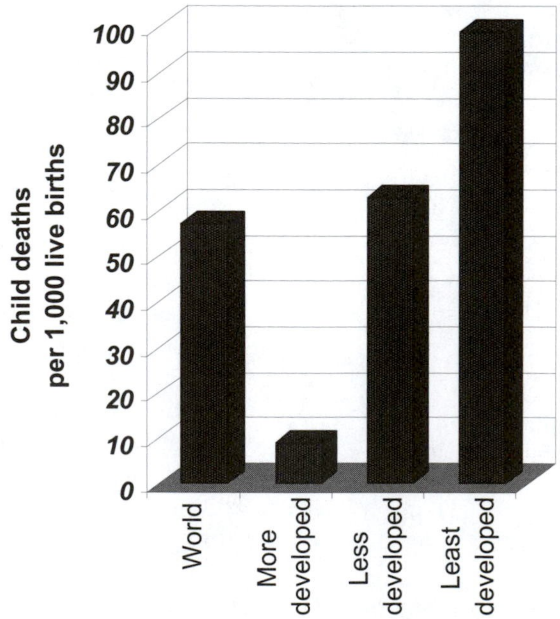

Infant Mortaility Rates by Level of Country Development

Source: United Nations, *State of the World Population 1999*

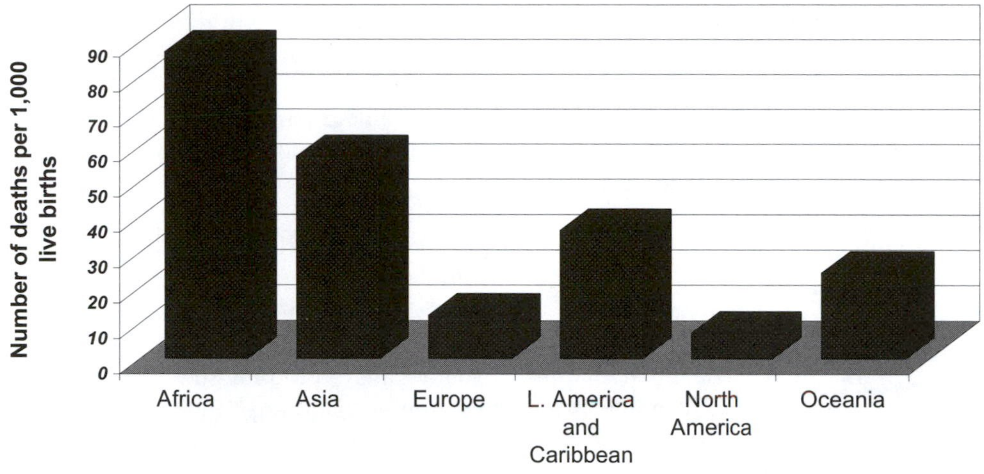

Infant Mortality Rates by Geographic Region

Source: United Nations, *State of the World Population 1999*

United States demonstrated that intervals of two years or more improved a child's health and survival rates. Studies in developing countries in the 1990s confirmed the benefits to children and mothers of spacing children more than the year or so apart that was common in poorer nations. A study conducted from 1990 to 1995 of children under one year old showed disparities even among developing countries. In Egypt, for example, 128 infants under age one per 1,000 live births died where only 46 of infants who where more than two years younger than their next older sibling died. In Egypt in 1994, 60 percent of births were considered high risk in part because of the short interval between births, the age of the mother, and the number of children she had born. In Pakistan, 135 children born close together died as infants, whereas 57 children with more than two years between siblings died.

Close birth spacing also jeopardizes the older child. With the mother needing her energy to carry, bear, and nourish the newborn, siblings younger than two are at greater risk for decreased attention and nutrition than are children over two.

Women under 20 are at greater risk of giving birth to low birth weight children than are women between 20 and 40 years old. Low birth rate babies are one-third more likely than full weight babies to die in infancy. The causes of this problem stem both from the young mother's own physical immaturity and her social immaturity, which can prevent her from gaining the prenatal help she needs to improve her child's chances of survival.

Children born to older women, over the age of 40, are also at higher risk of dying in infancy and early childhood. Many of the children born in developing countries to older women are the fourth, fifth, or even sixth child the mother has born. Frequent childbirth can weaken a woman and lead to birth difficulties and birth defects that threaten a child's life. Birth order also influences child mortality with younger children in larger families likely to suffer from competition for family resources.

Whether a pregnancy is planned or unplanned also has proven to be a factor in infant mortality. The impact of how much a woman wants to be pregnant has a strong influence on the care she seeks before and during pregnancy and that care influences the outcome of the birth with better care leading to healthier babies than those born to women with less care. The impact of a planned or unplanned pregnancy, however, varies significantly from developed to developing countries. In developed countries, women who plan pregnancies are more likely to seek the extra nutritional and medical help they need to increase the health of the child at birth. In developing countries, this pattern is harder to observe since so many children are born into poverty and health care services are much more scarce than in developed countries. Researchers, however, speculate that an unplanned child in a developing country is at greater risk from poverty and illness than a sibling the mother and father had planned for.

Patterns of infant mortality in developed countries show different concerns overall, since medical technology can overcome many of the health problems caused by low birth weight. However, racial, cultural, and economic conditions put some people at greater risk of higher infant mortality levels. In the United States, black infants are twice as likely to die in infancy as white infants. Falling numbers of teen pregnancies, especially among black teens, are expected to change these ratios, but infant mortality in the United States, which ranks 25 among developed nations, presents a challenge to that country. *See also* MATERNAL MORTALITY

Further reading: "Achievements in Public Health, 1900–1999: Healthier Mothers and Babies." *Morbidity and Mortality Weekly Report,* 1 October 1999, 849–858. Shane, Barbara. *Family Planning Saves Lives*. 3rd ed. Washington, DC: Population Reference Bureau, 1996. Wulfe, Deirdre. "Family Planning Improves Child Survival and Health." *Issues in Brief*. New York: Alan Guttmacher Institute, 1997. Online: http://www.agi-usa.org/pubs/ib20.html, 10 October 1999.

China

More than one-fifth of the world's people live in China, a huge country in east central Asia. Due to stringent family planning policies that the communist government of that country adopted in 1978, that population is growing at an ever slower pace. Chinese demographers estimate that China's official one-child policy helped slow world population growth enough to push the date of the birth of the 6 billionth child into late 1999. Without that policy demographers speculate that the Earth would have become home to 6 billion people by 1996.

China's huge population increase of the 1960s resulted from improved medical conditions and directives from early communist governments, especially that of Mao Zedong in the 1950s, that the people give birth to many children to build the resources of the communist state. By 1970, China's population had risen to 830 million and was growing at 2.8 percent annually. When China recognized the hazard of that growing population to its ability to feed its people and to develop a healthy economy, communist leaders began taking strong measures to change the nation's attitude toward large families. Through stringent, official state programs, China cut that rate of growth to 1 percent by 1998. In that year, women in China could expect to give birth to 1.8 children. Those decreases represented limited success for leaders who had hoped to cut population growth to zero and the birth rate to less than an average one child for every woman by 2000. Despite those shortcomings, China's government officials declared the one-child policy a success and promised to continue its efforts to persuade families to give birth to only one child.

Contraceptive use in China ranks very high, even compared to wealthy industrialized nations. More than 81 percent of China's women of reproductive age rely on a modern birth control method to prevent pregnancy. The vast majority have undergone tubal sterilization or have an intrauterine device (IUD) in place. In 1994, 37 percent of China's women had been surgically, permanently sterilized and 36.5 percent used IUDs. While the women who use IUDs do so voluntarily, many of the sterilized women, particularly those who underwent procedures in the 1980s, had been coerced by local government

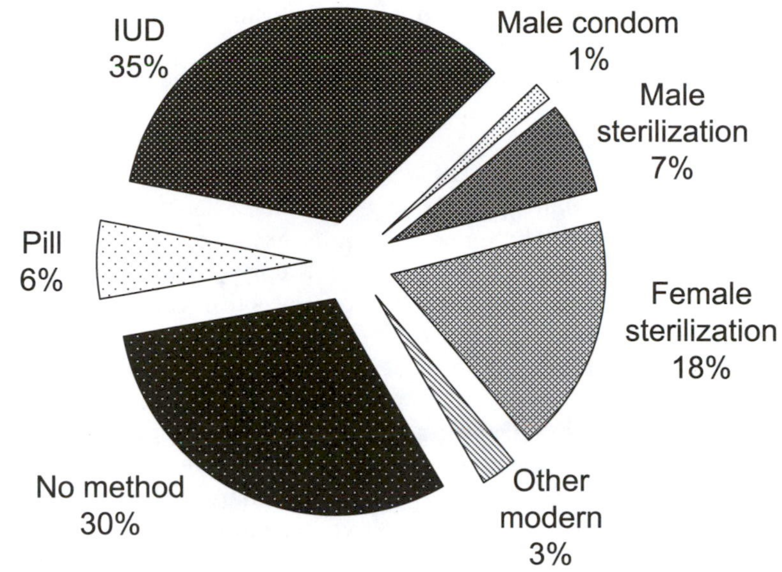

China: 1982 Contraceptive Use by Women Ages 15–49

Source: U.S. Census Bureau International Data Base

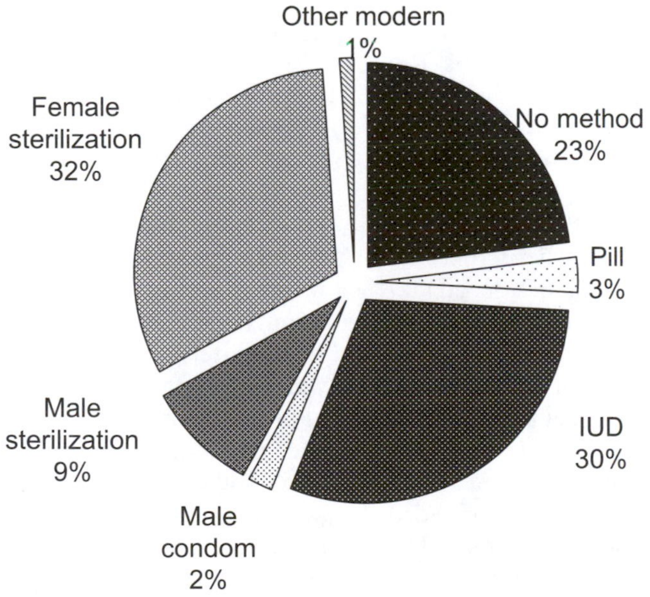

China: 1992 Contraceptive Use by Women Ages 15–49

Source: U.S. Census Bureau International Data Base

officials into undergoing the surgery according to official Chinese sources and outside observers. In efforts to meet government quotas for birth rates, health care workers would sterilize women after childbirth and without the woman's permission, these sources report.

The common use of IUDs developed as a result of China's scientific research into IUDs, work which began in the 1950s. Through 30 years of study, China developed several highly effective IUDs, some of copper and some containing levonorgestrel, both known to produce near sterilization rates of contraception.

Only one man in China has undergone a vasectomy for every four women who have had tubal sterilization. In Sichuan province, however, vasectomy is four times more common than tubal sterilization. In that province, scientists in 1974 developed the no-scalpel method of puncturing the skin of the man's scrotum and gently pulling the vas deferens outside where they can be severed or blocked. This method increasingly gained popularity around the world by the 1990s. China has also developed its own brands of condoms, hormonal pills, and hormonal implants. Research on the antifertility effects of gossypol, a substance found in cottonseed oil, which is often used in cooking in China, from the 1950s through the 1980s appeared promising, but side effects from that drug led researchers to suspend testing when fertility did not quickly return after the man stopped taking the drug. China has been involved in a variety of contraceptive research in cooperation with the World Health Organization and with private research organizations and universities to develop a wider variety of contraceptives for people to use.

Abortion is legal in China and is provided in the nation's family planning clinics. The official abortion rate stood at approximately 27 abortions for every 1,000 women in 1999. In 1997, that equaled about 8 million abortions, a figure that Chinese officials consider too high. Efforts to improve contraceptive use and to provide for chemical abortions increased in China in the 1990s. Mifepristone, a chemical abortifacient developed in France in the early 1980s, became available to Chinese doctors in 1986. China's chemists also developed a version of mifepristone, and now that drug and the French drug are frequently used in Chinese hospitals to perform very early chemical abortions. The use of chemical abortions is expected to reduce the cost that nation has paid since the late 1970s to provide women with abortions.

Young people in China appear not to use contraceptives as frequently as people in their later reproductive years. As China works to limit its population size, and to thwart a threat from sexually transmitted diseases that looms as more people contract acquired immunodeficiency syndrome, the government has begun taking action to increase teen and young adult access to contraceptives. In 1999, government workers installed 5,000 condom machines in China's cities and installed another 1,000 in smaller communities in the rural provinces.

China's population and family planning policy and the way local governmental officials administered that policy brought it under close international scrutiny during the 1980s and 1990s. Reports of coercion in forcing women to undergo abortions and surgical sterilization against their will surfaced in international media and foreign affairs reports, despite close government restrictions on access to information. People emigrating from China, reported on government clinics where doctors and nurses were forced through the threat of recriminations to abort even late-term fetuses and to sterilize women when the opportunity presented itself. Much of the coercion has been blamed by Chinese and international experts on officials at the local level of China's governmental system, which put regional officers in charge of maintaining local quotas of births. While the government had offered incentives to people to have one child and encouraged that family goal through education and public statements, local officials, some have argued, used unethical means to persuade women and families to limit their family size to one child.

The one-child policy, even according to the Chinese governments that have come into power since 1978, has not been highly successful at convincing people in rural China to limit their families. Seventy-one percent of China's people still live in rural areas. While fertility rates fell to near one child per family in the cities, rural fertility rates hovered near three children per family, a low figure by the standards of many countries, but still too high for China's hope to further limit its population growth.

In the late 1990s, in efforts to broaden the social acceptability of one-child families, China reportedly worked to emphasize reproductive health in its national family planning program and the ministers of the State Family Planning Commission began reform efforts to eliminate coercion from the state system. They also began working to provide greater access throughout the country to contraception and reproductive care. Cooperating closely and officially with the China Family Planning Association, China's affiliate of International Planned Parenthood Federation, the government has sought to help the volunteer doctors of that organization, many of them retired, improve instruction in reproductive health to rural women, and improve the quality of abortion services and insertion procedures for IUD use. China has not, however, backed down from its one-child policy and will continue efforts to persuade more people to accept the need for this policy, at least for the next two or three generations. *See also* ASIA; INDIA

Further reading: Kane, Penny. "Population Policy." In *The China Handbook,* edited by Christopher Hudson. Chicago: Fitzroy Dearborn, 1997. Peng, Xizhe. *Demographic Transition in China: Fertility Trends Since the 1950s*. Oxford: Clarendon Press, 1991. Xiao, B. L., and B. G. Zhao. "Current Practice of Family Planning in China." *International Journal of Gynecology and Obstetrics* 58 (1997): 59-67.

Coitus. *See* INTERCOURSE

Coitus Interruptus. *See* WITHDRAWAL

Combined Oral Contraceptives

Combined oral contraceptives (COCs), which contain artificial forms of the two primary female sex hormones, estrogen and progesterone, are manufactured as pills and represent the most often prescribed and used form of modern contraceptives. Taken daily throughout most or all of the menstrual cycle, these pills offer most women excellent protection from unwanted pregnancy. Modern combinations of the estrogen and progestin and modern "low-dose" pills have greatly reduced the risks of complications and side effects caused by altering the body's hormonal balance.

Each day when she is "on the pill," a woman ingests a dose of artificially created estrogen and progesterone in order to alter her natural hormone balance. The levels of these hormones must remain high enough to be contraceptively effective. Missing a day can cause the hormones to fall to a level that could in turn cause a woman's natural cycle to begin functioning and put her at risk of pregnancy.

By elevating estrogen levels above normal during a woman's cycle, the synthetic form of this hormone suppresses the actions of the pituitary gland and prevents it from producing the follicle-stimulating hormone (FSH), which acts upon immature eggs on a woman's ovaries. Synthetic estrogen levels also prevent the pituitary from producing luteinizing hormone (LH), which causes a mature egg to erupt from the ovary. The synthetic estrogen mimics the high levels of estrogen found in a woman's body after ovulation. Artificially sustaining these high levels in essence deceives the pituitary into functioning as if a pregnancy has commenced and thus suppressing the development of the next batch of eggs toward maturity.

Maintaining an artificially high level of progestin assists in the suppression of the manufacture of LH by the pituitary gland and reinforces that function of the estrogen. Together, the synthetic estrogen and progestin alter the endometrium, the inner lining of the uterus, making it incapable of supporting a fertilized egg in the unusual circumstance that ovulation does occur during a cycle.

The progestin also thickens a woman's cervical mucus. This natural substance, when dry, effectively plugs the cervix, the opening to the uterus, and slows the progress of sperm from the vagina into the upper portion of the reproductive tract. During ovulation, however, that dry plug moistens, becomes slippery, and actually assists the sperm in swimming into the uterus. High levels of progestin keep the mucus dry throughout the cycle. Scientists, however, still debate the contraceptive effect of the thickened cervical mucus.

Working together, the estrogen and progestin have proven to be 99.9 percent effective at preventing pregnancy when the woman takes the pills according to directions. With such a high success rate, only one woman out of every 1,000 using combined oral contraceptives is likely to become pregnant in the first year of use. That success is hampered by the "typical use" success rate which is much lower at 95 percent, where one out of every 20 women can expect to become pregnant.

Typical use reflects some of the difficulties that keep combined oral contraceptives from being the perfect contraceptive. Taking a pill every day, or 21 out of every 28 days, presents a challenge to women's memories. Knowing and following the directions should she forget to take a pill also presents a challenge. Proper counseling and education by health care providers greatly increases the success rate of oral contraceptives.

Women find combined oral contraceptives to be a very effective long-term, reversible means of preventing pregnancy. Contrary to a commonly held misperception of combined oral contraceptives, women's bodies do not need a break from the pills. In fact, women who take such a break put themselves at high risk of pregnancy since they often fail to use a back up contraceptive while not taking the pills.

Most women, if they decide to become pregnant, find that fertility returns within three months of stopping combined oral con-

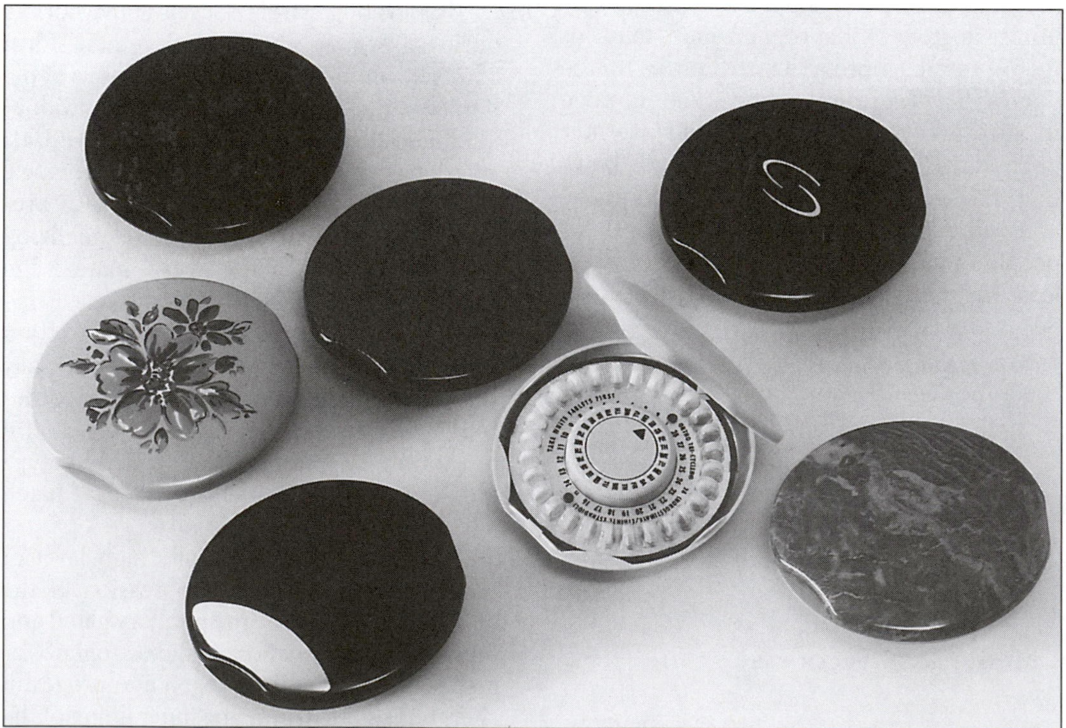

This line of discreet containers for birth control pills resemble a woman's make-up compact. © *Ortho-McNeil Pharmaceutical Cooperation 2000. Reprinted/reproduced with permission of copyright owner.*

traceptives. About 1 to 2 percent of women who have used the pill will not menstruate for six months after stopping this contraceptive.

Combined orals contraceptives have proven to be very safe for most women. Research has established that in the United States, taking COCs results in far fewer risks than delivering a baby for women younger than 35 years who do not smoke cigarettes. The development of very low dose oral contraceptives in the 1980s and 1990s has made COCs very safe and highly recommended for women up until the age of 50.

Women who smoke regularly receive advice not to use oral contraceptives. Research has established that smoking presents by far the greatest risk to women who are using combined oral contraceptives.

As they work to prevent ovulation, combined oral contraceptives alter a woman's menstrual cycle in ways that many women find advantageous, decreasing blood flow and the length of the period. COCs tend to reduce menstrual cramps and pain, suppress androgens, or male hormones, produced by the ovaries, and reduce abnormal hair growth. By suppressing androgens, combined oral contraceptives provide help in treatment of severe cases of acne and have been approved for that specific use also.

In addition to their reproductive advantages, combined oral contraceptives also protect women from pelvic inflammatory disease, ovarian and endometrial cancer, ectopic pregnancy, and benign breast disease.

Minor side effects of oral contraceptives are relatively common. Women report headaches, nausea and vomiting, and decreased sexual drive. These side effects can lead women to quit using the pill and reject it as their choice of contraceptive. With more than 50 brands of combined oral contraceptives on the market, doctors and health care providers are able to work with the woman to choose a COC with the fewest side effects. Counseling also prepares a woman for those side effects and makes them more tolerable and treatable should they occur.

Invented in the 1950s, the first COCs were high-dose products that carried with them high risks of deep vein thrombosis, dangerous blood clots, headaches, and nausea. The first marketed combined oral contraceptive, Enovid, contained 150 micrograms of estrogen, but studies soon revealed that such high estrogen levels caused high risk of blood clotting in the lungs, deep veins, and even the brain. Several studies conducted in the late 1960s showed that women taking combined oral contraceptives were eight to 12 times more likely to develop fatal blood clots than women who did not use oral contraceptives. More in-depth research revealed a greater risk for women who smoked and women more than 35 years old. Research also established that the estrogen compound in those early pills caused most of the problems and soon manufacturers and clinicians began making and prescribing COCs with lower estrogen doses. By the mid-1960s, estrogen amounts in combined oral contraceptives were lowered to 100 micrograms and then to 50 micrograms by the 1970s. By 1985 most prescriptions for oral contraceptives were written for products with 35 micrograms of estrogen. In the 1990s very low estrogen dose pills with only 20 micrograms of estrogen reached the market.

That first combined oral contraceptive also contained 10 milligrams of the progestin norethynodrel. Though early scientific study of combined oral contraceptives focused on elevated estrogen levels, progestins also received close scrutiny. Scientists recognized in the 1970s a connection between the progestin dose and hypertension, cholesterol levels, and blood glucose and insulin levels. Recognizing the need to use the lowest possible dose of both artificial hormones, manufacturers and doctors began creating and using products with increasingly lower progestin levels as well. By the late 1990s, combined oral contraceptives typically contained 1 milligram or less of a synthetic progestin.

Two artificial estrogens, ethinyl estradiol and mestranol, dominate the combined oral contraceptive market. They have proven the most successful at duplicating the effects of the large class of hormones known collectively as estrogen and have proven highly effective and safe as contraceptives. All COCs with 35 mcg or less of estrogen contain ethinyl estradiol, which is immediately available for use by the woman's body. Mestranol must be converted in the liver to ethinyl estradiol before becoming active.

Work with progesterone, the naturally occurring hormone that helps a woman's body prepare for and support a fertilized egg, has led to many different synthetic varieties. Nine progestins have been approved for use in the United States. The most commonly marketed and used progestins include levonorgestrel, norethynodrel, and norethindrone. Three progestins developed in the late twentieth century and known as new or third-generation progestins, desogestrel, norgestimate, and gestodene, offer refinements in the effectiveness of the progestin component of the combined oral contraceptive, though they have also been linked to greater risk of deep vein thrombosis or blood clots than the older progestins.

Available most commonly by prescription, combined oral contraceptives have proven so safe and effective that several countries in Europe have proposed making them available over-the-counter without a prescription. For years, COCs have also been prescribed in large doses for use as emergency contraception in the case of contraceptive failure and rape. Those high doses, however, increase the severity of side effects, including nausea and cramping.

The success of combined oral contraceptives led throughout the latter half of the twentieth century to the development of many contraceptive methods containing synthetic estrogen and progestin hormones. *See also* EMERGENCY CONTRACEPTION; MULTIPHASIC PILLS; ORAL CONTRACEPTIVES; PROGESTIN-ONLY CONTRACEPTIVES; RISK; SIDE EFFECTS

Further reading: Dickey, Richard P. *Managing Contraceptive Pill Patients.* 8th ed. Durant, OK: Essential Medical Information Systems, Inc., 1994. "International Medical Advisory Panel Statement on Steroidal Oral Contraception." *International Planned Parenthood Federation Medical Bulletin* 32.6 (1998): 1–6. Kaunitz, Andrew M., and Howard Ory. "Estrogen Component of OCs." *Dialogues in Contraception* 5 (1997): 1–6.

Comstock, Anthony (1844–1915)

Anthony Comstock spent his adult life publicly fighting pornography and obscenity. Through his personal and intense lobbying effort when he was 27, Comstock pushed through the U.S. Congress in 1873 a bill that tightened loopholes in older obscenity laws and made the mailing of birth control devices a federal crime. The law, which came to be known as the Comstock Laws, specifically outlawed any device intended to prevent conception or to cause an abortion. Birth control advocates in the early twentieth century struggled against those laws and worked toward having them rewritten.

Comstock was born in 7 March 1844, in New Canaan, Connecticut. As a teen and a young soldier in the Civil War, Comstock developed a strong antagonism to moral decadence and social vice. A man of strong moral convictions and a believer in the strict moral codes of the Victorian age, Comstock fought against people's increasingly easy access to obscene publications, which for him

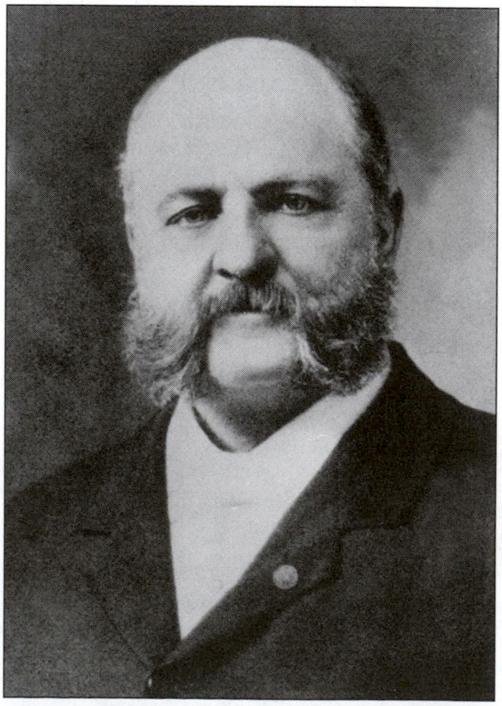

Anthony Comstock developed legislation to keep birth control information from the public. *Bettmann/Corbis*

ranged from postcards to serious scientific literature on sexuality.

Upon moving to New York City, in 1868, Comstock began fighting the corrupting influences of people's exposure to obscenity, and by 1872 had formed a close relationship with the city's Young Men's Christian Association (YMCA), which also fought against the moral depredation in young men. His opposition to contraception and abortion grew out of his belief that they allowed morally degenerate people to escape the consequences of their acts. Comstock wrote and published four books that discussed his view and advised his audience on moral behavior, including *Traps for the Young* (1883) and *Morals versus Art* (1887).

Frustrated that they had only weak legal tools to help them fight obscenity, Comstock's wealthy supporters in the YMCA financed a three-month effort on his part to write and pass legislation that would allow them to arrest and convict sellers, publishers, and distributors of obscene literature and that would give them the power to prevent the distribution of contraceptive and abortive techniques. In the last hours of 3 March 1873, as Congress was preparing to adjourn and after very personal lobbying that began in December 1872, Comstock saw passed the Federal Anti-obscenity Act, which gave them that power. Included in that bill was the enforcement provision that created special agents of the U.S. Post Office who could arrest people found in violation of that law. Three days after the law passed, Comstock became a special agent and, until his death in 1915, used his authority to confiscate more than 160 tons of literature and pictures. Comstock also served as secretary of the newly formed New York Society for the Suppression of Vice. He recorded the history of his work in the reports he made to that society.

Enthusiastically supported by the public and the courts during the early days of enforcing the Comstock Laws and finally derided for prudery and narrow mindedness in the later years of his career, Comstock remained convinced of the need for laws to protect people from society's eroding morals. From the beginning of his career until its end, however, people developed a more tolerant attitude toward healthy sexuality than that which Comstock advocated. The world changed so much around him that Comstock's efforts no longer even matched the efforts of the federal government which had supported him and even given him his job in 1873; during World War I, the U.S. government began issuing condoms to soldiers to help prevent venereal diseases.

Comstock's convictions remained consistent throughout his 42 years as an agent of the post office, but by the time Margaret Sanger began her career as an advocate of the right of women to information on birth control, Comstock had become what his critics often called a buffoon and a prude. In 1915, Comstock arrested William Sanger for distributing an explicit pamphlet on birth control written by Margaret, his wife. Society's attitudes toward sexuality had changed so much that an audience of birth control advocates booed and heckled Comstock during Sanger's trial.

Anthony Comstock died of pneumonia in New York City in 21 September 1915, during the middle of William Sanger's 30-day jail term. Not until 1970 did Congress rewrite the federal Comstock Laws and remove from contraception its legal classification as obscene. *See also* COMSTOCK LAWS; OBSCENITY

Further reading: LaMay, Craig L. "America's Censor: Anthony Comstock and Free Speech." *Communications and the Law* 19.3 (1997): 1–59. Weisberger, Bernard A. "Chasing Smut in Every Medium." *American Heritage* 48.8 (1997): 12–13.

Comstock Laws

On 3 March 1873, the United States Congress passed into law the Federal Anti-obscenity Act, commonly referred to as the Comstock Laws. The bill amended and updated the Federal Obscenity Act of 1872.

The new law made illegal the importing of obscene material into the United States, the mailing of any obscene matters within the United States, and advertising obscene material. The Comstock Laws also gave enforcement officials the authority to seize, condemn, and destroy obscene materials and threatened to punish any government official who helped mail such materials.

Essentially, the new law closed loopholes in the year-old version and provided a legal tool for enforcing obscenity laws. The 1873 act, however, went one step further. It specifically characterized as obscene "any article or thing designed or intended for the prevention of conception or procuring of abortion."

Moralist and public defender against vice and obscenity Anthony Comstock had guided the drafting of the legislation, supported by the anti-vice committee of the New York Young Men's Christian Association (YMCA). Comstock, a determined fighter for the traditional morals of the Victorian era, had been pursuing his own efforts to enforce the 1872 law and state laws in New York for several years before finding support in his efforts in the YMCA. With the financial backing of members of the board of that group, Comstock found a lawyer to write a new anti-obscenity bill that included the means to deal with the crimes he perceived taking place all around him in bookstores, newspapers, and even the public health sector.

In December 1872, Comstock traveled with the bill to Washington, DC, and the halls of Congress where he personally lobbied the legislature until the new law, amidst more than 250 bills, was passed on the last day of that session. The bill created the position of special agent of the U.S. Post Office and gave those agents the authority to raid places suspected of containing illegal material. Three days after the bill passed, Comstock applied to become an agent, and from that day until his death in 1915, he pursued the letter of that law.

The Comstock Laws remained part of the American legal system until 1970 when Congress rewrote the act and removed contraception and abortion devices from the list of obscene materials. During the years it was in place, however, birth control advocates fought against the constraints of the Comstock Laws.

Early in her years of advocating for birth control, Margaret Sanger, a nurse and founder of the United States's first birth control clinic, wrote in 1912 a series of articles in *The Call* magazine titled "What Every Girl Should Know" about sexuality, physiology, and reproduction. While postal officials ignored her articles at first, when the magazine attempted to publish her essay on sexually transmitted diseases, postal officials declared the magazine unmailable. In 1914, Sanger was arrested under the provisions of the Comstock Laws on charges of mailing and distributing her magazine *The Woman Rebel.* Rather than compromise her principles and face a trial or agree to plead guilty and negotiate a plea agreement, Sanger fled to Europe. In her absence, Comstock himself trapped William Sanger, Margaret's husband, into giving him one of the pamphlets, and Comstock arrested Sanger. After a very public and rancorous trial in September 1915, William Sanger was convicted and eventually served 30 days in jail. Comstock died two weeks after that trial, but his legacy lived on. Margaret returned to the United States after Comstock died, ready to face the charges against her. However, in February 1916 the prosecution chose to drop those charges.

In 1929, Mary Ware Dennett, another leader in the American birth control movement, was arrested for mailing obscenities in the form of her educational pamphlet *The Sex Side of Life.* Though she lost that case in state court, Dennett won the district court appeal. The judge there ruled that her intent had been to educate and not to arouse sexual interest and was therefore not obscene. *See also* COMSTOCK, ANTHONY; DENNETT, MARY WARE; OBSCENITY; SANGER, MARGARET HIGGINS

Further reading: Chen, Constance M. Introduction to *"The Sex Side of Life": Mary Ware Dennett's Pioneering Battle for Birth Control and Sex Education*. New York: New Press, 1996. Fowler, Dorothy G. *Unmailable: Congress and the Post Office*. Athens, GA: University of Georgia Press, 1977. LaMay, Craig L. "America's Censor: Anthony Comstock and Free Speech." *Communications and the Law* 19.3 (1997): 1–59.

Conception

While scientists and ethicists agree upon a definition of fertilization, no such clear agreement exists for the definition of conception.

Some people view conception as equal to fertilization, when a man's sperm penetrates the outer surface of woman's ova. Others see conception at the moment such a joined cell implants into the woman's uterine wall about six days after fertilization. For many people, conception means that a pregnancy has begun.

By the time of implantation, the two sex cells have been growing and dividing for six days and are a small ball of cells, called a blastocyst. After a two or three day trip through the fallopian tube, where the sperm and ova joined, the blastocyst spends two to three days floating in the uterus before beginning implantation.

Some people feel that the moment the sex cells join, a new human being has been created. Others argue that nature can disrupt that fragile biological process and many eggs that have been fertilized are not able to continue growth and are naturally shed from the woman's body after fertilization and before implantation. Spontaneous loss of a fertilized egg occurs often. Approximately 50 percent of fertilized eggs do not survive the first two weeks after fertilization. However, spontaneous loss of eggs is less common after the first two weeks when approximately 15 percent of pregnancies end in loss of embryo. These biological circumstances lead some people to define conception as the moment of implantation or soon after.

This uncertainty in the definition of conception leads debate over the ethics and morals of contraceptives, devices that are designed to prevent pregnancy. At the center of the debate is the question of whether a device that stops implantation is a contraceptive or an abortifacient, a substance that causes an abortion. Emergency contraception, a series of concentrated doses of hormonal contraceptive pills, works by preventing implantation should it occur after sexual intercourse where no contraceptive was used. Some see this device as an abortifacient since it would effect a fertilized egg. Others see it as a contraceptive since it prevents implantation, and thus a pregnancy, from occurring after intercourse. *See also* ABORTION; BIRTH CONTROL; CONTRACEPTIVE; FERTILIZATION; IMPLANTATION (OF EGG); LIFE (BEGINNING OF)

Further reading: "Fertility Control." In *Encyclopedia of Bioethics,* rev. ed., edited by Warren Thomas Reich. New York: Simon and Schuster/Macmillan, 1995. Hatcher, Robert, James Trussel, Felicia Stewart, and others. *Contraceptive Technology*. 16th rev. ed. New York: Irvington, 1994.

Condom—Female

A plastic lining for the vagina, the female condom was first sold in Switzerland and the United Kingdom in 1992 and approved for use in the United States in 1993.

About the size of a woman's hand, the soft, loose-fitting polyurethane sack, which is 6.75 inches long (17 centimeters) by 3.125 inches wide (7.8 centimeters), comes with two plastic rings fastened to each end. The woman inserts the first ring deep into her vagina, hooking it over her pubic bone. Polyurethane, a plastic, fills this ring and covers the woman's cervix, the entrance to her uterus. The second ring at the other end of this pouch re-

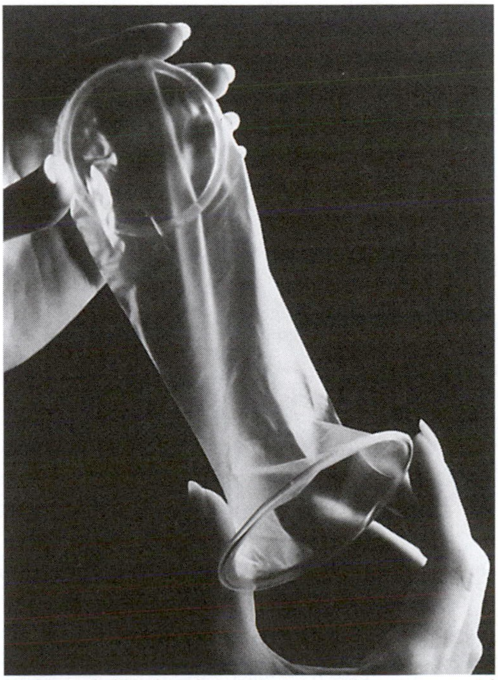

The pouch-like female condom provides women with another barrier method of contraception. *The Female Health Company*

mains outside of the woman's body and covers her labia. No spermicides are required with this device. Women may insert the condom up to eight hours before intercourse.

When used according to package direction, the female condom offers a 94 percent protection rate against accidental pregnancy. In typical use, where people may not properly follow the directions, the success rate is 79 percent. The female condom provides protection against sexually transmitted diseases at least as well as that offered by male latex condoms, perhaps better since polyurethane is known to provide excellent protection.

Each female condom may be used only once and, in 1997, cost about $3 in the United States. This cost factor, higher than for the male condom, has discouraged many people from choosing this contraceptive option, though users in test studies have found the device more comfortable than the tight-fitting male condom. Researchers are studying the possibility of developing a reusable female condom to help reduce the cost and increase its convenience.

Manufactured by the Female Health Company of Great Britain, the female condom is available without prescription primarily in Europe and North America. Marketing and sales efforts are underway in Brazil, Zimbabwe, Zambia, and other African countries. The World Health Organization and the United Nations, through an agreement with the manufacturer, have made the female condom available for less than US$1 in developing countries. *See also* BARRIER CONTRACEPTIVES; CONDOM—MALE; SAFE SEX; SEXUALLY TRANSMITTED DISEASES

Further reading: "Female Condom Becomes Available Nationwide." *The Contraception Report* 5 (1995): 11–13. Grimes, David A. et al. eds. *Modern Contraception: Updates from the Contraception Report.* Totowa, NJ: Emron, 1997. "The Polyurethane Vaginal Pouch: New Barrier Contraceptive May Give Women More Control over STD Prevention." *The Contraception Report* 3 (1992): 12–14.

Condom—Male

The condom, a covering that fits over a man's penis, prevents sperm from entering a woman's vagina. From ancient times, men have used various coverings from animal tissue to plant pods to act as such barriers. Modern condoms made of latex or animal skin provide men and women with protection against pregnancy and have become the most readily available and most often used barrier contraceptive.

The latex condom is the only contraceptive that adequately protects people against sexually transmitted diseases including the human immunodeficiency virus (HIV), which causes acquired immunodeficiency syndrome (AIDS).

Condoms need to be applied to the man's erect penis before sexual intercourse. They come packaged singly and rolled into a ring. Before intercourse, the man or the woman places the condom on the penis after full arousal and then rolls the plastic sheath down toward the base of the penis.

When used correctly with each act of sexual intercourse, the male condom results in a 3 percent pregnancy rate. The typical use, however, leads to a 14 percent success rate; this occurs when people forget or choose not to use the condom on all occasions. Condoms rarely break during intercourse and most failure is due to not properly using the condom.

People typically use condoms when they have sex infrequently or when they are shifting from one form of long-term contraception to another. Both men and women commonly make the choice to use the condom.

More than 100 brand names of condoms are manufactured, most of them made of latex, and several made of animal skin. Several brands include spermicides to increase the protection of the condom. All companies make several sizes and different textures, even colored condoms. In the late 1990s condoms made of alternative materials were being manufactured and were being studied for approval by the U.S. Food and Drug Administration (FDA). Condoms made of alternative plastic materials would provide alternatives to people sensitive to or allergic to latex. The FDA has given temporary approval to several non-latex condoms.

A "baggy" or flexible condom has been patented in the United States and is also under study for approval there. This model is reported to increase the sensations during intercourse compared to those experienced while wearing the snug, traditional condom.

Men react differently to wearing a condom. Some report that the device interferes with their enjoyment of intercourse, decreasing the sense of touch, hugging their penises too tightly, and slipping while the penis is in the vagina. Others complain that condoms are too snug.

Condom use has increased significantly since the early 1980s. In fact, from 1988 to 1995, condoms increased more in use than any other studied device, from 5.1 million users in 1988 to 7.9 million condom users in 1995.

Worldwide, condoms are the most accessible method of contraception. In developed nations, people have easy access to condoms, needing to spend little time and money on this protection. Condoms are also easily available to people in most developing countries. Twenty-one countries, however, have very poor access to condoms. Despite such widespread access to condoms, in many nations, most notably in Africa, people's use of condoms does not coincide with access, even though condom use can provide much needed protection against AIDS. *See also* ACQUIRED IMMUNODEFICIENCY SYNDROME (AIDS); BARRIER CONTRACEPTIVES; CONDOM—FEMALE; SAFE SEX; SEXUALLY TRANSMITTED DISEASES

Further reading: Hatcher, Robert, James Trussel, Felicia Stewart, and others. *Contraceptive Technology*. 16th rev. ed. New York: Irvington, 1994. Population Action International. *Contraceptive Choice: Worldwide Access to Family Planning*. Washington, DC: Population Action International, 1997. Online: http://www.populationaction. org/ programs/rc97.htm, 11 October 1999. Winikoff, Beverly, and Suzanne Wymelenberg. *The Whole Truth about Contraception*. Washington, DC: Joseph Henry Press, 1997.

Contraception

Contraception refers specifically to methods of fertility regulation and family size limitation that prevent the union of a mature male sperm with a mature female egg. As a social phenomenon, contraception refers to the concept of people, women and men, choosing to influence the biology of reproduction before fertilization, to separate sexual intercourse from pregnancy as an uncontrollable consequence of the expression of passionate emotions, and to decide for themselves when they wish to conceive children. Contraception is also a driving force to reduce abortion, eliminate infanticide, and increase the advantages for the children a couple does choose to conceive.

Contraception, in general, influences women's lives far more than men's since it is a woman who carries the child should intercourse result in pregnancy. The development of modern contraceptives in the twentieth century also focused mainly upon influencing egg and sperm within a woman's body. Of the modern contraceptive methods, only the condom and vasectomy are under a man's control. Women have access to spermicides in a variety of forms; three forms of vaginal contraceptives with research underway to provide several more; a wide range of hormonal contraceptives, including pills, injections, implants, and patches worn on the skin; and the more complex and frequently used surgical method of tubal sterilization. Together, women and men can use fertility awareness methods of contraception, which are based upon sexual abstinence around the time of ovulation, which in turn is determined by an increasingly precise observation of a woman's body functions.

Simple numerical calculations show that a woman who wishes to bear only two children, would spend 246 months of her adult life from ages 20 to 45 needing or using contraceptives. Increasingly worldwide, women are expressing the desire to have fewer children; this includes women who have borne more children then they say they wanted and women planning their families who say they want to bear fewer children than their mothers and grandmothers bore. Research shows that women will change the methods they use frequently during those times, depending upon their marital status, frequency of intercourse, financial circumstances, and quality of health.

Men's concern with preventing conception increased steadily in the last quarter of the twentieth century. Educators and researchers focusing on a man's role and responsibility in reaching his goals, his family's goals, or the goals of women in general of preventing unwanted pregnancies have found men to be very willing to share in the responsibilities for planning families and preventing unwanted pregnancies. Efforts with teenagers in the United States have shown that when educated about the consequences of sexual intercourse in their lives and in the lives of their female partners, men are willing to take greater responsibility in preventing pregnancy. Public opinion polls taken around the world suggest that between 60 and 80 percent of men would use new male contraceptive techniques, such as testosterone injections or patches, if they were available.

Studies by the Alan Guttmacher Institute, the World Health Organizaton, and other international health and research groups demonstrate that contraception also functions to reduce the need for abortion. As modern contraceptives become available to women, the number of abortions demanded by women slowly decreases. When women and men are given the opportunity, the education, and the social support needed for preventing pregnancy, a woman's need for abortion greatly diminishes. Learning the proper use of a contraceptive method leads to less failure of that method. Efforts by health professionals to improve a woman's understanding of the details of a particular method, such as the combined oral contraceptive pill, improves the success of that method. Less failure then leads to less need for abortion. Contraception, however, cannot eliminate the need for abortion, since no contraceptive is perfect and men and women do not use contraceptives perfectly.

Contraception, as a principal, functions in prevention of fertilization; it functions early in the reproductive cycle. Methods of fertility awareness, such as chemicals and hormones to induce menstruation after an egg has been fertilized, and of induced abortion, whether surgical or chemical, are not forms of contraception, while they are forms of fertility control and methods of reducing family size. *See also* ABORTION; CONTRACEPTIVE

Further reading: "Contraception for Men." In *A Research Agenda for the Reproductive Sciences Branch of the NICHD*. Bethesda, MD: National Institute of Child Health and Human Development, 1995. Online: http://www.nichd.nih.gov/publications/online_only/agenda/contents.htm, 8 September 1999. Cohen, Susan A. "The Role of Contraception in Reducing Abortion." *Issues in Brief.* New York: Alan Guttmacher Institute, 1998. Online: http://www.agi-usa.org/pubs/ib19.html, 11 September 1999.

Contraceptive

Specifically, a contraceptive device or chemical that works against the biological process of a male sperm fertilizing a female egg, a process known as conception. However, common use of the term generalizes contraceptive to include, perhaps mistakenly, any substance that prevents pregnancy.

People who believe that pregnancy begins when a fertilized egg implants itself in the woman's uterine lining hold a different definition of a contraceptive than do people who believe that pregnancy begins at the moment a sperm enters and joins chromosomes with an egg at conception or fertilization. The two events are generally six to seven days apart. The distinction between a product or process that prevents conception and a product or process that interferes with a pregnancy at a later stage in the reproductive sequence becomes an important distinction when people discuss the moral, ethical, and religious aspects of birth control.

Physical barriers designed to keep sperm away from eggs, such as condoms, diaphragms, cervical caps, and spermicides, are contraceptives. All attempt to prevent sperm from entering the uterus; all attempt to keep the sperm from traveling beyond a woman's vagina, the beginning of her reproductive tract.

Current synthetic female hormones, such as those found in oral contraceptives, injectables, and implants, influence several different stages of the female reproductive system. Their most powerful influence is to prevent ovulation. The artificial hormones mimic the actions of progesterone and estrogen and prevent the pituitary gland from secreting the follicle-stimulating hormone (FSH) that would cause eggs to mature on the woman's ovaries. Progestins (artificial forms of progesterone) also help maintain the natural block of dry mucus found in a woman's cervix when she is not close to the time of ovulation; this cervical block also prevents sperm from reaching mature eggs. Because they actually prevent conception, these hormones are generally considered contraceptives.

A third effect of synthetic hormones, however, confuses that classification. In addition to preventing ovulation and thickening the cervical mucus, synthetic hormones also interfere with and prevent the implantation of a fertilized egg, should an egg rupture from the woman's ovaries despite the influence of the chemicals. Scientific knowledge of hormonal contraceptives shows that their dominant action is to prevent ovulation, but because they have this added action, some people consider them to have characteristics of an abortifacient, a substance or device designed to interfere with a pregnancy after the egg has settled into the lining of the uterus.

Recent studies have shown the intrauterine devices (IUDs) also work mainly by interfering with conception, though it was long thought that IUDs worked only by preventing implantation of a fertilized egg. Long seen as an abortion-inducing device, IUDs are now more commonly classified as contraceptives, especially those than contain progestins.

Chemicals currently under study that would influence sperm while they are still in the man's body would be contraceptives, since they clearly prevent conception.

Except for chemicals such as mifepristone and devices such as vacuum aspiration that stop a pregnancy well after implantation, which are clearly seen as abortifacients or abortion inducers, most chemicals and devices are referred to as contraceptives. The distinction becomes important to a person whose moral, ethical, and religious beliefs hold that a new human life begins at fertilization. Such a person may be willing to use a chemical or object to prevent the union of an egg and a sperm but not be willing to use a device that disrupts the natural product of that union.

The term "birth control" has even broader meanings than "contraceptive." Since first used by Margaret Sanger in the 1914, birth control has come to refer to a person's ability to determine when or if he or she wished to have children. The control that contraceptive methods give a person over her or his reproductive processes, allows them choices that Sanger and other early social advocates saw as solving many of the problems of poverty and reproductive diseases. Contraceptives became the means by which people achieved birth control. *See also* ABORTIFACIENT; BARRIER CONTRACEPTIVES; CONCEPTION; FERTILIZATION; HORMONAL CONTRACEPTIVES; MALE CONTRACEPTIVES; MIFEPRISTONE; REPRODUCTIVE SYSTEM—FEMALE; REPRODUCTIVE SYSTEM—MALE

Further reading: Knight, James W., and Joan C. Callahan. *Preventing Birth: Contemporary Methods and Related Moral Controversies.* Ethics in a Changing World 3. Salt Lake City: University of Utah Press, 1989. Nordenberg, Tamar. *Protecting Against Unintended Pregnancy.* Rockville, MD: U.S. Department of Health and Human Services, 1997.

Contraceptive Research and Development Program (CONRAD)

The Contraceptive Research and Development Program (CONRAD), funded through the United States Agency for International Development, conducts research to develop new or improved contraceptives and protection from sexually transmitted diseases. Based at the East Virginia Medical School, in Arlington, Virginia, CONRAD itself funds explorations into safe, effective, and acceptable contraceptives for use in the United States and around the world. It aims to provide contraceptives that fit people's cultural and social needs and desires.

Staff at CONRAD work with scientists at domestic and international universities, research institutes, and private companies. Program administrators devote their attention to methods women can control themselves, to methods that provide breastfeeding women with protection from unwanted pregnancy and disease, to long-acting contraceptives, and to processes that interfere with the function of the ovum, the sperm, and the union of the two.

CONRAD-funded teams worked with Family Health International to develop the female "Reality" condom, which reached the European market in 1992 and the U.S. market in 1993. That collaboration also developed the Lea Contraceptive and FemCap, two new vaginal barriers that are expected to reach U.S. markets early in the 2000s.

Projects in early stages of research include barriers and intrauterine devices that contain a synthetic progestin to increase their effectiveness and a single rod hormonal implant. CONRAD also continues to support studies of a male condom made from a new thermoplastic.

More speculative CONRAD research involves contraceptive methods for women and men that work in ways similar to immunizations, and hormonal contraceptives for men.

To provide people with protection from AIDS and other sexually transmitted diseases, CONRAD also invests in research into microbicides, products that kill bacteria and viruses. *See also* FAMILY HEALTH INTERNATIONAL; U.S. AGENCY FOR INTERNATIONAL DEVELOPMENT

Further reading: *Contraceptive Advances,* http://www.reproline.jhu.edu/english/1contech/1advances/1advance.htm, 11 October, 1999. Contraceptive Research and Development Program (CONRAD) Web site. htpp://www.conrad.org.

Contraceptive Use

How and if contraceptives are used depends on a variety of factors, from the users' personalities and personal goals to the effort they need to put into obtaining the contraceptives. Economics, geography, religion, society, upbringing, and even the shapes of their bodies and their biochemistry influence how women and men choose to use contraceptives. Involved in the equation of contraceptive use are the types of relationships adults and adolescents might find themselves in and the circumstances under which they engage in sexual intercourse.

In the early days of the modern contraceptive age, as barriers and condoms slowly became socially acceptable, finding information on birth control methods and gaining access to those few methods provided the greatest obstacles for the use of devices that could help them prevent pregnancy during intercourse. In the United States and Europe in the early twentieth century, laws that regarded birth control as an obscenity and public discussion of human sexuality as unacceptable prevented people from learning of diaphragms and condoms, the two oldest forms of modern contraception. With a small number of buyers, manufacturers made few of these contraceptives.

As laws broke down under changing social norms, new obstacles to the use of contraceptives began exerting influence. Religions, notably the Christian churches, resisted the public acceptance of birth control as did medical doctors. Until the 1940s, doctors and clerics alike discouraged women and men from taking steps to prevent pregnancy. As both of those groups became more accepting of the social change toward the personal enjoyment of sexuality without the risk of pregnancy, contraception gained greater credibility and greater acceptance. Birth control clinics opened slowly across the United States and Europe and opportunities for women and men to find birth control grew.

Science, too, provided obstacles to contraceptive use. Until hormonal contraceptives, first in pill form, were developed in the 1950s and marketed in 1960, people had only limited barrier contraceptives and, increasingly, access to sterilization operations. Though researchers had experimented with intrauterine devices, none had proven widely effective or readily acceptable to women. With the development of artificial hormones and the discovery of their ability to block pregnancy, the world experienced its first contraceptive revolution.

In the 1960s, world attention also began turning to what appeared to many as a dangerous increase in the size of the human population. During that decade world population for the first time exceeded 2.5 billion people and was growing at a rate of more than 2 percent each year. For the rest of the twentieth century, scientists, social and political policy analysts, and the funds from developed nations, nonprofit organizations, and the United Nations began supporting the widespread, worldwide use of modern contraceptives. Continuing research into hormonal contraceptives led to the development of a variety of contraceptives, including implants, injectable contraceptives, modern intrauterine devices, a wide variety of condoms, and new vaginal barriers. Most methods were designed for use with women's bodies, and easy access by women to modern contraceptives became the issue that organizations worked to overcome.

By the late 1980s, researchers had come to understand that, more than roads and supplies, personal preferences made a greater difference to the use of contraceptives. While living close to affordable contraceptives still helped determine if most people used modern birth control, researchers learned that side effects, convenience, and personal preference, as much as affordability and the need for a prescription, helped women, and men decide if they would use contraceptives.

With the development of hormonal contraceptives, the use of modern birth control methods has spread around the world. In Europe and the United States, more than 90 percent of fertile, sexually active women now use modern contraceptives to prevent pregnancy. In the developing nations of Africa, Asia, Latin America, and the Caribbean, contraceptive use is also increasing. Though rates vary, from nearly 70 percent of married women in China to less than 5 percent in Ethiopia, contraceptive use worldwide through the mid-1990s rose steadily to more than 20 percent of married couples.

In the face of increasing world population, which reached 6 billion in 1999, doubling since 1960, and with more women worldwide expressing interest in using contraceptives but not doing so, researchers have turned their attention to understanding the difficulties women, and men, face in limiting the number of children they produce. Those barriers to contraception may include local attitudes of family planning providers to a woman's or man's not wanting to jeopardize a new romantic involvement by discussing birth control.

In some countries, specific methods of contraception are unavailable to women. In Japan, hormonal pills were approved for use in 1999, in the United States, Depo-Provera, an injectable hormonal contraceptive that had been widely used in Europe and Asia since the late 1970s, only received government approval in 1992. In other countries, geography hinders access to contraceptives. The scattered islands that form the Philippines and Indonesia make contraceptive delivery difficult. In some nations, religion slows access to contraception. Until 1980, people in the Republic of Ireland, where more than 75 percent of the population are Roman Catholics, could not buy contraceptives in their country. In the Philippines, the Catholic Church discourages modern contraceptive use and influences the government to discourage family planning programs.

Side effects of contraceptives are as likely as availability to limit a person's willingness to use a contraceptive. Women have turned away from hormonal contraceptives when they experience weight gain, nausea, or irregular bleeding. Men have stopped using condoms when they found condoms to interfere with the pleasure of intercourse.

Science, too, has kept people away from using contraceptives by, experts suggest, not providing people with enough options from which to choose when considering family planning. Population growth seems to have begun to slow, according to 1999 estimates from the United Nations; however, any further slowing would depend upon giving a greater variety of contraceptive options to more people. By the year 2000 the number of women of reproductive age, generally considered to be 15 to 44, though younger girls and older women can become pregnant, was larger than at any time in history and increased the demand for contraceptives. To maintain the current use rate, the actual number of couples using contraception would need to increase by between 20 and 110 percent from 2000 to 2025. To help all of those women, science will need to develop new, more acceptable contraceptives, and health care providers in all societies will need to work with women and men to meet their contraceptive use goals. *See also* ACCESS (TO CONTRACEPTIVES)

Further reading: Biddlecom, Ann E., and Bolaji M. Fapohunda. "Covert Contraceptive Use: Prevalence, Motivations, and Consequences." *Studies in Family Planning* 29 (1998): 360–372. Rosenberg, Michael, and Michael S. Waugh. "Causes and Consequences of Oral Contraceptive Noncompliance." *American Journal of Obstetrics and Gynecology* 180.2, Part 2 (1999): S276–S279. Stanback, John, Andy Thompson, Karen Hardee, and Barbara Janowitz. "Menstruation Requirements: A Significant Barrier to Contraceptive Access in Developing Countries." *Studies in Family Planning* 28 (1997): 245–250.

Costs (of Birth Control)

Two aspects of the monetary costs of birth control determine its immediate value. The first is the price of a specific method of contraception, birth control, or pregnancy termination. The second is the health care cost savings to individuals, insurance programs, societies, and nations created by a contraceptive's ability to prevent unplanned or unwanted pregnancies.

In assessing the value of birth control, policy makers and reproductive health advocates examine the price paid for birth control compared to the medical costs of not using contraception. Those prices vary from country to country, and from method to method. In many developed countries, insurance plans help individuals pay for prescriptive drugs and surgical procedures, such as combined oral contraceptive pills and vasectomy. Government programs in these nations also pay for part of the price of contraceptives for people with poverty or near-poverty incomes. In most developing nations, the cost of a birth control method may be provided free by the government or provided at a greatly reduced price by government subsidies or funds from nonprofit organizations, such as the United Nations Population Fund or a local Planned Parenthood affiliate. This assistance provided to the person using the contraceptive helps the organizations and governments avoid the costs of abortion, or post-abortion medical needs, or of prenatal care, delivery, and postnatal health care for the mother and the child.

The male condom is by far the least expensive method available for preventing pregnancy for each act of sexual intercourse. The male condom success rate with perfect use is 97 percent. Its added benefit of protecting people from sexually transmitted diseases has made it a rapidly increasing method of choice around the world. Its availability over-the-counter provides a benefit of privacy to condoms that improves its value to people. The fact that each condom, which typically costs less than US$1, may be used only once, raises its annual cost, and that cost can become a deterrent to its use.

In contrast, surgical sterilization of men and women carries a significantly higher one-time cost than the condom. The procedure for men is far less expensive than the procedure for women. In the United States in 1993 the prices of a tubal sterilization cost between $1,200 for surgery in a publicly supported clinic and $2,500 in a private medical practice. That year a vasectomy cost between $325 in public clinics and $750 in private clinics. Sterilization, however, is a permanent form of contraception. If a person counted the number of times she or he had sexual intercourse after being sterilized and divided it into the price of the procedure, a difficult calculation to make, the cost per act of sexual intercourse rivals the cost of a condom.

Other forms of contraception—intrauterine devices, implants, injectable, and pills—fall within the cost range of condoms and tubal sterilizations. They each have a higher initial cost. Each also requires a prescription to permit the person to purchase it, and that person would need to factor the cost of the visit to a doctor's office or a clinic into the cost of the procedure.

Estimates show that the price of contraceptives is far smaller than the cost of pregnancy and treating sexually transmitted diseases. A woman experiencing an unwanted pregnancy in 1995 would have incurred costs for prenatal care and delivery of approximately $1,173 for private health care and $609 for public supported health care. Had that woman's partner used a condom for one year to prevent that pregnancy, she would have saved $946 in a private health care setting and $525 in a public health care setting. More effective contraceptives save more on health care fees the longer the woman uses them.

Accuracy of use also influences the value of a contraceptive. All contraceptives work more effectively with perfect use—no forgotten pills, or misplaced diaphragms. *See also* INSURANCE COVERAGE (FOR CONTRACEPTIVES)

Further reading: Hatcher, Robert, James Trussell, Felicia Stewart, and others. *Contraceptive Technology*. 17th rev. ed. New York: Ardent Media, 1998. Trussell, James, Jacqueline Koenig, Felicia Stewart, and Jacqueline E. Darroch. "Medical Care Cost Savings from Adolescent Contraceptive Use." *Family Planning Perspectives* 29 (1997): 248–255. Trussell, James, et al. "The Economic Value of Contraception: A Comparison of Fifteen Methods." *American Journal of Public Health* 68 (1995): 494–503.

D

Dalkon Shield

Problems associated with the Dalkon Shield, an intrauterine device (IUD) designed in the United States in the 1960s, first marketed in 1970 and removed from the market in 1974, led to a steep plummet in the worldwide use of IUDs in the 1970s. The huge number of lawsuits filed against the company that marketed the Dalkon Shield and the damages paid by that company have been blamed by many birth control researchers and advocates for the decline of interest in the United States in contraception research and development by major pharmaceutical companies.

The flat, crab-shaped, plastic device, designed by doctor and inventor Hugh Davis, featured small fins that projected out from the sides, and a string made up of many micro-filaments that attached to a loop in the base of the device. This string eventually proved to be a hazard to wearers of the shield. Designed to allow for easy removal of the Dalkon Shield, the strings passed out of the uterus through the cervix and hung in the vagina when the device was in place.

In the late 1960s, Davis and his partner sold the device to the A.H. Robbins pharmaceutical company, which then went on to market the device, based upon the testing Davis had done during his invention and modification of the shield. At that time, the U.S. Food and Drug Administration (FDA) did not have the authority to require that companies prove the safety of medical devices before putting them on the market. The Dalkon Shield appealed to many doctors who realized their patients wanted highly reliable alternatives to contraceptive pills, which in the late 1960s and early 1970s were under close scrutiny for their safety. A.H. Robbins heavily promoted the Dalkon Shield to those doctors.

Eventually, hundreds of thousands of women in the United States and around the world had the device inserted, believing that the device offered them almost a 99 percent success rate at preventing pregnancy. About 235,000 women in the U.S. suffered from injuries caused by the Dalkon shield, including pelvic inflammatory disease (PID), unwanted pregnancies, spontaneous, septic abortions of those pregnancies, and even deformities in children born to wearers. Eventually, scientific research established that many of the complications were associated with the many fibers in the tail. These fibers allowed naturally occurring bacteria in a woman's vagina to wick up into the otherwise sterile uterus, causing serious infections that could and did lead to sterility and death. The flat, disk-like design also seemed to cause the device to pass through the walls of the uterus and cause complication in the woman's abdomen that also had life threatening consequences. In the United States, 20 women died from injuries caused by the Dalkon Shield.

A.H. Robbins stopped selling the shield in 1974 though it did not recall those devices that women were already wearing. Patients began suing first their doctors and then A.H. Robbins in 1972. The first case went to trial in 1974. Court documents showed that Davis was aware of design problems with the device before the pharmaceutical company bought it. Those same documents also showed that A.H. Robbins knew the pregnancy rate was at least five times higher than Davis had claimed for the shield.

Under the weight of thousands of law suits, A.H. Robbins filed for Chapter 11 bankruptcy protection in 1985, 10 years after the first suit against the company settled for $85,000 in damages. In 1989, American Home Products purchased the company. Not until May 1996 did the Dalkon Shield trust fund pay out its last payments to women injured by the device.

Faulty research and corporate greed receive much of the blame for the damage done to women and the reputation of IUDs by the Dalkon Shield. However, the roll of the FDA in allowing a faulty device to remain on the market has also been seriously challenged by public health and safety advocates. In 1976, during the trials of the lawsuits against A.H. Robbins, the FDA received congressional responsibility for approving medical devices for use in the United States. Under laws passed that year, companies carried the burden of proving their devices were safe and effective before the FDA would approve them. Had the Dalkon Shield been brought to market under the rules passed in 1976, its dangers and the weakness of the studies used to promote its effectiveness and safety would have been discovered in the approval process.

Intrauterine devices designed and invented since 1976 have undergone close and careful scrutiny and layers of scientific testing before they were approved for the market. Only the copper T380a and the ParaGard T380a devices have received approval since the Dalkon Shield failure. Testing has shown modern IUDs to be highly safe and effective devices, providing protection against pregnancy better than that of surgical sterilization. Still less than 1 percent of U.S. women used IUDs as of 1995. Worldwide, between 85 and 100 million women rely on IUDs for contraception. Medical practitioners have struggled to overcome the shadow caused by the Dalkon Shield, including holding international conferences on these devices.

Modern devices rely upon monofilament tails that do not cause the problem with bacteria traveling up the sting as did the Dalkon Shield. Their narrow T-shape makes insertion much easier than the painful insertion of a Dalkon Shield. This single-thread tail greatly reduces a woman's risk of suffering a pelvic inflammatory disease. Recent studies show that PID risk is greatest shortly after an IUD is inserted into the uterus and device instructions include improved sanitary conditions during insertion and monitoring of patients for symptoms during those early days.

Doctors, nurses, clinicians, and contraceptive advocates find themselves still discussing perceptions of IUDs that linger from the problems in the 1970s with the Dalkon Shield. Researchers also point to that device for causing a dramatic decline in the number of large pharmaceutical companies willing to take the legal risk of developing and marketing new contraceptive devices. The legacy of the Dalkon Shield has influenced both the effective use of IUDs and the rapid development of modern, effective, scientifically proven contraceptives. *See also* INTRAUTERINE DEVICE

Further reading: "The Dalkon Shield Story: A Company Rewarded for Its Faulty Product." *Health Facts,* May 1996, 1. Mintz, Morton. *At Any Cost: Corporate Greed, Women, and the Dalkon Shield.* New York: Pantheon, 1985. Mishell, Daniel R., and Patricia J. Sulak. "The IUD: Dispelling the Myths and Assessing the Potential." *Dialogues in Contraception,* 2nd ser., 2 (1997): 1–4. Perry, Susan, and Jim Dawson. *Nightmare: Women and the Dalkon Shield.* New York: MacMillan, 1985.

Dennett, Mary Ware (1872–1947)

Mary Ware Dennett, birth control activist, suffragist, and legal reformer, struggled for women's rights and peace during most of her adult life. As a leader in the American birth control movement of the early twentieth century, and mother of two sons, she found herself in 1930 involved in a legal battle over obscenity that would tear away at laws prohibiting sending obscene material, including information on sexuality, contraception, and abortion, through the U.S. mail.

Mary Coffin Ware was born on 4 April 1872, in Worcester, Massachusetts. She married William Hartley Dennett in January of 1900. In December, their first son, Carleton, was born. Mary nearly died during a difficult delivery and remained ill for several months after Carleton's birth. Three years later, Mary gave birth to her second son. The delivery left her so ill that she could not feed her child, who died within three weeks. Then in May of 1905, another son, Devon, was born. Again, a difficult delivery, Mary remained ill for an extended period and doctors recommended that she and her husband abstain from sexual intercourse to protect her health. After the birth of Devon, however, Mary's ill health prevented her from working as an interior designer in her husband's business, and he intensified a friendship with the wife of a client that would eventually lead to the very public dissolution of the Dennett marriage. When doctors discovered in 1907 a tear in Mary's reproductive tract, the result of Devon's rapid birth, they recommended surgery to repair the damage. Mary spent three weeks in a New York City hospital and returned from surgery to find her marriage in jeopardy, a situation she fought unsuccessfully to remedy.

The legal battles that followed, first for the custody of her sons, which she won in 1909, and then for the divorce in 1913, drew significant newspaper attention and gave Mary and her eccentric husband public attention that she found extremely uncomfortable. Her desire to regain her privacy after those scandals led directly to Mary Dennett shying away from publicity during the years of social advocacy that followed her return to health and the dissolution of her marriage.

While facing turmoil in her home life, Mary turned to activism in the local and state suffrage movements. In 1910, in an effort to support her children, Mary accepted the job as corresponding secretary of the National Woman Suffrage Association and moved to New York. Dennett worked simultaneously for many causes—suffrage, peace, birth control, and even the arts and crafts movement. A strong organizer and talented writer, Dennett gained a reputation as a woman who could achieve success for the organizations with which she worked. In 1914, Dennett attended a meeting where a young nurse, Margaret Sanger, discussed poor women's needs for contraception and the need for women of greater means to fight the battle for this right. Dennett found in the issue a resonance with her own experience. Fighting for birth control, Dennett realized, would provide her with a way to help improve the lives of women, a cause she believed in since her own childhood.

Early in 1915, faced with the task of answering her 14-year-old son's questions about sex, Dennett wrote her son, Carleton, a long essay, including diagrams of the female and male reproductive systems. She titled the essay "The Sex Side of Life: An Explanation for Young People." After giving her son the essay, and learning from him that it had done an excellent job of answering his questions, Dennett shared that essay with friends facing the same challenge.

Meanwhile, in the end of 1915, Dennett helped form the National Birth Control League, the first such organization. Dennett's approach to the struggle followed her belief that change in society needed to come from the top down and through this organization and the Voluntary Parenthood League, which she helped form in 1919, after the financial collapse of the NBCL, aimed at repealing or rewriting the 1873 Comstock Laws.

Dennett's career as a birth control activist was often in conflict with that of the more well-known Sanger. Dennett believed in working through the legal and legislative systems to bring about change, where Sanger believed in publicly challenging the law. Sanger sought attention; Dennett shunned it. Dennett also believed in the individual's right to knowledge concerning birth control and refused to compromise her principles as she felt Sanger had in agreeing to work through medical doctors as a way to provide contraception to needy women.

Dennett devoted her efforts in the 1920s to lobbying Congress, and even the U.S. Post Office, seeking senators and representative who would sponsor bills to rewrite the nation's anti-obscenity laws. In those years, her sex-education essay, which she'd made into the pamphlet *The Sex Side of Life,* had become very popular among women, and she freely distributed it to anyone who asked for it. In 1918, it had been published in the professional journal *Medical Review of Reviews* and in *The Modern School*. Its success there lead Dennett to self-publish the pamphlet.

Unable to convince Congress to seriously address birth control, Dennett, 57, was ready to remove herself from social advocacy and retire to a life as an artist, when in 1929 she was indicted on felony charges for mailing obscene materials. She had for several years been mailing her sex-education pamphlet to people upon request, having concluded that the tremendous rise of advertising for ineffective contraceptives and feminine hygiene products had rendered the old obscenity laws ineffective. That year, however, federal prosecutors, disguising their identity, sent for a pamphlet, and when it arrived at a Virginia mailbox, issued the indictment.

The case of *United States v. Mary Ware Dennett* went to trial in March 1929 and ended in a guilty verdict in April. Fined $3,000, which she refused to pay, Dennett faced willingly the prospect of jail in defense of young people's right to information on sex education. In the tremendous public support she received, Dennett recognized the social change in attitudes toward sex and birth control brought about by years of advocacy by members of the birth control movement. With the backing of the American Civil Liberties Union and a committee organized to raise money for her defense, Dennett, 58, and her attorney, Morris Ernst, appealed the conviction.

In January 1930, the U.S. Court of Appeals heard the case. The majority opinion reversed the lower court's conviction and found that Dennett's intent had been to educate and to inform, not to appeal to impure thoughts, and that the intentions of the author were not obscene and therefore the material was not obscene. The prosecutors chose not to further appeal this decision. Dennett's legal victory and the stand the appellate judges took set the stage for the legal defeat of federal and state laws banning contraception, abortion, and obscene material. That legal battle culminated in the right to privacy cases of the 1960s and early 1970s that made access to contraception and abortion legal for people across the United States.

In her years as an activist, Dennett struggled for women's right to vote, which was granted in the United States in 1920, for world peace, and for political reform. After her obscenity trial, Dennett retreated from public life. She died 25 July 1974, in Valatie, New York. *See also* COMSTOCK LAWS; OBSCENITY; SANGER, MARGARET HIGGINS

Further reading: Chen, Constance M. *"The Sex Side of Life": Mary Ware Dennett's Pioneering Battle for Birth Control and Sex Education*. New York: New Press, 1996. Craig, John M. " 'The Sex Side of Life': The Obscenity Case of Mary Ware Dennett." *Frontiers* 15 (1995): 145–166. Dennett, Mary Ware. *Birth Control Laws: Shall We Keep Them, Change Them, or Abolish Them?* 1926. Reprint, New York: Da Capo Press, 1970.

Depo-Provera

Known commonly as "the shot," Depo-Provera provides a women with a hormonal contraceptive through injection. Depo-Provera, the trademarked name of the contraceptive manufactured by the Upjohn Company, has come to commonly refer to the progestin-only contraceptive depot medroxyprogesterone acetate also known as DMPA.

Women receive Depo-Provera through a deep injection into the upper arm or buttock. Each injection contains 150 milligrams of the progestin in the form of microscopic crystals. Depo-Provera prevents pregnancy by suppressing the production of mature eggs, by preventing ovulation, by thickening the mucus which blocks the woman's cervix, and by changing the inner surface of the endometrium to prevent implantation of an egg should fertilization occur. DMPA levels remain high enough to be effective for 14 weeks.

To be most effective, a woman's first injection is given at a clinic or doctor's office within five days of the beginning of a normal menstrual period. If she begins the regimen later than that day in her cycle, the woman is advised to use an alternative contraceptive for two weeks following the injection. Follow-up shots are given at three-month intervals. Patients new to this birth control method are advised to follow strictly this schedule; women who remain on Depo-Provera for several years build up hormone levels that provide a two-week grace period.

Success rates for this progestin-only contraceptive are very high, even higher than for surgical sterilization. Because the woman receives injections—she need take no other action, such as remembering to take a daily pill—the actual success rate and the perfect success rate are identical. Unintended pregnancies occur rarely, only with 0.3 percent of the women who use Depo-Provera, less than 1 pregnancy for each 100 women each year. Fertility typically returns within six to 12 months after a woman discontinues using DMPA.

Side effects may include some disruption of the menstrual cycle, decreasing the amount of blood flow, and amenorrhea, the complete suppression of menstruation. Most women using DMPA report irregular menstrual cycles in the first year of use and others have reported irregular bleeding, spotting, or changes in the duration of their periods. Women have also reported weight gain while taking Depo-Provera, though research shows that women using progestin-only contraceptives such as Depo-Provera experience less weight gain than do women on oral contraceptives that combine amounts of synthetic progestins with synthetic estrogen.

More than 70 percent of the women who begin to use DMPA continue using it after one year. Many women who stop using DMPA do so because of concerns with their menstrual cycles. While DMPA increases the days that a woman has light spotting, the longer a woman uses Depo-Provera, the greater the likelihood she will develop amenorrhea.

Studies by the World Health Organization (WHO) in the early 1990s established that women taking DMPA are not at greater risk of developing breast cancer than the overall population, though early reports of this contraceptive suggested such a link.

Researchers developed depot medroxyprogesterone acetate as a contraceptive hormone in the early 1972. Since than women in more than 90 countries have used this convenient, private form of contraception. Great Britain approved use of Depo-Provera in 1978, but concerns by the U.S. Food and Drug Administration involving a connection to breast cancer kept it from use there until approval in 1992. The WHO study, however, convinced regulators that such risk did not exist. Canada approved Depo-Provera for use in 1997. *See also* HORMONES—SEX; HORMONES—SYNTHETIC; INJECTABLE CONTRACEPTIVES; PROGESTIN-ONLY CONTRACEPTIVES; SIDE EFFECTS

Further reading: "DMPA at a Glance." *The Population Reports* 23 (1995): S1–2. Grimes, David A., et al., eds. *Modern Contraception: Updates from the Contraception Report.* Totowa, NJ: Emron, 1997. Stehlin, Dori. *Depo-Provera: The Quarterly Contraceptive.* Rockville, MD: U.S. Department of Health and Human Services, 1993.

Diaphragm

The small, round, dome-shaped rubber diaphragm, a reusable barrier contraceptive, fits over the woman's cervix and blocks the path of sperm. This device blocks the sperm, but does not kill it. The diaphragm combined with an over-the-counter cream or gel spermicide, blocks and kills sperm, which can survive as long as 3 to 5 days in the vagina and cervix, once the woman removes the diaphragm. Together, the rubber diaphragm and the chemical spermicide provide very effective contraception.

Diaphragms are available worldwide in a variety of shapes and sizes. The diameter of the round, rubber dome ranges from 50 millimeters to 105 millimeters (about 2 to 4 inches). All diaphragms have a flexible outer ring that the woman pinches together before she inserts the device into her vagina. Once she fills the cup with spermicide, the woman pushes the diaphragm, bowl down, deep into her vagina and hooks the rim over the back of her pubic bone. The cup then fits fully over her cervix, extending slightly down into the vagina. Because the diaphragm needs to fit snugly, a medical professional needs to examine the woman and determine the proper size diaphragm. For this reason, diaphragms require prescriptions.

The diaphragm can be inserted up to six hours before intercourse. If several hours elapse between putting it in place and having intercourse, fresh spermicide can be inserted into the vagina without removing the diaphragm. To be fully effective, the diaphragm must remain in place for six hours after intercourse, and, to prevent the risk of side effects, it must be removed no more than 24 hours after insertion.

Leaving the diaphragm in longer than 24 hours can expose the woman to risk from toxic shock syndrome. Other risks from diaphragms include minor problems due to sensitivity to spermicides and risk of urinary tract infections if the woman does not use the diaphragm properly.

The overall success rate of diaphragms at preventing unintended pregnancy with perfect use, that is with every occasion of intercourse and following directions precisely, is 94 percent. With typical use, however, when women may forget to use the diaphragm, not position it properly, or forget to use spermicide, is 82 percent. Younger women, who are likely to have intercourse more frequently than older women and who are more fertile than older women, and women who have intercourse three or more times a week, according to studies, experience a higher failure rate, even with perfect use, than women over 30 and women who have intercourse less often than once a week. This higher failure rate for younger and very sexually active women represents a statistical variance.

Diaphragms are the oldest female-controlled form of contraception and were once very popular in the United States. Their use has dwindled in recent years, due primarily to the fact that diaphragms offer no protection from sexually transmitted diseases. In 1982, 8 percent of the women using contraceptives relied upon diaphragms for their protection. By 1988, the percentage had fallen to 5.7 percent and in 1995, the diaphragm was used only by 1.9 percent of women between ages 15 and 44. By this time, many couples had replaced the diaphragm with condoms to give themselves greater protection from disease in addition to protection from unwanted pregnancy. *See also* BARRIER CONTRACEPTIVES; CERVICAL CAP; CONDOM—FEMALE; SPERMICIDES; TOXIC SHOCK SYNDROME; VAGINAL SPONGE

Further reading: Lieberman, E. James, and Karen Lieberman Troccoli. *Like It Is: A Teen Sex Guide.* Mefferson, NC: McFarland, 1998. Speroff, Leon, and Philip Carney. *A Clinical Guide for Contraception.* Baltimore: Williams and Wilkins, 1992.

Disability, Developmental

Developmental disabilities can be those of a physical, cognitive, or psychological nature that prevent normal physical or emotional development. People with these disabilities may be challenged in finding adequate birth control information and access, and health care providers may be challenged in delivering it.

Women and men, in their teen years and older, who have physical disabilities or chronic disease often fail to receive sexuality education and reproductive counseling, because the commonly held belief that they do not engage in sexual intercourse still influences health care providers and families. Research shows that people with physical disabilities often desire help meeting their reproductive needs but do not know where to turn to find that help.

The specific nature of an individual's physical disability can significantly influence which modern birth control methods may be most effective for that person. Women for whom a pregnancy may be difficult or life threatening may need a permanent form of sterilization. Women with difficulty using their arms or hands would find vaginal barrier contraceptives impossible or awkward to use. Norplant may cause irregular bleeding, a difficult side effect for some physically disabled women to deal with.

Intrauterine devices can also cause irregular bleeding, enough that excessive blood loss could cause anemia, which would be a problem for women with respiratory problems or with rheumatoid arthritis. Menstrual bleeding can also cause hygiene problems for women with impaired dexterity. A woman who has lost sensation in her pelvis would have difficulty feeling the pain that can signal pelvic inflammatory disease or an IUD that has moved out of position.

Modern methods may also have a positive benefit to disabled women. Early studies of combined oral contraceptives (COCs) on multiple sclerosis suggest these birth control pills may stabilize some of that disease's symptoms, which include tremors and speech disturbances and eventually can lead to paralysis. Other studies, however, show no long-range effect on the disease.

Studies show that teens with disabilities are at the same risk from unwanted pregnancy as their non-disabled classmates, yet parents, teachers, and health care providers often mistakenly assume they are not sexually active. A study of Minnesota high school students showed that the sexual activities of disabled teens were little different from the activities of their peers.

The need for reproductive health of women and men with disabilities in developing countries is likely to be even greater than for those in developed countries. In some societies, cultural attitudes may lead people to consider their disabled relatives and neighbors as invisible or as not worthy of reproduction.

Casualties of war and violence may also go overlooked by reproductive health care providers.

All of these factors contribute to a rising effort by family planning practitioners and medical experts to pay closer attention to the reproductive needs and wants of disabled adults. Research has confirmed a need and desire for contraception among the disabled population that matches, or more often exceeds the population at large.

Women who suffer from psychological disabilities also often receive inadequate attention to their reproductive health needs. Social stereotypes and deficiencies in the medical system that such women rely upon often lead to a low level of attention to sexuality and contraception for women who suffer from depression, drug abuse, and a wide variety of mental disabilities.

Concern arose among mental health advocates and family planning experts that women who suffered from disorders that prevented them from adequately caring for themselves were not receiving reproductive care from medical professionals. Psychiatric clinicians also may pay too little attention to the birth control needs of their patients. Consumed by dealing with the woman's mental health needs, these medical professionals overlook or underestimate the sexuality of their patients. In study programs where care givers recognized and discussed contraceptive needs with their patients, patients received information and counseling tailored specifically to them, and the women were then better able to meet their own contraceptive needs.

Pregnancy and motherhood poses added risks to a mentally ill woman and a child to which she might give birth. A pregnancy can create new stress for a woman already finding difficulty coping with her mental illness. If she becomes pregnant, the developing fetus could be at risk from inheriting the illness or prenatal abuse of drugs by the mother. Once born, the child would be at risk from the mother's inability to cope with the infant's needs. Studies released in 1999 showed that infants of clinically depressed mothers developed their learning skills more slowly than children of healthy women and were at greater risk of developing learning disabilities.

The drug treatments for mental disorders complicate the choice of a contraceptive. Hormonal contraceptives may conflict with drugs that treat depression, though synthetic estrogen and progestogen may actually work to help alleviate some of the causes of depression. An intrauterine device may appear to be a good choice for a woman since it requires little effort on her part to remember to use it, but women with more than one sexual partner, as can be the case with women who abuse drugs and who use an IUD, are at greater risk from sexually transmitted diseases than women who do not use IUDs. In some situations, the treatment a woman receives for a mental disorder can help her choose a contraceptive method; she may find a long-term hormonal method fits the same schedule as the medicines she receives for her illness.

Discussing contraceptives with a mentally disturbed patient also creates time constraints for psychological clinicians. The depth of knowledge a health care provider needs to fully discuss the benefits and risks of a contraceptive method can be significant, and psychological clinicians may not have the time to develop that knowledge. Despite these limitations, psychological clinicians infrequently refer patients to reproductive health care providers for such help. Recognizing the reproductive health needs of their patients is the first step psychological health care providers must take in increasing the help they give their patients to help them protect themselves from unwanted pregnancies and reproductive tract infections.

The mental health of men also influences issues of pregnancy prevention. As are mentally ill women, mentally ill men who become fathers are less likely to provide infants with necessary daily care and emotional nurturing. Studies also show that men with mental disabilities, including drug and alcohol abuse, are less likely to use condoms to protect against disease and pregnancy than are men without psychological disabilities.

Researchers involved in international efforts to provide people with the contraceptives they demand and need worry that if concern is rising in developed countries for the care of mentally disabled women, then a greater need must exist for such people in developing countries where women's mental illnesses often go undiagnosed and untreated.

Solutions to the problems of women and men with developmental disabilities or who abuse drugs involve a greater network of health care providers and elimination of stereotypes that suggest such patients rarely express their sexuality. The best solution, experts recommend, is for mentally ill patients to direct their own reproductive choices with the help, education, and expertise from their mental health care and reproductive health care providers.

Further reading: Best, Kim. "Disabled Have Many Needs for Contraception." *Network* 19 (1999). Online: http://resevoir.fhi.org/en/fp/fppubs/network/v19-2/nt1924.html, 25 June 1999. Best, Kim. "Mental Disabilities Affect Method Options: Many Factors Involving a Psychiatric Condition or Mental Retardation Influence Contraceptive Decisions." *Network* 19 (1999). Online: http://resevoir.fhi.org/en/fp/fppubs/network/v19-2/nt1925.html, 25 June 1999. Hankoff, Leon D., and Philip D. Darney. "Contraceptive Choices for Behaviorally Disordered Women." *American Journal of Obstetrics and Gynecology* 168.6, part 2 (1993): 1986–1989. Leavesley, Gwen, and John Porter. "Sexuality, Fertility, and Contraception in Disability." *Contraception* (Australia) 26 (1982): 417–441. Suris, Joan-Carles, Michael D. Resnick, Nadav Cassuto, and Robert W. Blum. "Sexual Behavior of Adolescents with Chronic Disease and Disability." *Journal of Adolescent Health* 19 (1996): 124–131.

Douching

Research has proven postcoital douching (flushing the vagina clean with an acidic fluid after sexual intercourse) to be an ineffective form of contraception. It also appears to have a significant relation to increased rates of pelvic inflammatory diseases, ectopic pregnancies, infertility, and cervical cancer.

Sperm move very quickly along the vagina, through the cervix, and into the uterus. Within as little as 15 seconds of a man ejaculating into his partner's vagina, most of his sperm have traveled through this route and are no longer in the vagina, the only place that the douching solution reaches. While an acid-based solution, such as vinegar or lemon juice, will kill some sperm, a woman cannot douche fast enough to kill more than a small percentage of sperm. Even spermicides mixed with the solution are not effective for the same reason.

Also, if while using spermicide women douche sooner than six hours after intercourse, they wash away any spermicide and prevent it from effectively destroying sperm. Douching also washes away cervical mucus, making it practically impossible for women using the Billings Method of observing cervical mucus to notice changes in their cervical discharge.

Studies have established a connection between women who douche and the instances of pelvic inflammatory diseases (PIDs). Though douching is not known to cause these diseases, researchers have found that pelvic inflammatory diseases were twice as common among women who douche regularly as among women who do not douche. The connection to cervical cancer is less clear, though researchers have found an association between frequent douching and diseases such as vaginitis and cervicitis, which themselves have a high risk of leading to cancer.

Douching as a hygiene practice is declining in the United States. The 1995 National Survey of Family Growth showed that only 27 percent of women ages 15 to 44 douche regularly. That's down from 37 percent in 1988. Douching is still more common than average among Hispanic women (34 percent), black women (55 percent), women who did not finish high school (53 percent), and those who had pelvic inflammatory diseases (41 percent). Black college graduates were four times more likely to douche regularly as white college graduates (40 percent compared to 9 percent).

Because douching provides little or no contraceptive protection and is linked to pelvic diseases and some cancers, many doctors and scientists recommend that women not douche. *See also* SPERMICIDES

Further reading: Abma, J., Chandra, A., Mosher, W., Peterson, L., and Piccinino L. *Fertility, Family Planning, and Women's Health: New Data from the 1995 National Survey of Family Growth.* Vital and Health Statistics 23, 19. National Center for Health Statistics, 1997. Zhang, Jun, A., George Thomas, and Etel Leybovich. "Vaginal Douching and Adverse Health Effects: A Meta-Analysis." *American Journal of Public Health* 87 (1997): 1207–1211.

E

Education (of Women)

Social science and population researchers have found a strong relationship between the level of education of women and contraceptive use. Generally, the more education a woman has, the more likely she is to decide to limit the number of children she bears and the more likely she is to use modern contraceptives to prevent unplanned pregnancies. This relationship can be seen most clearly in the less developed nations of the world that are at greatest risk from the stresses of overpopulation, but it is also visible in developed nations where contraceptive use is high and the number of children to which women give birth is low.

In general, girls who regularly attend school and stay in school into and throughout adolescence most often delay marriage and childbearing. This association assumes that the girl will not become sexually active while in school. Research into teen pregnancy shows that if girls believe that education has a value to them personally, they are more likely than girls who see little future value to education to delay their first sexual intercourse and to delay frequent intercourse. Girls who see the value of education are also likely to use contraceptives, if they are available, during those educational years if they become sexually active.

Education exposes women to knowledge and information about ways to prevent pregnancy or to limit their own fertility. Women with education have been shown to make informed choices between types of contraceptives, to successfully follow directions, and to take action if a contraceptive fails. They demonstrate a better ability to understand the actual risks, as opposed to the rumored risks, of contraceptives and the ability to find medical help in achieving their goals. Studies also suggest that formal education allows women to better communicate their wishes and desires to a man within a sexual union and through this communication choose when and if they wish to have children.

Reproductive health professionals and researchers and human rights activists have established that education also influences a woman in abstract ways that influence her family planning choices. Through education, women gain greater aspirations and learn to recognize options other than bearing children.

Access to education, for girls and boys, has risen steadily since the 1970s. As in the developed world, primary education for children ages 6 to 11 is nearly universal in east Asia and Latin America, with literacy rates of women and men correspondingly high. Access to primary education has risen to near universal levels in the Middle East and northern Africa, too. Sub-Saharan Africa, however, saw increases in access to education into the 1980s and then a sharp decline. By 1995, approximately 65 percent of children in southern Africa were enrolled in primary school.

Enrollment in secondary schools has also increased steadily worldwide. In east Asia in the late 1990s more than 55 percent of the children ages 12 to 17 were enrolled in secondary school. In sub-Saharan Africa that rate was about 15 percent. College enrollments worldwide are also increasing as more children gain the elementary and high school educations they need to prepare them for further study. Almost all children in developed countries receive high school educations and increasingly they receive postsecondary educations.

In all settings around the world, well-educated women tend to have fewer children than do uneducated or less educated women. This observation has led to significant numbers of studies into the relationship between women's education and population growth and fertility rates. Studies have shown that education of women has a much stronger impact on changing fertility behavior than does education of men and than do other factors in the woman's life, such as economic or social status *See also* REPRODUCTIVE RIGHTS

Further reading: Jejeebhoy, Shireen. *Women's Education, Autonomy, and Reproductive Behavior: Experience from Developing Countries*. Oxford: Clarendon Press, 1995. McClamroch, Kristi. "Total Fertility Rate, Women's Education, and Women's Work: What Are the Relationships?" *Population and Environment: A Journal of Interdisciplinary Studies* 18 (1996): 175–186.

Effectiveness (of Contraceptives)

The effectiveness of a contraceptive at preventing pregnancy depends in part on its characteristics and in part on how accurately the person using the method follows its directions. All contraceptives are studied to determine their effectiveness rates with perfect use, when people follow the directions precisely in all aspects of use, and with typical use, when people do not follow directions precisely.

Studies reveal that even people who have chosen a specific contraceptive often have mistaken understandings of how effective a contraceptive method actually is. Rumor, incorrect information, and word of mouth from people who had poor success with a method cause people to inaccurately use a method or to believe that a method they would prefer to use is not as effective or safe as they would like it to be. Such misinformation itself results from the misuse of the contraceptive by the person sharing the information. A story about a friend who became pregnant while taking hormonal pills, for example, will lead others to believe the method is ineffective though they may not understand or know the reason for the friend's failure.

Knowledge of the effectiveness of modern birth control methods varies around the world depending on a person's access to contraceptives and access to accurate information. Worldwide, people receive most information from friends, relatives, and family members, the least well informed of people with access to contraceptive information. In general, however, simply being aware of a method, having heard of it from a friend or through the mass media, does not mean that a person accurately understands the method in question. Knowledge of contraceptive pills, for example, varies so greatly that in some countries and cultures people do not understand that this method, though used daily, influences a woman's monthly menstrual cycle.

Frequently, people have low expectations of the effectiveness of methods that are scientifically very effective. Conversely, they have high expectations of methods that are scientifically proven to be much less effective than other methods. Surveys revealed that people understood the near perfect effectiveness of long-acting methods such as hormonal implants and injectable contraceptives. They were less aware of the effectiveness of daily pills and emergency contraceptive methods. Americans, in general, believe contraceptive pills to be less effective than do people in western Europe and Canada. Far less effective methods such as fertility awareness and withdrawal are seen by Americans as more effective than scientific study reveals them to be.

To increase the overall effectiveness of new contraceptives, researchers focus on human traits that tend to lead to imperfect use. Memory and opportunity offer the two main challenges to the effectiveness of current contraceptives, and researchers are working to develop systems that can overcome these human failings. Contraceptive pills require that women remember to take a daily tablet; researchers are at work on pills with time-release formulas that would require a woman to take one each week or one a month and thus require less constant attention to memory. Barriers require that women or men carry contraceptives with them so that when they find themselves in an intimate setting they have the opportunity to use the device. Researchers have developed female barrier methods that can remain in place in the vagina for hours and perhaps days and ease the need for women to interrupt a romantic setting to insert a barrier. They expect that developing contraceptives that suit a person's lifestyle and improving access to a variety of contraceptives will improve the overall effectiveness rate of current and future contraceptives.

Hormonal contraceptives of all varieties, which prevent ovulation and create a form of temporary sterility, were by far the most effective temporary contraceptive methods available in 2000. Implants prevent pregnancy 99.91 percent of the time. Injectables work 99.7 percent of the time. These two hormonal methods were developed after the invention of contraceptive pills in attempts to ease the burden of memory on women who prefer hormonal birth control. Neither method requires daily effort by the person using them and both have perfect and typical use rates that match each other. Hormonal pills with perfect use range from 99.9 percent to 99.5 percent for combined estrogen and progestin pills and progestin-only pills respectively. They're typical use rates are lower, at 95 percent. The difference is attributed to women forgetting to take a pill and being unclear on the directions to follow when they do forget. Clinicians who explain these directions in detail, rather than relying on the woman to read and understand manufacturers' instructions, find that women more effectively use contraceptive pills.

Only permanent surgical sterilization rivals hormonal contraceptives for effectiveness, but these methods do not easily allow people to change their minds and are most often used by people who have completed their childbearing. The typical use effectiveness rates for male vasectomies is slightly lower than perfect use, at 99.85 percent compared to 99.9 percent, due to the fact that some men engage in sexual intercourse too soon after the procedure, while sperm are still in their reproductive tracts. Female sterilization is 99.5 percent effective with perfect and typical use.

Intrauterine devices (IUDs), some of them containing synthetic hormones, also provide near-surgical levels of contraceptive effectiveness. Manufacturers and designers have developed modern IUDs that eliminated problems with the uterus expelling the IUD and with IUDs that some how moved outside of the uterus. Eliminating these failures of early IUDs resulted in highly effective modern devices that are easy for doctors and practitioners to insert and remove.

Barrier methods, such as condoms and diaphragms, and spermicides offer the least effective forms of modern contraception. All have the potential to slip out of place or to be incorrectly positioned before intercourse. Perfect use effectiveness for these devices ranges from 97 percent to 74 percent. Typical use ranges from 86 percent to 60 percent.

Natural forms of birth control such as withdrawal and fertility awareness techniques, also known as periodic abstinence, have effectiveness rates similar to those of barrier methods for both perfect and typical use. Modern refinements of these methods involve charts and thermometers designed to make charting monthly bodily changes easier. Learning the precise method and following the procedures also make these methods more effective.

To improve understanding of contraception, reproductive health care workers and advocates recommend that medical professionals and clinic workers spend increasing amounts of time teaching their clients how to use the various methods and discussing with them the effectiveness rates and side effects. Further education, they argue, will lead to more fact-based decisions concerning contraception and help people more effectively prevent pregnancy.

See also BIOLOGICAL METHODS OF CONTRACEPTION; FAILURE RATES; HORMONAL CONTRACEPTIVES; INJECTIBLE CONTRACEPTIVES; INTRAUTERINE DEVICE

Further reading: Delbanco, Suzanne, et al. "Public Knowledge and Perceptions about Unplanned Pregnancy and Contraception in Three Countries." *Family Planning Perspectives* 29 (1997): 70–75. Hatcher, Robert, James Trussel, Felicia Stewart, and others. *Contraceptive Technology*. 17th rev. ed. New York: Ardent Media, 1998.

Egg. *See* OVUM AND OVARIES

Egypt

Since the mid-1950s, the government and people of Egypt have struggled to slow its rapidly growing population. In 1953, Egypt's first elected government established the National Council for Population Affairs to study and propose policy for influencing population growth. In 1955, the government opened eight clinics to provide family planning services to women who qualified for the program. 1958 brought the foundation of the Population Studies Association, which would in 1996 become the Egyptian Family Planning Association. These political and social efforts achieved little in slowing the number of people born in Egypt each year. Not until the mid-1980s did Egypt's efforts begin to work and the rate of growth begin to slow.

The unusual geography of Egypt provides an added challenge to population and family planning efforts in that nation. Located at the delta of the Nile River in northern Africa, Egypt has very fertile soil along the river and desert throughout the rest of the country. Approximately two-thirds of Egypt's land is desert and essentially uninhabitable and incapable of supporting farming. The great majority of Egypt's population, 97 percent, live on only 4 percent of the land. Egypt's cities are growing rapidly. More than half of the population lives in or near Cairo, the nation's capital. While statistics suggest that Egypt has plenty of land to grow into, the presence of the desert covering so much of its land makes Egypt's fertile areas very heavily populated and increasingly crowded.

To ease that crowding, the Egyptian government since the late 1980s has worked to encourage families to have only two to three children. The leveling off of Egypt's growth suggests that people have accepted this advice. In 1980, Egyptian women could expect to give birth, on average, to 5.5 children, the nation's total fertility rate. By 1998, that fertility rate had fallen to 3.6 children. While that fertility decline is greater than reported in other north African countries, it is still much higher than the 2.0 fertility rate that would mean a stabilization of the growth of the population. With that average, Egyptians expect their population to continue growing well into the twenty-first century. In 1998, that growth rate was 2.2 percent each year.

The use of contraceptives rose steadily in the last decades of the twentieth century, with 46 percent of women of reproductive age using modern contraceptives. Half of those women rely on intrauterine devices for pregnancy prevention and one-quarter use hormonal contraceptive pills. Condom use, female sterilization, and other modern method use are increasing slowly in Egypt and few people, less than 5 percent, rely upon traditional birth control methods to limit family size.

Egypt's official policy and social policy also support greater education for women. The number of women who can read and who attend primary and secondary schools and college is increasing also, though in the late 1990s the gap between men and women was still one of the widest in north Africa and the near east. In 1998, 39 percent of Egypt's women were literate, compared to 64 percent of Egypt's men. Educating women is seen by the world community as important to lowering a nation's total fertility rate and decreasing a nation's rate of population growth. With greater education, women find more options in their lives than marrying and

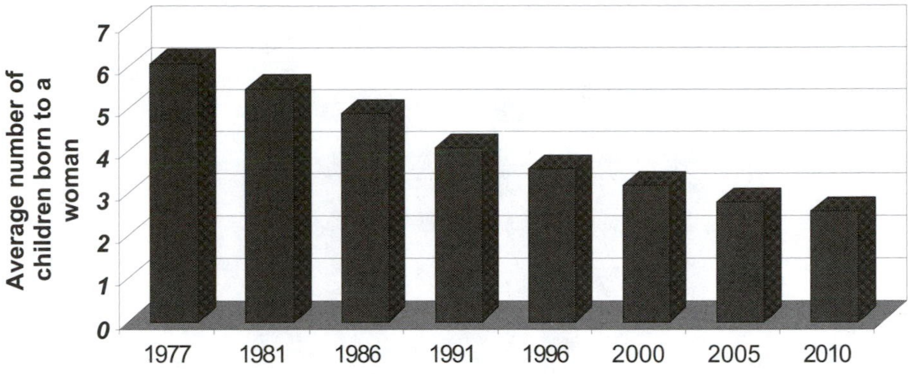

Egypt: Total Fertility Rate: Actual and Projected

Source: U.S. Census Bureau International Data Base

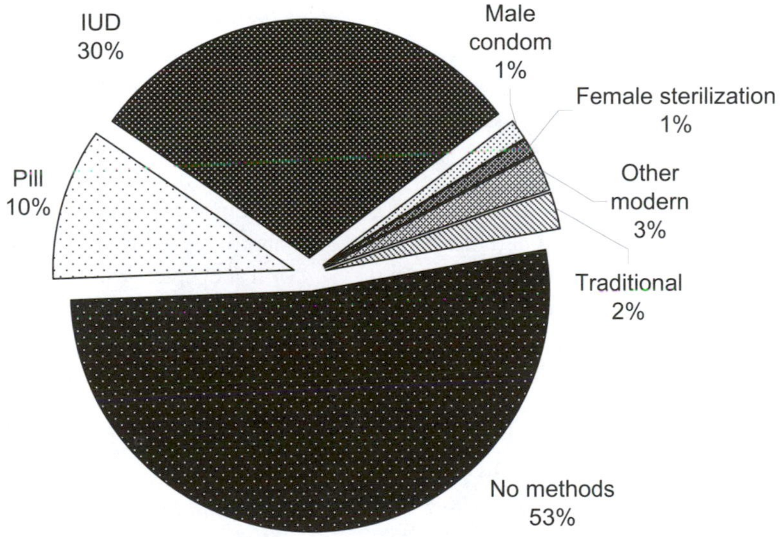

Egypt: 1995 Contraceptive Use by Married Women Ages 15–49

Source: U.S. Census Bureau International Data Base

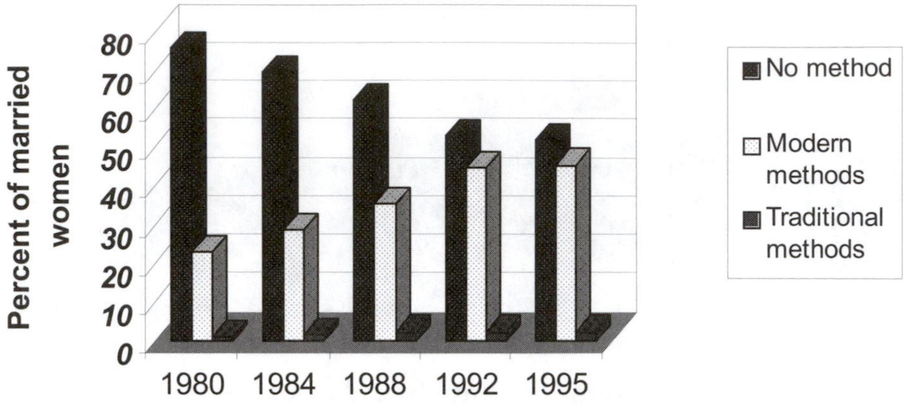

Egypt: Changes in Contraceptive Use by Married Women Ages 15–49

Source: U.S. Census Bureau International Data Base

having children. Egypt's government is actively involved in promoting the education of girls and women.

As a nation where Islam is the dominant religion, Egypt stands out in history as the home of the first Islamic leader to issue a *fatwa*, religious opinion, in support of men and women using scientific means for preventing pregnancy.

Egypt has also worked in the late 1990s to decrease the incidence of female genital cutting, also known as female genital mutilation and female circumcision, the cutting of some or all of a girls external genitalia, a traditional practice usually performed before a girl reaches 13 years old. Efforts by the government since the 1994 United Nations International Conference on Population and Development held in Cairo to decrease the incidence of this procedure seem to be having an influence on the public. A 1997 national survey of adolescents showed that 86 percent of girls 13 to 19 had undergone this procedure, down from the nearly universal use of the practice in Egypt before 1994. Among the daughters of families where at least one parent had completed secondary school, only 48 percent had undergone female genital mutilation.

Egypt law allows abortion only to protect the health of the mother. Estimates show that about 25 for every 1,000 women aged 15 to 44 undergo an abortion each year; many of these are performed illegally.

With current growth rates and current population size, experts see Egypt's population growing steadily into the 2000s. It is likely to reach 96 million by 2025. By educating teens and encouraging people to have fewer children, governmental and nongovernmental organizations expect to curb that growth, and increasing the use of modern contraceptives will be an important tool in achieving that goal. *See also* AFRICA

Further reading: Bureau of the Census. *Population Trends: Egypt*. Washington, DC: U.S. Department of Commerce, Economics and Statistics Administration, Bureau of the Census, 1994. Fargues, Philippe. "State Policies and the Birth Rate in Egypt: From Socialism to Liberalism." *Population and Development Review* 23 (1997): 115–138.

Eisenstadt v. Baird

In 1972, the United States Supreme Court, ruling in *Eisenstadt v. Baird* removed the crime of providing contraceptives to unmarried people. By deciding that unmarried people had the same private right to contraception that the courts had granted to married people in 1965 in *Griswold v. Connecticut*, the Court overturned laws in 23 states that denied birth control methods and information on contraception to unmarried couples. The court issued its ruling on 22 March 1972, less than a year before its pivotal ruling in *Roe v. Wade* which made abortion legal in the United States.

On 6 April 1967, birth control activist William Baird presented a lecture on people's right to privacy in their sex lives, including their right to contraception, at Boston University to an audience of more than 2,000 people. The lecture was part of an effort to test Massachusetts law, which at that time held as a felony the providing and exhibiting of birth control and abortion information and devices. During his lecture, Baird gave condoms and spermicidal foam, both nonprescription contraceptives, to a group of students including a 19-year-old woman. In part, the charge against Baird stemmed from the fact that he was neither a physician nor a pharmacist; both professions were permitted under Massachusetts law to distribute contraceptives to patients and customers. Though birth control advocates had been winning reform in state legislatures, Massachusetts lawmakers had resisted changing their eighteenth-century laws which were aimed at protecting people from obscenity.

Found guilty in Massachusetts Superior Court on 17 October 1967, Baird appealed the decision. The appellate court, however, ruled in 1 May 1968, in favor of the state on the charges of distributing contraceptives, though it overturned the charge of discussing contraception. Baird served a 30-day jail sentence in 1970 while his appeal to the U.S. Supreme Court went forward.

By a vote of six-to-one on 22 March 1972, the Supreme Court overturned the lower courts' decisions in *Eisenstadt v. Baird*. In issuing its decision, the majority opinion, written by Justice William Brennan, argued that the right of privacy established for married individuals in *Griswold v. Connecticut* in 1965 clearly extended to unmarried individuals. People, regardless of marital status, had the right to be free of unwanted pregnancies and from unwarranted intrusion by the government into their lives on such fundamental levels as when to "bear or beget a child."

Three months before ruling in Baird, the seven justices then sitting on the court had heard the arguments in the *Roe v. Wade* and *Doe v. Bolton* cases, which the court had earlier combined. Those cases involved a woman's right to privacy in choosing an abortion. As the court waited to issue its ruling in *Roe v. Wade*, it decided the Baird case. Its language in *Baird*, specifically the phrase "to bear or beget a child," seemed to signal that some of the justices had formed legal opinions on abortion. To "beget" a child referred to contraception, the topic of *Eisenstadt v. Baird*; however to "bear" a child seemed to refer to the private choice to terminate a pregnancy. *See also* GRISWOLD V. CONNECTICUT; ROE V. WADE

Further reading: Baird, Bill. "The People Versus Bill Baird: Struggling for Your Right to Privacy." *The Humanist*, March–April 1997, 39–40.

Ejaculation

The process that forces semen through the urethra and out of a man's body is known as ejaculation. This expelling of semen, which in a fertile male contains several million sperm cells, results from sexual stimulation. If ejaculation occurs while the man's penis is inserted in a woman's vagina, the sperm enters the woman's body where it may fertilize a mature egg. Sperm can also enter the woman's body if the semen is ejaculated while the penis is touching the woman's genitals.

Ejaculation is the end of the process that moves sperm from the testicles, where a man's body creates the sperm, through the body to the base of the penis, and finally out through the urethra. During sexual arousal, pleasurable signals from the man's spinal cord trigger muscles in his reproductive organs to contract rhythmically and to move the sperm from the testicles through the vas deferens and to the prostate gland where the sex cells mix with the semen. Similar contractions in the prostate and seminal vesicles move the semen into the urethra. At the culmination of intercourse, muscles at the base of the penis contract and shoot the semen from the man's body.

Covering the penis with a condom, a widely used and effective form of birth control, prevents semen from entering a woman's body. Stopping the sperm from mixing with the semen by severing the vas deferens, a surgical procedure known as a vasectomy, provides a form of sterilization.

Though a man withdrawing his penis from the woman's vagina before ejaculation may prevent most sperm from entering her body, if some semen touches the woman's external sex organs, the sperm can enter her body and survive long enough to fertilize an egg. *See also* CONDOM—MALE; REPRODUCTIVE SYSTEM—MALE; VASECTOMY; WITHDRAWAL

Emergency Contraception

Emergency contraception offers women the means of preventing an unwanted pregnancy within days of having unprotected intercourse. Women who feel that they need contraceptive help within 72 hours of a barrier method failing during intercourse, who have been raped, or who have missed a contraceptive pill or have not used a contraceptive during intercourse, have several options available to them.

Three approaches to what has been known as postcoital contraception, or the "morning-after" pill, and now is most commonly referred to as emergency contraception, have been known and used to a minor degree since the 1970s. During the 1990s, however, reproductive health care providers and women around the world have been working to provide emergency contraception and to make it more widely known and used. Until the mid-1990s in the United States, emergency contraception was often referred to as the "best kept secret" of the modern contraceptive age. Methods of emergency contraceptives were available at hospitals for rape victims who reported the assault, though unavailable to women who had been forced into having sex and did not seek medical help. Reproductive health specialists concentrated efforts in the 1990s on educating women, physicians, and pharmacists of the need for and availability of emergency contraceptive methods. By the end of that decade, with encouragement by the U.S. Food and Drug Administration (FDA), oral contraceptives packaged specifically for emergencies had reached the U.S. market. PREVEN, manufactured by Gynetics Inc., received FDA approval in September 1998. Packaging of emergency contraceptives was also readily available to women in Great Britain, eastern Europe, and the former Soviet Republics. Worldwide, emergency contraception became of key concern for health professionals providing services to victims of politically motivated rape. Projects were also underway to provide the contraceptives without prescriptions or without a visit to a doctor's office.

If women use emergency contraception after they have had unprotected sexual intercourse, if they suspect the birth control method they are using did not work, or if they have been raped they can effectively prevent pregnancy more than 75 percent of the time, depending on the method they choose. Two methods rely on forms of oral, hormonal contraceptives. The third involves the insertion shortly after intercourse of a Copper-T intrauterine device.

In the early 1960s shortly after birth control pills were first available to women, researchers discovered that high doses of synthetic estrogen pills, when taken close together, rather than every day, also effectively prevented pregnancy. However, those high estrogen doses caused side effects that made estrogens unworkable as emergency contraceptives. In 1974, A. Albert Yuzpe, a Canadian physician, showed that the new formulations of oral contraceptives, which combined lower doses of estrogens and progestins than those used in the 1960s, worked up to 75 percent of the time at preventing unwanted pregnancies. Since then, high doses of oral contraceptives have been used for emergency contraception, though it was not always a convenient solution. In the 1990s, however, beginning in Europe, companies began marketing products aimed specifically at emergency contraception and containing only the number of pills needed. Most of these early formulas followed the estrogen-progestin regimen that Yuzpe studied and described.

Studies of progestin-only oral contraceptives in the 1990s suggested that this synthetic hormone would more effectively prevent pregnancy in emergencies than combined oral contraceptives. Levonorgestrel, a commonly used chemical that imitates the function of progesterone, a natural hormone involved in the development and support of a pregnancy, underwent comparative testing with combined emergency contraceptives by the World Health Organization (WHO) in 1998. Results showed that the combined contraceptives prevented 76 percent of the pregnancies, while the levonorgestrel-only pills prevented 89 percent of pregnancies. The levonorgestrel also caused fewer side effects, including nausea, vomiting, tiredness, and dizziness. The progestin-only pills used in the tests contained higher doses of levonorgestrel than were packaged in marketed contraceptives. Since then, drug companies have developed emergency contraceptive products that do contain the higher levonorgestrel doses.

In January 1999, Women's Capital Corporation, a privately held U.S. company, submitted a new drug application to the FDA for approval of a progestin-only emergency contraceptive product containing 0.75 milligrams of levonorgestrel, the dosage used in the WHO study. On 1 June 1999, the French government approved the sales of Norlevo, a progestin-only emergency contraceptive, for sale without a prescription.

Emergency contraceptives based upon pill forms of synthetic hormones seem to work by disrupting ovulation if taken early in a woman's menstrual cycle, or by disrupting fertilization or even implantation if taken later in the cycle. The exact method would depend upon when in the cycle the woman takes the pills. Emergency contraceptive doses of hormonal contraceptives do not work after a fertilized egg has successfully implanted in the uterus.

In addition to hormonal contraceptives, a Copper-T intrauterine device inserted into the woman's uterus within seven days of ovulation in a cycle during which a woman has had unprotected sexual intercourse can also interrupt the pregnancy process. Studies have revealed that IUDs are extremely effective in preventing pregnancy in emergency situations. This system is far less frequently used, though, since IUDs represent a long-term contraceptive option. Few women who have experienced unprotected intercourse and are concerned with possibly becoming pregnant find themselves capable of making a long-term decision.

Though available in much of Europe as a specifically packaged product and labeled for emergency contraception, hesitation by pharmaceutical companies in the United States, under pressure from antiabortion groups, delayed the marketing of emergency contraceptives in the United States. The FDA had approved in June 1996 the use of six different brands of birth control pills for emergency contraception and in February 1997 publicly announced that it encouraged manufacture of products designed specifically for emergency contraception.

Researchers and health policy experts expect that once women learn of their options, emergency contraceptives will play a major role around the world in decreasing the numbers of unwanted pregnancies and abortions that occur each year. In the Unites States, nearly 3 million women experience unintended pregnancies each year, half due to contraceptive failure and half to people not using contraceptives. Estimates suggest that emergency contraception could reduce unintended pregnancy in the United States alone by 1.7 million and could reduce the number of abortions by 800,000. In Great Britain, politicians have sought to make emergency contraceptive products available over-the-counter, without a prescription, in an effort to encourage women to use this option.

Availability of emergency contraceptives also influences how effective these products are at reducing the number of unwanted pregnancies. The findings of a 1998 pilot project in the state of Washington conducted by the Program for Appropriate Technology in Health (PATH), showed that women who must first visit a doctor to receive a prescription are less likely to seek help than women who have the contraceptive pills available to them at a pharmacy. In that state more than 100 pharmacists who have been specially trained are working in state-approved and -regulated drug collaborations with medical professionals licensed to prescribe drugs. The project agreement allows the pharmacists to fill emergency contraceptive prescriptions for women without the woman needing to have consulted her doctor. These services are available on weekends and at night, when most medical offices are closed. Pharmacists filled more than 2,700 prescriptions for emergency contraceptive pills in the first four months of the pilot project.

Also a part of the education process for women about emergency contraceptives has been the availability of information on emergency contraception through the Internet. Princeton University in Princeton, NJ, maintains a site at http://opr.princeton.edu/ec that discusses emergency contraceptive methods and how users can obtain those contraceptives. The Population Council's regional office for Latin America and the Caribbean also maintains a site in Spanish at http://www.en3dias.org.mx.

In countries where Roman Catholic influences are strong, however, some advocates of emergency contraception fear that church's objection to birth control devices will slow and even prevent the use of emergency contraceptives by women who seek them. In the United States, for example, mergers between Catholic-owned hospitals and sectarian hospitals have led to Catholic principals determining if rape victims brought to emergency rooms would receive the emergency contraceptive pills that would prevent a pregnancy. Advocacy groups are challenging these religious-based infringements on women's rights, especially in communities where a Catholic hospital is a woman's only option for emergency medical treatment.

Few people see any form of emergency contraception as a viable alternative to regular, planned, and consistent, contraception. With its side effects and success rates significantly below those of hormonal methods, including daily oral contraceptives, implants, and injectables, emergency contraceptives are not likely to become, as opponents suggest, once-a-month contraceptives. *See also* HORMONAL CONTRACEPTIVES; ORAL CONTRACEPTIVES; ROMAN CATHOLIC CHURCH; YUZPE REGIMEN

Further reading: Ellertson, Charlotte, Beverly Winikoff, Elizabeth Armstrong, Sharon Camp, and Pramilla Senanayake. "Expanding Access to Emergency Contraception in Developing Countries." *Studies in Family Planning* 26 (1995): 251–263. Glaser, Anna. "Levonorgestrel for Emergency Contraception." *International Planned Parenthood Federation Medical Bulletin* 32.6 (1998): 6–7. Van Look, Paul F. A., and Felicia Stewart. "Emergency Contraception." In *Contraceptive Technology,* 17th rev. ed., edited by Robert Hatcher, James Trussel, Felicia Stewart, and others. New York: Ardent Media, 1998. Wells, Elisa S. "Using Pharmacies in Washington State to Expand Access to Emergency Contraception." *Family Planning Perspectives* 30 (1998): 281–82.

Endometrial Ablation

Endometrial ablation, a procedure that removes the inner lining of the uterus, most often leads to infertility, and medical specialists have speculated that it might be a form of surgical sterility. However, though rare, pregnancy can occur in women who have undergone the procedure and such a pregnancy can cause serious complications.

Endometrial ablation developed as a nonintrusive replacement for hysterectomy, the surgical removal of the uterus, to stop unusually heavy bleeding from which some women suffer. Sixty percent of the patients completely stop menstruating. The menstrual flow for another 30 percent significantly decreases, and the procedure does not work for 5 to 10 percent of the patients.

To remove the endometrium, a doctor inserts a viewing scope through the vagina and the cervix and into the woman's uterus. Once able to see the inside of the uterus, the doctor uses an electrical device or laser to cut away the inner lining. This lining is responsible for holding the blood that gradually fills the uterus during the first portion of the menstrual cycle and for providing a place for a fertilized egg to implant and grow. The procedure takes between 20 and 40 minutes and is most often performed on an outpatient basis in a surgical center or hospital.

Without this thick inner lining, a fertilized egg has nowhere to implant, and infertility results for most women who undergo successful endometrial ablations. Removal of the lining does not alter the woman's hormonal system, however, and ovulation still occurs. While only 0.8 percent of the women who undergo this procedure become pregnant, those who do are at serious risk of rupturing their uteruses, or miscarriage and spontaneous abortion as well as abnormalities to the placenta. For these reasons, gynecologists recommend that women choosing endometrial ablation also undergo tubal sterilization. *See also* ENDOMETRIUM; HYSTERECTOMY; TUBAL STERILIZATION

Further reading: McLucas, Bruce. "Pregnancy after Endometrial Ablation: A Case Report." *Journal of Reproductive Medicine* 40 (1995): 237–239.

Endometrium

The inner layer of the uterus, the mucus-producing tissue of the endometrium, fills with blood and thickens during each month of a woman's menstrual cycle.

Should a woman's egg be fertilized by a man's sperm, the thickened endometrium provides a cushioned place for the zygote to rest, to connect to the woman's body, and to grow. If no fertilization occurs or if the fertilized egg fails to implant, the endometrium sheds its stored blood during the three to five days of the woman's monthly period.

Part of the effectiveness of hormonal contraceptives comes from the changes that altered levels of estrogen and progesterone cause in the endometrium. Essentially, the lining fails to develop a consistent or adequate thickness to support a fertilized egg should one be produced, despite the other inhibiting factors created by such contraceptives. The specific changes to the endometrium depend upon the specific artificial hormone the woman takes.

Recently, endometrial ablation, a procedure used to eliminate or ease problems that some women have with heavy menstrual bleeding, has been studied as a possible permanent or long-term method of birth control. Though is it not recommended for birth control purposes by medical specialists, researchers, or approval agencies, such removal of the lining, often by laser or electric current, often results in permanent infertility. *See also* ENDOMETRIAL ABLATION; REPRODUCTIVE SYSTEM—FEMALE

Further reading: Seeley, Rod R., Trent D. Stephens, and Philip Tate. *Anatomy and Physiology*. 5th ed. Boston: McGraw Hill, 2000.

Estrogens

Estrogens, the primary female sex hormones, are manufactured in a woman's ovaries, though small amounts are made in the cortex of the adrenal glands located on the top of her kidneys. Though commonly talked of as one substance, a woman's body manufactures several forms of estrogen, most notably estradiol and estrone, all of which are important in developing her reproductive system during puberty and in supporting the function of that system during her reproductive years. Estrogen levels decrease during perimenopause. After menopause, the ovaries steadily secrete small amounts of these hormones.

When a woman reaches puberty (about age 13), hormones from her pituitary gland trigger the ovaries to begin making estrogens. These hormones trigger the development of the female reproductive system and the secondary female sex characteristics such as breast development and changes in body shape. In adulthood, estrogen levels increase and decrease during the phases of a woman's menstrual cycles. Increasing levels in the beginning of the cycle cause to resume growing the immature eggs that had formed but had stopped growing during the woman's own fetal development. At this point in each cycle, estrogens also trigger changes in the woman's uterine lining causing it to begin to thicken with blood.

These higher levels of estrogens prevent the pituitary gland from releasing the hormone that signals eggs to resume development. After a mature egg is ejected from the ovary, the remaining follicle wall secretes much larger amounts of estrogens and progesterone, another major female sex hormone. When the egg does not fertilize or implant in the uterine wall, estrogen levels begin to decrease, causing the uterus to shed its lining. This decrease in estrogens allows the pituitary gland to once again secrete the hormones that signal eggs to resume growing.

The scientific discovery and analysis of estrogens in the late 1800s and early 1900s led in the 1950s to the discovery of ways to artificially create substances that mimic natural estrogen. These manufactured versions of this sex hormone allowed scientists to develop ways to keep estrogen levels in a woman's body just high enough to stop the pituitary gland from secreting the hormones that cause a woman's eggs, or sex cells, to mature. With estrogen levels always as high as those found during ovulation, a woman's body does not know when it is time to mature another egg and ovulation does not occur. Understanding the function and cycle of estrogen has lead to one of the most effective contraceptives, the oral contraceptive pill.

Men also produce small amounts of estrogen in their testicles and synthesized forms of these hormones are used to treat some cancers in men and are being studied for their roles in developing male contraceptives. *See also* HORMONAL CONTRACEPTIVES; HORMONES—SEX; HORMONES—SYNTHETIC; MALE CONTRACEPTIVES; MENSTRUAL CYCLE; ORAL CONTRACEPTIVES; REPRODUCTIVE SYSTEM—FEMALE

Further reading: United States Food and Drug Administration. *Estrogens*. Rockville, MD: U.S. Department of Health and Human Services, 1993.

Ethics

The ethics of birth control, the standards by which methods would be developed, tested, and used, caused many in the late twentieth century to question the focus of family planning programs. Emphasis on controlling population growth had caused reported abuses of contraceptives, sterilization, and abortion. Coercion by governments, health care providers, and even judges in courtrooms, led in the last quarter of the twentieth century to international agreements that shifted the family planning emphasis to human and reproductive rights and the ethical use of birth control methods and away from governments reaching numerical population goals.

In the medical profession, practitioners and ethicists extended the requirements of informed consent to the process of providing individuals with contraception. To ethically and morally provide contraception, medical professionals and clinic workers would be obliged to wait until clients came to them before beginning a discussion of methods. Under informed consent, medical professionals could not attempt to unduly influence people to have fewer children, and they would be obliged to provide clients with full and complete information, in the language of the client. Highest standards would call for providers to ascertain that the clients had understood the information. With this full information and understanding, people would then be able to give clear judgment to their decisions to prevent pregnancy.

In the United States, members of the medical profession worked to incorporate discussions of informed consent into a woman's or man's visit to the gynecologist or urologist. Efforts to educate doctors and nurses extended to the length of discussion they could have with clients and to the documents doctors may give to their patients. In many cases, doctors provide their clients with handouts, videos, and displays that specifically identify the nature of the contraceptives, their effectiveness, and side effects, and the risks the person may have in using the method. The medical professionals also give the client time to consider all of the implications of their choices and to ask enough questions to make the client feel comfortable with his or her understanding.

Ideally, maintaining a high ethical standard would preclude government workers, clinicians, and health care workers from causing a person to use contraception against his or her will. Doctors could not sterilize women or insert intrauterine devices while the woman was undergoing or recovering from childbirth. People could not be misled or even lied to concerning the permanency of surgical sterilization. Clients who had had hormonal contraceptives implanted under their skin could not be denied the removal of those devices at their request. Advocates for improving the ethical use of modern contraceptives argue that even the behavior of husbands who prevent their wives from gaining access to the contraception they desire demands attention from human rights policies and workers.

As population control became an increasing issue for many nations in the twentieth century, reports of forced sterilization became common. Several governments developed policies that did not specifically call for deceiving people about contraception but that led to, some critics say encouraged, local officials and clinic staff members to perform tubal sterilization on women when they gave birth through cesarean sections. Unethical forms of forcing people to limit their family sizes, of denying people their informed consent to procedures, have been reported around the world, from clinics in the United States to hospitals in India, China, and Peru.

Coercion and incentives, using the power of the government to enforce strict population policies, such as those found in China and Vietnam, challenge the ethical validity of population and family planning programs. In some nations, families have been denied basic services, such as power and water, if they defied the policies concerning the number of times they became pregnant. Programs that reward people for having few births and punish people for having many births also violate a high ethical use of modern birth control methods. Such was the case, some critics argue, when welfare reform in the United States in the late 1990s led to fewer benefits to welfare mothers who had more than one or two children. The more children the women gave birth to, the fewer government-supported benefits they received.

Medical research faces challenges from ethicists as scientists work to develop and discover still more effective methods of birth control. The testing of new contraceptives, for example, where the results are unknown, may prove an ethical dilemma. Do you risk a woman's health for the possibility of developing a new contraceptive? Such questions surfaced during the testing of the first hormonal contraceptive pills in the 1950s, when researchers turned to poor women to learn of the pill's effectiveness beyond the laboratory. While researchers used early forms of informed consent to attract participants in their studies, critics suggest that doctors rushed the pill to market too soon and exposed millions of women to risks from circulatory illness and cancer. Many argue that the refinement of hormonal contraceptives that took place once they were being sold around the world should have been done before the first pills were approved.

Recent international agreements, like the program of action signed by 180 nations at the 1994 International Conference on Population and Development held in Cairo, Egypt, aim to improve the ethical use of contraception, to improve the reproductive health of women, and to make human rights, rather than numbers of people, the goal of population programs.

Beyond contraception, abortion and religious beliefs also challenge the ethical aspects of modern birth control. *See also* ABORTION; LIFE (BEGINNING OF)

Further reading: Curran, Charles. "Fertility Control: Ethical Issues." In *Encyclopedia of Bioethics,* rev. ed., edited by Warren Thomas Reich. New York: Macmillan, 1995. Faden, Ruth R., and Tom L. Beauchamp. *A History and Theory of Informed Consent*. New York: Oxford University Press, 1986. Knight, James W., and Joan C. Callahan. *Preventing Birth: Contemporary Methods and Related Moral Controversies.* Ethics in a Changing World 3. Salt Lake City: University of Utah Press, 1989.

Europe

The countries that make up the continent of Europe represent a wide variety of experiences with family planning and birth control. As of the end of the twentieth century, in virtually all of Europe's nations, women could expect to give birth to fewer than two children. Most nations, as a result of these very low fertility rates, were not growing in population and some actually had negative population growth figures.

Modern contraceptive use was widespread in western Europe at the end of the twentieth century. In most of these nations, from the United Kingdom to Switzerland and Norway to Spain, use of modern contraceptives generally exceeded 65 percent of women between the ages of 15 and 49. In many nations that figure exceeded 70 percent. The citizens of Germany, Spain, Sweden, and Switzerland had the most access to all major forms of contraception, including male and female sterilization. Other nations ranked close behind those four. Availability and use of hormonal implants and injectable contraceptives was growing steadily in western Europe.

Abortion on demand also characterized the laws of most of western Europe during this time. The exceptions stood out. In the Republic of Ireland only abortions to save the life of the woman were legal. Northern Ireland, Portugal, Spain, and Switzerland allowed abortion to save the woman's life and to protect her physical and mental health. Great Britain and Finland allowed abortion for those reasons and also permitted abortion for social and economic reasons. In all of the other nations of western Europe, abortion on demand was legal at least through the first trimester.

In eastern Europe, contraceptive use and abortion rates changed rapidly during the 1990s, following the breakup of the Soviet Union early in that decade. Policies of the former communist governments that ruled most of the eastern European countries discouraged contraception but encouraged abortion. Those countries retained their reliance upon abortion, but with the opening of trade with western Europe and the United States, all modern forms of contraception became increasingly available. In Slovakia, the availability of hormonal contraceptive pills increased five-fold between 1990 and 1999. The abortion rate decreased by more than half in that same time. In the Czech Republic, use of modern contraceptives rose steadily also and the abortion rate decreased by 55 percent.

In Latvia, a former Soviet Republic, quality contraceptives at affordable prices slowly became available through pilot programs, and the government in the end of the twentieth century was drafting a national reproductive health policy and new abortion law. Poland alone among the former Soviet allies saw little increase in the use of contraceptives. Influenced by the Roman Catholic Church, the government of that country did not support the use of modern birth control methods. Changes in the nation's abortion law after the communist party lost control of Poland resulted in making abortion illegal except for health and family hardship reasons. In the late 1990s that law was revised to allow abortion only for the protection of the woman's health.

Across Europe women on average currently give birth to fewer than two children in their lives. The highest birth rate at the end of the twentieth century was found in Ireland where women averaged 1.9 children. The lowest birth rate for all of Europe was 1.2 children in Italy and Spain.

Most of the nations across Europe in the late 1990s experienced little if any population growth, the result of widespread contraceptive use and abortion. Some nations even experienced decreases in their population size. Great Britain grew at a rate of 0.2 percent in 1998, Greece and Sweden's population did not grow, and Bulgaria's population decreased by 0.5 percent and Latvia's decreased by 0.6 percent.

The Roman Catholic Church, with its international headquarters in the Vatican in Italy, exerted varying levels of influence in Europe's dominantly Catholic countries. In Italy itself Catholics by and large ignored the church's official ruling against the use of

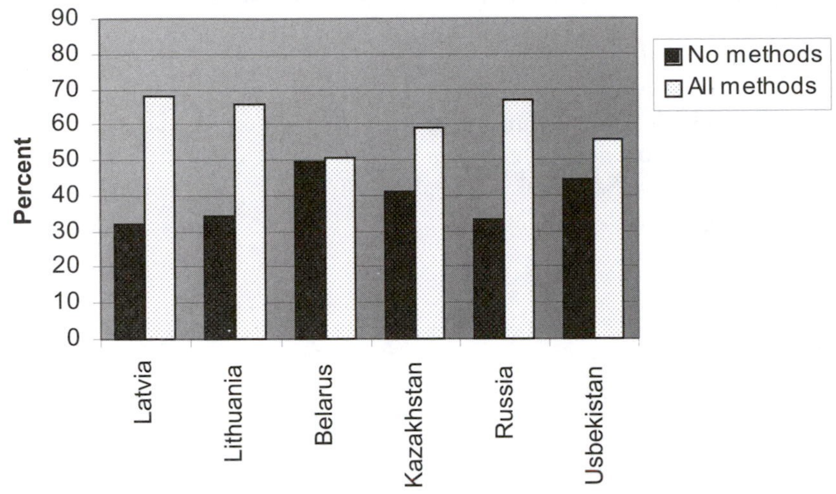

Newly Independent States: 1994–1996
Married Women Using Contraception Ages 15–49

Source: U.S. Census Bureau, *World Population Profile 1998*

modern contraceptives. Economic and social institutions and a lack of government support for families influenced Italian parents' decisions to use contraceptives more than did the Catholic Church's ban on all but fertility awareness methods of birth control. In Ireland, the Catholic influence appeared to some analysts to be declining as more people traveled to nearby Great Britain to undergo abortions in private clinics and where contraceptive use rose through the 1990s. In Poland, however, the Catholic Church successfully influenced the government to tightly restrict abortion and discourage the availability of contraceptives.

The amount and nature of sex education in schools across Europe also varies greatly from country to country. In many nations sex education is mandatory from age seven on in the nations' schools. Countries such as Sweden and the United Kingdom have written books and provided curriculum materials for the teaching of the biology and the psychology of reproduction. In other nations, again due in part to the influence of the Roman Catholic Church, sex education is not taught in the schools, but is left to the families. As a result of this variety, teens in 1999 still reported that they learned little about sex education in schools and most teens across the continent still relied upon friends for their knowledge of reproduction.

A greater proportion of teens in the eastern European countries gave birth each year than in the western European countries. With the exception of the United Kingdom, western European nations had teen birth rates below their eastern counterparts from 1990 to 1995. Switzerland, with a rate of five births for every 1,000 women between the ages of 15 and 19, had the lowest European birth rate, and, except for Japan at four births, the lowest in the world. Bulgaria had the highest teen birth rate in Europe at 59 for every 1,000 women. The United Kingdom's birth rate stood at 33. Only Albania's teen birth rate at 14 rivaled those of western Europe. Statistics suggest that many teen pregnancies in eastern Europe end in abortion.

As Europe entered the twenty-first century, governments and nongovernmental organizations focused their reproductive health attention on teen pregnancy rates and on providing more consistent access to contraception for people in all geographic areas and across all economic levels. The growing numbers of people older than reproductive age, as the nations' populations aged due to those low levels at which children were being born, began offering Europe more policy challenges than did family planning. *See also* ADOLESCENTS; FRANCE; ROMAN CATHOLIC CHURCH

Further reading: Chenais, Jean-Claude. "Fertility, Family, and Social Policy in Contemporary Western Europe." *Population and Development Review* 22 (1996): 729–739. David, Henry P. "Abortion in Europe, 1920–1991: A Public Health Perspective." *Studies in Family Planning* 23 (1992): 1–222.

F

Failure Rates

A contraceptive fails when, despite its use, a woman becomes pregnant. The *failure rate* for a contraceptive is the percentage of women who become pregnant while using that contraceptive. The failure rates that scientists and statisticians calculate take into consideration the number of women likely to become pregnant over time when not using a contraceptive and those likely to become pregnant when using that contraceptive. Most statistics are based upon clinical studies conducted during the approval phases of developing specific contraceptives. Research concerns in the 1990s focused on whether these numbers accurately represented how people not involved in a study would actually use a product. At best, some researchers suggest, the often published and utilized failure rates for contraceptives are overestimates of how effective a specific contraceptive is in use.

Failure rates attempt to take into consideration the actual dysfunction of a device, such as a condom breaking or a diaphragm slipping out of place, and the human dysfunction involved in using a device, such as a woman forgetting to take a contraceptive pill or a man not withdrawing his penis from the woman's vagina before ejaculation. The numbers listed for contraceptive methods, then, represent the ideals of contraceptives based upon their success during closely scrutinized testing and the actual success during the private use of the devices. Figures of actual success are based heavily upon accounts from people during surveys and interviews.

A woman's or man's ability to follow package directions and the directions given by health care professionals, a concept known as contraceptive compliance, greatly increases her or his success with a contraceptive device and improves the effectiveness rate while decreasing the failure rate of that device. The greater a person's compliance with directions, the greater the success of the device and the more closely actual use statistics will match ideal use statistics. Ease of use of a product, making products whose directions are easy to follow, has thus become an important feature in designing and developing contraceptives.

Each of the modern contraceptives offers its own difficulties as couples attempt to follow directions. A woman may have trouble inserting a vaginal barrier or in remembering what to do when she forgets to take a daily pill. Differences between typical and perfect use failure rates for modern contraceptives range from 2 percent to 16 percent. For contraceptive pills, the typical use failure is 3 percent and the perfect use rate is 0.1 percent. For the new female condom, the typical use failure rate is 21 percent and the perfect use failure rates is 5 percent. Some of the newer implantable and injectable hormonal contraceptives offer methods of use that require very little effort on the couple's part. Implants need be tended to only on insertion and removal, actions which may be as many as five years apart. Injectable contraceptives require that a woman remember and keep quarterly or monthly health care appointments. This ease of use keeps the perfect and typical use failure rates for the implant Norplant at 0.09 percent and for the injectable Depo-Provera at 0.3 percent.

Published failure rate estimates generally focus on a person's first year of use of that product. Over time, as she continues to use a contraceptive, a woman faces less risk of contraceptive failure than during the first year of use. The average annual risk over years of use falls significantly as a woman or man becomes accustomed to using the method.

Reproductive health professionals discuss another failure rate, the rate at which women decide not to continue using a specific contraceptive method. Successful use of a contraceptive depends heavily on how that product fits into a woman's or man's lifestyle and how she or he reacts to the possible side effects of the contraceptive. Though most modern contraceptives require that a woman visit a doctor's office or medical clinic to receive a prescription to purchase the device, a woman may decide after trying a product, such as a diaphragm or combined oral contraceptive pill, that the product does not suit her personality, upsets her physically, or offers greater risk than anticipated. In this case, the woman may reject the contraceptive and decide not to use it, risking pregnancy during unprotected intercourse. Studies in the mid-1990s suggest that overall, 31 percent of women discontinue using a reversible contraceptive within three months of beginning its use, while 44 percent will stop using a method within one year. However, studies also revealed that of those women who quit using a contraceptive, 68 percent will resume using a method within one month and 76 percent will resume within three months.

Failure rates, or their opposite, success rates, are influenced by several factors beyond the test results researchers obtain in tests. Failure rates take into account the fallibility of the human beings who turn to the products for help in preventing pregnancies. While biological scientists work to develop products with high clinical success rates and low failure rates, such as implants and injectable contraceptives, social scientists work to develop methods for improving the human understanding of the products and the use of those products. Improved education of medical professionals and their clients aims at decreasing the typical failure rates of methods. By helping clinicians properly teach clients how to insert a diaphragm, for example, or by encouraging companies providing package instructions that clearly warn people that age influences the durability of a latex condom, reproductive health specialists work to improve the ways people use contraceptives and to decrease the failure rates of those methods.

In addition to working with current contraceptives, biological and social science researchers also work to develop new products, such as the contraceptive patch and the hormone-containing vaginal ring, that combine ease of use with methods that have proved highly effective during research. Study also continues into understanding why and how people choose contraceptives, why they stop using a specific method, and why and how their concerns and choices vary over their reproductive years. By combining all of the factors that lead to contraceptive failure, researchers and advocates hope to provide more efficient, effective ways to meet individuals' family planning goals. *See also* EFFECTIVENESS (OF CONTRACEPTIVES); RISK; SIDE EFFECTS

Further reading: Matteson, Peggy. *Advocating for Self: Women's Decisions Concerning Contraception*. New York: Harrington Park Press (Imprint of the Haworth Press), 1995. Trussell, James, and Barbara Vaughan. "Contraceptive Failure, Method-Related Discontinuation and Resumption of Use: Results from the 1995 National Survey of Family Growth." *Family Planning Perspectives* 31 (1999): 64–72.

Fallopian Tubes

The two fallopian tubes, each about 10 centimeters (2 to 4 inches) long and about 0.7 centimeters (1/4 inch) in diameter, open and connect on one end to the upper part of the uterus, one on the right and one on the left. The other open end of each tube hovers near one of the two ovaries, the egg producing and primary female reproductive organs.

Also known as oviducts or uterine tubes, the fallopian tubes transport eggs from the ovaries to the uterus. They also carry sperm, the male sex cell, up from the uterus toward the ovaries. Most often, fertilization of an egg by a sperm occurs within a fallopian tube.

In a tubal ligation, a common form of sterilization or permanent birth control, these tubes are surgically cut or fused. This prevents mature eggs from traveling to the uterus and prevents sperm from reaching the mature eggs. *See also* OVUM AND OVARIES; REPRODUCTIVE SYSTEM—FEMALE; TUBAL STERILIZATION; UTERUS

Family Health International

Family Health International (FHI), a nonprofit organization, conducts research aimed at developing new contraceptives and works with groups around the world to improve reproductive health and provide safe, effective, and affordable family planning services. FHI also trains scientists around the world in how to conduct clinical trials of contraceptive methods and in how to improve health care. From its headquarters in North Carolina, FHI works in more than 40 countries, mostly in Africa, Asia, and Latin America.

The organization, which now has more than 400 employees, began in 1971 at the University of North Carolina at Chapel Hill as the International Fertility Research Program. Funded initially by a grant from the United States Agency for International Development (USAID), that original group involved a network of 40 scientists and physicians from 18 countries. Four years later, the group ended its affiliation with the university and became an independent nonprofit group. In 1982, having grown to more than 100 employees, the fertility research group changed its name to Family Health International in an effort to better describe its expanding areas of concern.

Among its early projects, FHI researched and established the safety of vasectomies in developing countries and demonstrated that outpatient female sterilization methods were more advantageous than procedures that required hospitalization. In the early 1980s, FHI began researching natural family planning methods, including the lactational amenorrhea method (LAM), which with strict guidelines, offers breastfeeding mothers a biological method of contraception. In 1995, FHI research led to international endorsement of this method as effective and beneficial, especially in developing countries.

FHI research also developed barrier contraceptives including the "Today" vaginal sponge, a non-latex male condom, and the female "Reality" condom. Research in the 1980s and 1990s demonstrated the effectiveness of the Filshie Clip, a removable clamp that, once inserted, blocks the fallopian tubes and provides a reversible form of surgical sterilization.

Research into the prevention and spread of acquired immunodeficiency syndrome (AIDS) also receives attention from FHI, which in 1987 began scientific study to help slow the AIDS epidemic. In 1997, FHI began a five-year project to prevent the spread of AIDS and care for infected people in developing countries in Africa, Asia, Latin America, the Caribbean, and Europe.

Funding for FHI now comes in part from USAID, but also from the National Institutes of Health and private foundations. Funds from the sale in 1991 of a for-profit corporation that had been formed by FHI in 1986 now also underwrite FHI programs. That money supports the work of two divisions, Family Health Institute and Health Futures. The institute works on public health projects around the world, including developing and developed countries. Health Futures works with companies that develop pharmacology products, medical devices, and biotechnology approaches to family health. *See also* U.S. AGENCY FOR INTERNATIONAL DEVELOPMENT

Further reading: Family Health International Web site. http://www.fhi.org. "FHI Receives USAID Contract for Research in Africa." *Africa News Service,* 15 December 1999.

Family Planning

Family planning involves the choice by parents to give birth to the number of children they perceive as important to complete their families. The concept differs from birth control in its focus on family and reproductive health rather than upon the narrower focus of preventing pregnancy. It has a broader connotation than contraception, which focuses on the biology of reproduction.

By the end of the twentieth century, the expression "family planning" was often used interchangeably with "birth control." In precise discussions, family planning refers specifically to people having the children they want as well as not having the children they do not want, and usually centers around the context of marriage or similar social relationships. Women who find themselves in danger of unwanted pregnancy outside of marriage or a family commitment would likely be included in a discussion of birth control and pregnancy prevention rather than family planning. The needs of teens, too, are more precisely included in a discussion of contraception and birth control. These distinctions, however, are often blurred as the discussion moves from the specific scientific realm to more general public health and social welfare discussions. Culture, too, blurs these distinctions.

The phrase "family planning" came into popular vogue when in 1942, the American Birth Control League, which had recently merged with the Birth Control Federation of America, changed its name to the Planned Parenthood Federation of America, the name the organization maintains to this day. The members of that new organization believed that a shift in attention to families and reproductive health and away from the individual woman involved in controlling birth would make the concepts of family limitation more acceptable to a broader range of financial supporters who could help the organization further its goals of helping women prevent unwanted pregnancies.

Margaret Sanger had helped create the Birth Control Federation and had been given and taken credit for coining the expression "birth control" in 1914. At heart, this social reformer felt most strongly about providing women with the means of preventing pregnancy and protecting their health from giving birth to too many children spaced too closely together. She felt that "birth control" accurately put the emphasis on a woman's choice. As the Planned Parenthood Federation worked to provide services broadly across the United States, its organizers advocated that the family, and not the mother alone, benefited from access to effective contraceptive knowledge and techniques. Sanger resisted that change, but the evolution in the movement came about anyway. This adjustment of the focus from controlling births to planning families allowed the federation to reach out to more people.

Organizations around the world, as they began to develop, often included the expression in their titles. Great Britain's National Birth Control Association changed its name to the Family Planning Association. The Family Planning Association of India formed in 1949. The Japan Federation of Family Planning formed in 1954. Many of the members of the International Planned Parenthood Federation, which began in 1952, after a conference in Bombay, incorporated "family planning" in their titles.

Family limitation, by choice, had always been part of Sanger's message and had been the focus of other birth control advocates around the world, including the founders of Hull House in Chicago and birth control organizations in Los Angeles. Adapting this broader term allowed people to discuss more issues than preventing pregnancy. Family planning, then, includes discussions of a couple's desire for any children, for the spacing of those children if they decide to have more than one child, of the health and welfare of the mother, the children, the father, the entire family unit, and efforts to deal with infertility and sexually transmitted diseases. This broadened scope eventually reached the point where reproductive health researchers, demographers, social scientists, and public policy makers around the world began exploring how social relationships of families within communities influenced a woman's use of contraceptives. By the 1990s, "family planning" had become a commonly used expression for the complicated issue of choosing, by a woman, a family, and a people, when, if, and even how to have children. *See also* BIRTH CONTROL; CONTRACEPTION; FAMILY SIZE; INTERNATIONAL PLANNED PARENTHOOD FEDERATION

Further reading: Barnett, Barbara. "Family Planning Use Often a Family Decision: Better Ways Are Needed to Involve Relatives, Who May Influence Contraceptive Choices." *Network* 18.4 (1998). Online: http://resevoir.fhi.org/en/fp/fppubs/network/v18-4/nt1843.html, 8 October 1999.

Family Size

Contraceptives allow women and men to choose the number of children they have and control their family size. While research suggests that, given the technical means to make this choice, women and men will do so, other studies suggest that determining the ideal size for a family varies greatly from culture to culture and even within cultures. As demographers, economists, health scientists, environmentalists, and family advocates debate the issues of population growth, family size often becomes a point of conflict and disagreement.

Research shows that in developed countries, people generally want smaller families. These nations tend to be more urban with greater access to jobs for mothers as well as fathers. In cities, children do not contribute to the economic support of the family as they do in rural homes. In developed nations, average desired family size is typically small. In developing countries, people most often live in rural areas where land is important to family status and where children are likely to contribute to the economic support of the family. In rural areas, families have a preference for more children than do families in urban areas.

Cultural issues, such as parents looking ahead to their old age, influence people's decisions concerning the number of children they want. Where parents know they can rely on social programs to help them in their senior years, they are likely to want and have fewer children. Where parents believe they will need to rely on their children, especially sons, to support them, they are likely to want more children. The total fertility rate for a country, or the average of the number of children a woman is likely to have over her reproductive life, can indicate a society's family size preference on a large scale, while not always revealing the cultural reasons for higher fertility among some portions of that society.

Surveys conducted by the World Health Organization and nonprofit population and family planning research organizations, such as the Alan Guttmacher Institute, suggest that in many parts of the world, including developing and developed countries, women actually want fewer children than they conceive. This desire to give birth to fewer children leads to high rates of unwanted pregnancy around the world. In developed countries, estimates in the late 1990s showed that of the 28 million pregnancies that occurred each year, 49 percent were unplanned; 36 percent of all pregnancies in developed nations end in abortion. In the developing countries, 182 million women become pregnant each year. Of those 36 percent are unplanned and 20 percent end in abortion.

World population growth has policymakers around the world concerned with the role of family size in contraceptive use. While some experts argue that improving people's access to affordable contraception will allow couples to have the number of children they say they want, other experts argue that the only way to decrease family size in developing countries is to educate women, who will then see other opportunities for themselves and their children and effectively choose to provide those opportunities more effectively to fewer children than did their parents. *See also* CHILD MORTALITY; FAMILY PLANNING

Further reading: Alan Guttmacher Institute. *Hopes and Realities: Closing the Gap Between Women's Aspirations and Their Reproductive Experiences*. New York: Alan Guttmacher Institute, 1995. Wulfe, Deirdre. *Sharing Responsibility: Women, Society, and Abortion Worldwide*. New York: Alan Guttmacher Institute, 1999.

Fecundity

Fecundity refers to the biological potential of a woman, man, or couple to create a living child. The term is closely related to fertility, but *fecund* relates most specifically to a person's potential and *fertility* relates to the actual children a person conceives and carries through to birth.

In actual use by scientists, scholars, and researchers, even linguists, the terms often become confused and interchanged. Where some publications refer to the fertility of a couple, others refer to fecundity.

When most precisely used within the scientific community, a woman is said to be fecund if she retains the potential to become pregnant, if she has no physical barriers to prevent pregnancy. A woman who has not undergone an operation to cause permanent sterility or who has no known physical condition that inhibits either the transport of eggs or sperm through her reproductive system is considered to be fecund. Age decreases a woman's fecundity with perimenopause, the years that immediately precede menopause, slowing the production of fertile eggs on the woman's ovaries.

Similarly, a man is considered fecund if he has the potential to eject active, potent sperm into a woman's vagina, if he has not undergone a sterilizing procedure, if he has no physical barrier to moving sperm to the outside of his body, and if his body produces an adequately high number of well-formed, highly mobile sperm—according to some studies more than 50 million for each milliliter of semen.

A fertile woman, in contrast, has actually given birth to a living child and a fertile man has actually conceived a child. Fertility, then, proves fecundity but fecundity does not prove fertility.

According the the National Survey of Family Growth, 37 percent or 6.1 million women between the ages of 14 and 49 in the United States in 1995 were not fecund, or did not have the potential to become pregnant. That figure rose slowly from 1982 to 1995, spurred by larger numbers of women of childbearing age and more women choosing to delay childbearing into their later reproductive years, when fecundity and fertility naturally begin to decline. *See also* FERTILITY

Further reading: Chandra, Anjani, and Elizabeth Hervey Stephen. "Impaired Fecundity in the United States: 1982–1995." *Family Planning Perspectives* 30 (1998): 34–42. Thibodeau, Gary A., and Kevin T. Patton. *Anatomy and Physiology*. 4th ed. St. Louis, MO: Mosby, 1999.

Female

Female refers to the basic designation of the members of a species that produce the ovum or egg, a cell containing one half of the genetic material to reproduce that species.

In human biology, female refers to a member of this species for whom most of the reproductive organs, two ovaries, two fallopian tubes, the uterus, and the vagina, are located inside the abdomen.

The word "female" distinguishes these members of the species from males, who provide the sperm, a cell containing the other half of the genetic material needed to reproduce a species. The genetic material in the female egg and male sperm join to begin the process that can lead to a new individual of either sex. A female carries the developing offspring in her uterus during the nine-month gestation period.Because the egg remains within the female's body even after it is fertilized or penetrated by the male's sperm cell, females are said to bear offspring rather than to beget offspring. *See also* MALE; REPRODUCTIVE SYSTEM—FEMALE

Female Genital Mutilation

Female genital mutilation, the cutting or removal of a woman or girl's external sex organs—the clitoris, labia majora and labia minora, and surrounding tissue—for cultural or religious but not medical reasons, dramatically alters a woman's reproductive health as it alters her body.

The procedures are performed most frequently by cultural groups in 28 African countries, but as those people migrate to other parts of the world, they often take the practice with them. Reports of women undergoing such procedures also arise in Middle Eastern and Asian countries, as well as Europe, Australia, Canada, and the United States. Many nations, where the cultural practice still exists, have made all forms of female genital mutilation illegal, including Egypt, Kenya, and Senegal, where medical, governmental, and women's groups struggle to persuade people to abandon the procedure and to protect women's reproductive health.

All forms of female genital mutilation, also known as female circumcision, alter a woman's genitalia. The women or girls undergo the procedure as a protection of their virginity and to limit their enjoyment of sexual pleasure. In cultures where the practice is strong, men often require that the women they agree to marry undergo the cutting, if the cutting has not already been commanded by the father or a dominant male relative, before the marriage takes place. Most often the cutting is performed in homes by traditional "cutters," usually women, who use common objects such as razor blades and knives to remove the woman's organs. Rarely are the surroundings sterilized.

While traditionally women underwent cutting in their teens, more frequently young girls and toddlers have their immature genitalia cut to prevent them from resisting the procedure when they are older. Some families and groups have abandoned or are considering abandoning the practice out of consideration of the health and well-being of their daughters. Others consider abandoning the practice to keep their girls and women from fleeing the towns and village to protect themselves from the cutting.

All forms of genital mutilation cause the woman or girl severe pain during the procedure. Women must pin down and even sit upon an older teenage woman's chest to keep her still while the cutter removes the genitalia and sews up the skin without anesthesia and with nonmedical thread.

In its simplest form, female circumcision involves a small cut in the clitoris or the labia. In involved procedures, the cutter removes: the fold of skin that covers the clitoris and the tip of the clitoris; and the entire clitoris and some surrounding tissue. In its most extreme form, known as infibulation, a woman's clitoris and all surrounding tissue are removed and her vaginal opening is sewn securely shut, leaving a small opening, sometimes no bigger than an eighth-inch for urine and menstrual fluid to flow through. All procedures, even the least destructive, can cause damage to the urethra, located below the clitoris, and lead to urinary incontinence and infection.

During the procedure, women suffer from shock, hemorrhage, retention of urine or painful and slow urination, slow menstruation that can lead to infection from uncleanliness, and infection. Many women die. Lasting effects, however, often cause health problems throughout the woman's life. Infibulation impedes vaginal sexual intercourse, causing pain and sometimes causing someone to need to cut the woman open, usually her husband, with each act of intercourse.

Women who have been sewn shut cannot insert female barrier contraceptives and a condom would increase the pain of intercourse. In many women, the infections and complications that can result from female genital mutilation, even many years after the procedure, can lead to infertility. The procedure and the way in which it is performed also frequently cause psychological damage to the woman that itself damages her sexual life.

More than 130 million living women have undergone some form of genital mutilation, according to World Health Organization estimates. Nearly 2 million girls are likely to undergo the procedure each year. Efforts begun in the 1990s by nations around the world and by international organizations to reduce the incidence of female genital mutilation have had a slow but steady impact on decreasing the procedure world wide. While female genital mutilation is not a religious tradition, many Muslim people practice female circumcision. In a effort to curb its cultural use, many teachers of the Islamic faith have ruled that the practice does not follow the holy teachings of the Prophet

Muhammad. Those teachers have ruled that infibulation is a crime against the faith and that all procedures are dangerous to the person and of no benefit to woman or man. In 1997, the United Nations, and the World Health Organization, working with groups around the world, set a 10-year program to dramatically reduce female genital mutilation and to completely eliminate the practice within three generations. *See also* REPRODUCTIVE RIGHTS

Further reading: Brady, Margaret. "Female Genital Mutilation." *Nursing* 28.9 (1998): 50–51. "Female Genital Mutilation." *Fact Sheets*. April 1997. World Health Organization. Online: http://www.who.int/inf-fs/en/fact153.html, 26 March 2000. Rosenthal, M. Sara. *The Gynecological Sourcebook*. 3rd ed. Los Angeles: Lowell House, 1999.

FemCap. *See* CERVICAL CAP

Feminism

People who support feminism in its broadest sense, the belief that women should have rights equal to those of men, reshaped the discussion of and development of birth control and contraception in the later quarter of the twentieth century. Among the achievements of people arguing and even fighting for such equality was the agreement reached by the world's nations at the International Conference on Population and Development in Cairo, Egypt, in 1995. That agreement focused population issues on the rights of women, and men, to control their reproductive lives, put world attention on health issues that endangered women's lives, and supported efforts to educate women and grant them the social, political, and economic rights that have been granted to men around the world.

Feminism, however, is a many-faceted concept and within the philosophy of equality for women, individuals have taken different stands on issues of birth control and contraception. Women have fought for complete and easy access to all modern contraceptives; they have fought for the development of natural family planning, which is based on a woman's reproductive physiology; they have sought greater equity in scientific experimentation and for the end of using women as test subjects, as some argue women were used in the first marketing of hormonal, oral contraceptives.

Feminist arguments and the struggle for gender equality have also influenced research into future contraceptives where scientists are working to alter the male reproductive system in the hopes of developing products that will allow men to participate more equitably in the planning of families and in the avoidance of unwanted pregnancies. As researchers undertake work on sperm-suppressing agents, other advocates of women's rights encourage the continued research into methods that bring to women fewer side effects than modern hormonal contraceptives in the hopes of increasing a woman's options in controlling and determining her own reproductive life, especially for women around the world who find their partners reluctant to participate in planning pregnancy.

As women in the industrial nations of Europe and North America succeeded in the early 1900s in increasing women's political and economic rights—the right to vote and to own and inherit property—and as concerns with birth control spread around the world, women's advocates began addressing issues of gender bias and rights infringement by organizations that advocated for population control. Some feminists have argued that organizations such as the United Nations Fund for Population Activities and International Planned Parenthood Federation, based in London, have ignored women's rights while emphasized the need to reduce the growth of the world's population. Other feminists have pointed out changes within these organizations in the later half of the twentieth century that place women's sexual and reproductive health and family needs ahead of world population growth needs.

In nations such as Brazil, India, and Bangladesh, feminist advocates have developed programs and policies, as well as organized strikes and civil unrest, to increase women's access to quality reproductive care, including the right to birth control methods and methods for ending unwanted pregnancies. Women's organizations in those countries have had direct political impact on the laws of their nations that relate to family health, women's well being, and the testing by scientists of new reproductive methods. In many nations, such as Japan, where low-dose contraceptives were approved in 1999, though they had been in wide use around the world for nearly 40 years, women have had to struggle for decades against strong cultural forces to gain access to a broad selection of contraceptives. *See also* EDUCATION (OF WOMEN); FERTILITY AWARENESS; MALE CONTRACEPTIVES; REPRODUCTIVE RIGHTS

Further reading: Ginsburg, Faye D., and Rayna Rapp, eds. *Conceiving the New World Order: The Global Politics of Reproduction*. Berkeley: University of California Press, 1995. Jiggins, Janice. *Changing the Boundaries: Women-Centered Perspectives on Population and the Environment*. Washington, DC: Island Press, 1994.

Fertility

Essentially, fertility is the ability to bring together the biological elements needed to create a child. Those elements include the human egg, or ovum, which is carried by a woman on her ovaries, and the human sperm, which is created daily throughout his adult life in a man's testicles.

A woman is said to be fertile if her ovaries contain the necessary eggs and if her body goes through the cycle of hormone production that matures those eggs and sends them through her reproductive system. A man is said to be fertile if his testicles manufacture enough sperm, usually in the millions, and if his reproductive system is capable of moving that sperm out through his penis and into the woman's vagina. A couple is fertile if sexual intercourse can result in the egg and sperm uniting.

While science has explained much of the human reproductive cycle and while much of that knowledge has been used to design highly effective contraceptive devices, the variety of the reproductive cycle from one woman to the next and the variety of circumstances a person encounters throughout her or his life makes determining an individual's fertility at any given time difficult. While ovulation generally occurs in a woman 14 days before the onset of her menstrual period, that timing is an estimate. Men, though their bodies generally make sperm steadily, may experience emotional or physical circumstances that alter their ability to make sperm.

This basic uncertainty over fertility should lead adults to assume that they are fertile and can conceive children whenever they have sexual intercourse. *See also* BIRTH CONTROL; FERTILITY AWARENESS; INTERCOURSE; REPRODUCTIVE SYSTEM—FEMALE; REPRODUCTIVE SYSTEM—MALE

Further reading: Reich, Warren Thomas, ed. "Fertility Control." In *Encyclopedia of Bioethics*. Rev. ed. New York: Simon and Schuster/Macmillan, 1995.

Fertility Awareness

The birth control method of fertility awareness, also known as natural family planning or periodic abstinence, takes advantage of increased scientific understanding of the female reproductive cycle to allow a woman to anticipate the timing of ovulation. By the late 1990s, three methods of fertility awareness showed strong results at preventing pregnancy if couples followed the rules diligently.

The "rhythm" method, the oldest form of natural family planning, became widely regarded as ineffective by scientists and birth control professionals who advised women against using it. However, confusion between that old method of estimating dates and modern methods of relying on physiological signals have limited people's knowledge of the effectiveness and methods of fertility awareness.

Ovulation, the moment an ova or mature egg ruptures from the surface of the ovaries, occurs quite consistently at 14 days before the onset of a woman's menstrual period. The timing from the beginning of her period to ovulation however varies from 7 to 21 days from woman to woman. The length of the portion of the cycle that precedes ovulation can also vary from month to month for one woman, under the influences of exercise, stress, illness, and medication. Several consistent and observable bodily changes in the first stages of her cycle allow a woman to estimate when ovulation may occur.

On average, a woman is fertile from one to three days following ovulation. Hormonal changes before ovulation create corresponding changes in the woman's reproductive organs that allow a man's sperm to survive longer in her cervix, from two to seven days, than it would at other times during her menstrual cycle. These two time spans, the number of days an egg travels through the fallopian tubes and the number of days sperm can survive in a woman's reproductive tract, give a couple an estimate of the woman's average fertile period of from three to 10 days. The length of this fertile period, combined with measurable or noticeable changes, provides the basis of modern natural family planning techniques.

The thermal, or basal body temperature, method of fertility awareness involves a woman recording her temperature each morning immediately after she awakens. Approximately four-fifths of adult women see a noticeable spike in their morning temperature after ovulation has occurred. Increased levels of progesterone, the sex hormone released by the follicle that remains on the ovaries after the egg has left, cause the higher temperature. This increase occurs only after the ova leaves the ovary. The change in body temperature cannot anticipate ovulation; it only occurs after ovulation if it occurs at all. If a woman keeps a temperature chart for several months before beginning to rely on this method as a contraceptive, and if her cycles are regular and she sees a noticeable temperature rise, she may be able to estimate the days she would be fertile.

The Billings, ovulation, or mucosal, method of fertility awareness relies on consistent changes in a woman's cervical mucus to anticipate ovulation. Once an egg begins maturing on an ovary, it produces increasing amounts of the sex hormone estrogen, which alters the thick mucus that blocks the cervix during much of her cycle. As an egg matures, the cervical mucus changes from a dry substance that a woman might not notice, to a watery, slippery substance that resembles egg whites. This change signals to the woman that an egg is preparing to erupt from the ovary. From the day she first notices a change in her mucus to three to four days after ovulation, a woman would avoid sexual intercourse to prevent pregnancy.

Combining the thermal and Billings methods in what is known as the "sympto-thermal method" helps women and men achieve greater protection against an unintended pregnancy. Recording changes in mucus and temperature on the same chart allows a couple to bring more information about the woman's bodily changes into their decision of when to have sexual intercourse.

The calendar method of natural family planning, known most commonly as the "rhythm" method, is the most unreliable method and relies on assumptions about ovulation rather than observed physical features. It involves charting the number of days in a woman's menstrual cycle for several months to determine her shortest and longest cycles. The woman then subtracts 20 days from her shortest cycle to find her first unsafe or fertile day and subtracts 10 days from the length of her longest cycle to find her last unsafe or fertile day. While this method is the oldest known form of fertility awareness and is still a commonly used method, it is also the most ineffective since it relies only on estimates of the woman's cycle. This method used alone fails frequently since the numbers of days in the pre-ovulatory portion of her cycle can change radically and under many circumstances. Clinicians advising people on birth control methods rarely recommend this method be used alone. Methods of fertility awareness do not protect people against sexually transmitted diseases, including HIV.

All methods of fertility awareness require a commitment to the method by both the man and the woman to be effective in preventing pregnancy. Both partners need to be willing to abstain from sexual intercourse during a woman's fertile period, which can range from 1/2 to 2/3 of her monthly cycle.

Estimates of the effectiveness rate for typical use of all fertility awareness techniques vary considerably. If a couple follows the rules by avoiding sexual intercourse during a woman's fertile days, carefully charts the woman's body signals, and combines several methods, the success rate can be as high as 97 percent. However, many couples do not follow those rules and risk having sexual intercourse while not using another form of contraception during the fertile days. Each act of sexual intercourse during a woman's fertile days has as much chance of resulting in pregnancy, 85 percent, as the chance of a couples who are trying to conceive a child. Fertility awareness methods of contraception leave little room for error and couples often find abstinence for a week to two and a half weeks each cycle to be challenging.

Approximately 2.3 percent of American women use a form of fertility awareness as a contraceptive method. That percentage has remained steady since 1988, according to results of the 1995 National Survey of Family Growth. Worldwide, steadily decreasing numbers of people rely on periodic abstinence and other forms of traditional contraception, such as withdrawal and folk methods, to meet their contraceptive needs. Often, however, people turn to natural contraceptive methods when they choose not to use chemicals or devices to prevent pregnancy. Many also cite religious reasons for choosing this method since the policies of the Roman Catholic Church do not approve of the use of modern contraceptive methods. *See also* BASAL BODY TEMPERATURE METHOD; BILLINGS METHOD; OVULATION; ROMAN CATHOLIC CHURCH

Further reading: Stanford, Joseph B., Janis C. Lemaire, and Poppy B. Thurman. "Women's Interest in Natural Family Planning." *Journal of Family Practice* 46 (1998): 65–71. Weschler, Toni. *Taking Charge of Your Fertility: The Definitive Guide to Natural Birth Control and Pregnancy Achievement.* New York: HarperCollins, 1995. Winstein, Merryl. *Your Fertility Signals: Using Them to Achieve or Avoid Pregnancy Naturally.* Saint Louis: Smooth Stone Press, 1994.

Fertilization

Fertilization involves the complex series of steps that follow the contact of a healthy male sperm cell with a healthy female egg cell. This union usually takes place in the woman's fallopian tube. The egg, or ovum, arrives in that tube soon after erupting from its follicle sac on the woman's ovary. The sperm arrives in that tube after being ejected from the male's penis when it is inserted into the woman's vagina, then swimming through her cervix, and uterus.

Though millions of sperm leave the man's penis in one ejaculation, only one will actually penetrate and fertilize the egg. During this process, the 23 chromosomes from each sex cell meet, join, and prepare to begin the process of cell division and cell creation.

Many contraceptives prevent fertilization. Hormonal contraceptives prevent eggs from maturing on and leaving a woman's ovaries. Barrier contraceptives prevent sperm cells from reaching the uterus or the fallopian tubes. Intrauterine devices seem to alter the chemical balance in the woman's reproductive system and change the sperm and egg so that they are incapable of joining.

Many people believe human life begins with fertilization, with the union of those chromosomes. Others believe that human life begins with the implantation of the fertilized ovum in the uterine lining. Debates over the moment at which human life begins surround the ethical and moral issues of contraception and abortion. *See also* BIRTH CONTROL; CONCEPTION; CONTRACEPTION; LIFE (BEGINNING OF)

Further reading: Hatcher, Robert, James Trussel, Felicia Stewart, and others. *Contraceptive Technology*. 16th rev. ed. New York: Irvington, 1994. Winikoff, Beverly. *The Whole Truth about Contraception*. Washington, DC: Joseph Henry Press, 1997.

Food and Drug Administration. *See* U.S. FOOD AND DRUG ADMINISTRATION

France

The decline in fertility noted in modern, industrialized countries in the nineteen century began, according to historians, in France in the mid-eighteenth century. By the beginning of the twenty-first century, the French total fertility rate stood at 1.7, the average number of children to which a French woman would give birth. From the eighteenth century to the present, birth control and family planning has played an important role in the lives of the people of France.

The French government made legal in the mid-1960s the provision, use, importation, manufacture, and marketing of contraceptives. Since then, French women turned quickly to the use of modern contraceptives in planning their families.

By 1998, 69 percent of all women of reproductive age reported using modern contraceptives. Another 7 percent relied upon natural methods, such as fertility awareness and withdrawal, to prevent pregnancy. For those using modern contraceptives, the hormonal contraceptive pill and intrauterine devices provided most women with their contraceptive needs. Use of hormonal pills increased in the mid-1990s as new "mini-pills" and new progestin formulas entered the market. More than 31 percent of women ages 35 to 39 used hormonal pills as of 1994. For women ages 20 to 24 the use of the pill stood at 58.6 percent.

French women turned next to intrauterine devices. With these devices, use patterns show that older women are more likely to accept the insertion procedure and the long-term effectiveness of IUDs. More than 27 percent of women ages 35 to 39 chose IUDs in 1994 where only 2.9 percent of younger women did so.

French men and women rarely undergo surgical sterilization as a birth control method, and again, older women were more likely to choose this method than were younger women in the 1990s. Women are far more likely to undergo the more dangerous and costly female sterilization procedures than are men, at a rate even higher than the 2 to 1 worldwide ratio of tubal sterilization to vasectomy. In 1994, 4.1 percent of women,

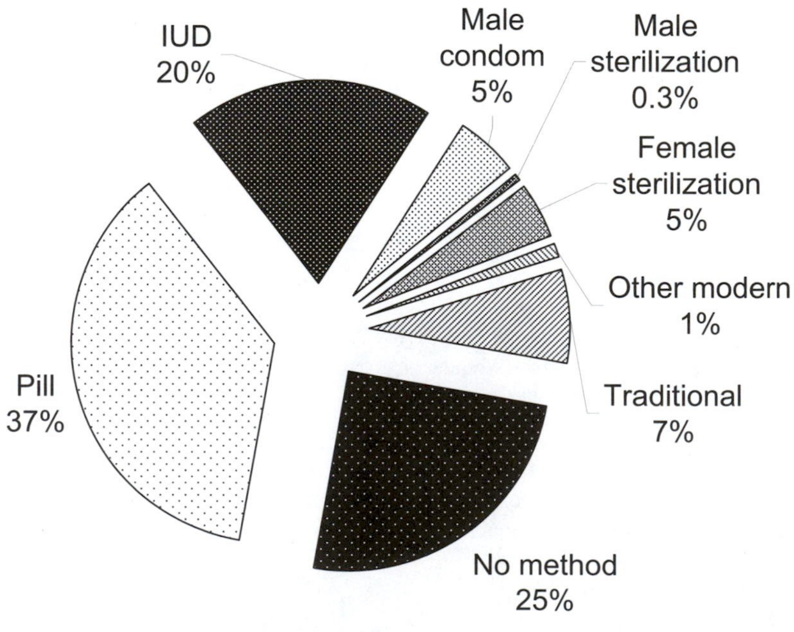

France: 1994 Contraceptive Use by Women Ages 15–49

Source: U.S. Census Bureau, *World Population Profile 1998*

most of them older than 30 years, had undergone surgical contraceptive sterilization. Only 0.2 percent of French men had undergone a vasectomy.

In general, French couples in a cohabiting union seem to see contraception as a joint effort and work together to obtain and use contraceptives. Single men and women also rely heavily on contraceptive pills for protection from unplanned pregnancy. Younger people are turning more often to condoms, though use is still below 10 percent for all age groups. Reproductive health care providers expect condom use in France to rise as the risk from sexually transmitted diseases, particularly acquired immunodeficiency syndrome, increases.

Abortion became legal in France in January 1975 when the government adopted a statute leaving the decision to end a pregnancy in the first trimester to the woman and her physician. This law was part of a lenient attitude toward abortion that spread across most of Europe from the late 1960s to the early 1990s. In France by 1998, approximately 13 women for every 1,000 underwent an abortion.

In 1988, France approved the use of mifepristone, then known as RU-486, for chemical abortions. The drug was developed by French chemists during the 1980s. It blocks the action of progesterone, a natural hormone that supports and continues a pregnancy. Though protests from the Catholic Church and antiabortion groups led the developers, Roussel Uclaf, to announce a month after approval that it would not market the drug, France's minister of health threatened to give the patent rights to another company, citing French women's moral right to the drug, and Roussel Uclaf recanted its decision and made RU-486 available. Since then mifepristone has become readily available in French hospitals and clinics.

Even teens have very easy access to contraceptives in France, and the nation's teen pregnancy rate is very low. With prescriptive contraceptives easily available in pharmacies and condoms available throughout the country, teens, like adults, can easily avoid pregnancy. In fact, a teen girl in France does not need her parents' permission to receive contraceptives. Only in abortion is she limited by the need for parental consent. *See also* MIFEPRISTONE

Further reading: Toulemon, Laurent, and Henri Leridon. "Contraceptive Practices and Trends in France." *Family Planning Perspectives* 30 (1998): 114–120. Walle, Etienne van de, and Helmut V. Muhsam. "Fatal Secrets and the French Fertility Transition." *Population and Development Review* 21 (1995): 261–280.

Future Methods of Contraception

An expanded variety of barriers, hormonal products for men, new biochemical and molecular methods for influencing reproduction, ovulation predictors, and vaccines that treat substances involved in fertilization as invaders fill the agenda of researchers working to develop future methods of controlling fertility, for men as well as women.

Some products, such as the Lea Contraceptive and FemCap, both barrier contraceptives, are in the late stages of development and targeted to reach the U.S. market in the early 2000s. Others, such as vaccines, though researched for more than 25 years, still have not yielded a specific product that can begin the regulatory approval process. Detailed research to understand and manipulate the outer surfaces of both egg and sperm also showed long-range promise of yielding contraceptive techniques that would create long-term reversible sterility. Indeed, researchers, scholars, and futurists speculate that advances in medical and biological technology could find very precise methods for disrupting the reproductive process at the molecular level that would allow people even more effective, convenient contraception with fewer side effects than products currently on the market, some of which have a 99.5 percent or better success rate when used perfectly.

Researchers anticipate the development of a greater variety of contraceptives, chemical abortifacients, and sterilization methods that would give women more choice and allow men to participate more fully in the planning of family size and pregnancy. Such variety would allow people to choose from a wide range of products, long-term methods, or one-use methods; hormonal, chemical, or barrier methods—different family planning methods to meet their needs at particular times in their reproductive lives.

Decreasing the number of side effects and medical risks also drives the study of future methods of contraceptives, since the non-contraceptive aspects of birth control often lead people to reject methods, the menstrual disruption of progestin-only hormonal contraceptives lead women to stop using that method after trying it for a brief time, and nausea and headaches often lead women to discontinue use of contraceptive pills.

Each contraceptive method and work underway on them is discussed below (listed alphabetically).

Abortifacients: While most research is focused on contraceptive development, work is also underway to study and develop forms of chemical abortifacients, such as mifepristone, which was developed in France and received approval for testing and research in the United States in 1996. Moral objections and strong social movements against abortion in many countries, however, have slowed research and development of products for terminating pregnancies, especially those that work after a fertilized egg has implanted in the uterus.

Barrier contraceptives: A nonprescriptive, one-size-fits-all diaphragm, a snugly fitting cervical cap, and a vaginal sponge containing new spermicides are planned to be made easily available in the United States and much of the world by the early 2000s. New varieties of condoms, made of thin synthetic materials, were arriving on the market by the late 1990s with more improvements under development and due on the market by the mid-2000s. Work was underway to add synthetic hormones to vaginal barriers as a way to improve the effectiveness of barriers.

Fertility Awareness: Research is underway to develop two types of products that would assist people using the fertility awareness method of birth control. Kits are being developed to provide the information, tools, and charts a woman needs to monitor the changes her body goes through during her menstrual cycle to determine when ovulation was most likely to have occurred. Scientists also hope to develop in-home tests, much like pregnancy tests, that react to the hormonal changes that occur at ovulation to tell a woman just when ovulation occurred. However, all such methods work after ovulation and because mature sperm can live for several days in a woman's reproductive tract, to be fully effective, such predictors would need to tell women when ovulation was about to occur so that they could know ahead of ovulation when to abstain from sexual intercourse. While kits designed to help people use fertility awareness were arriving on the market by the end of 1999, actual predictors were more of an expectation of the results of further understanding of the biochemistry of reproduction.

Hormonal contraceptives: Progestin-laden vaginal rings and intrauterine devices underwent testing during the 1990s as researchers attempted to develop contraceptives that offered both barrier and hormonal protection against unintended pregnancy. Refinements of long-lasting contraceptive injections and implants also are under development. They included new versions of Norplant that would require fewer rods, biodegradable implants, and injections of microscopic pellets that would slowly release synthetic hormones and then dissolve into the bloodstream, and development of male contraceptives that would interfere with sperm production.

Early testing of transdermal patches, worn like Band-Aids, that slowly release synthetic hormones through the skin, showed promise in preliminary research. Through-the-skin systems of administering chemicals had been tested and were under development in the late 1990s for administering testosterone to men involved in tests of male hormonal contraceptives. Products for women showed promise in early testing during 1999 of meeting the needs of convenience and ease of use and could quickly reach the market.

Development of more emergency contraceptive products, available in much of Europe since the 1980s and approved for specific packaging and marketing in the United States in the late 1990s, that would allow women to take large doses or hormonal contraceptives after having unprotected intercourse also offered promise for expanding contraceptive options.

In more speculative than directed research, scientists continued work on exploring monthly contraceptives, and hormonal and chemical means of bringing on menstruation as a woman's planned form of regularly used birth control.

Spermicides: New compounds that would kill sperm in the vaginal tract would offer women and men a choice less irritating than nonoxynol-9, the leading spermicide of the late twentieth century, which often causes irritation whether used with barrier contraceptives or alone. Many compounds under investigation showed promise at protecting people from sexually transmitted diseases, including the human immunodeficiency virus.

Sterilization: Research involving sterilization methods for women and men focuses on injecting or inserting substances into the fallopian tubes or vas deferens, including plastic plugs and chemicals that would expand and block the tubes without the need for surgery. Scientists are also experimenting with chemicals that would damage the tubes enough to cause scarring. The scar tissue would then block the tubes and prevent eggs or sperm from traveling further into the reproductive tract. Some of these methods could be reversible with simple medical procedures.

Vaccines: Work began in the 1970s in India and the United States to develop methods that encouraged a man or woman's immune system to treat chemical reproductive components like invading organisms. Research targeted gonadotropin-releasing hormone in men and women and human chorionic gonadotropin in women.

Time lines for the development of new contraceptive and fertility control products depends greatly on funding available for the primary research needed to discover biological processes and for the testing needed to develop viable consumer products. Despite rapid progress in the 1960s and early 1970s in the United States, pharmaceutical companies in the 1980s and 1990s gradually decreased their investments in the development of contraceptive products. Faced with public and religious objections and concerns with abortion and birth control, and threats of law suits such as those that removed the Dalkon Shield intrauterine device from the world market in the 1970s and slowed the use of Norplant, the companies responsible for the basic scientific research that leads to new products shifted funds from contraceptive research to more socially accepted, and profitable, products. Without the huge pharmaceutical companies at work, contraceptive research in the late twentieth century shifted to other countries or to university and nonprofit organizations. Until private business returns to the contraceptive market, scholars and public health officials fear that the development of new contraceptives will remain slow and people will continue to have limited access to a relatively small variety of birth control methods that changed little in the last quarter of the twentieth century. *See also* INTRAUTERINE DEVICE; MIFEPRISTONE; PATCH (CONTRACEPTIVE); QUINACRINE; RESEARCH (CONTRACEPTIVE); VAGINAL RING

Further reading: Alexander, Nancy J. "Beyond the Condom: The Future of Male Contraception." *Scientific American Presents: Men,* Summer 1999, 80–84. Harper, Michael J. K. *Birth Control Technologies: Prospects by the Year 2000.* Austin: University of Texas Press, 1983. Mastroianni, Luigi. "Future Contraceptive Methods." *The Contraceptive Report* 5 (1994): 4–12. Population Council. "Contraceptives and Other Reproductive Health Products Under Development by the Population Council." Online: http://www.popcouncil.org/faqs/contia97.html, 15 June 1999.

G

Griswold v. Connecticut

On 5 June 1965, the U.S. Supreme Court ruled in *Griswold v. Connecticut* that married people have the right to privacy within their marriage and that the state of Connecticut, in passing a law prohibiting the use of contraceptives, infringed upon that right. Ruling seven to two, the court overturned Connecticut's law and any others that still made contraceptive use among married people a crime, as did laws in Massachusetts. In its ruling the court was continuing the legal effort to undo state and federal laws written in the late 1800s banning the use and dissemination of contraceptives as obscene and immoral that birth control advocates had been fighting since the early 1900s.

On Thursday, 2 November 1961, Estelle Griswold, executive director of the Planned Parenthood League of Connecticut, with her staff opened a birth control clinic at 79 Trumbull in New Haven, Connecticut. The league had been struggling against Connecticut's restrictive law, sending people who requested contraceptives to New Jersey and Rhode Island, and fighting the issue in court and the state legislature. The clinic, they expected, would provide the state with the opportunity to arrest Griswold and Dr. C. Lee Buxton, a Yale gynecologist and obstetrician who was director of medical services at the clinic. By 2 P.M. the next day, police officers had arrived at the clinic to investigate whether the league was indeed committing a crime. Griswold and Buxton, acting on behalf of the league, were prepared with the evidence the police would need and even arranged for married women to give testimony to the police that they had received contraceptives at the clinic, diaphragms, and the new birth control pills, and had used those contraceptives.

On November 10, Griswold and Buxton were arrested. The legal proceedings that followed included a state trial on 2 January 1962, by a judge who that same day found the two guilty and fined them $100. Lawyers for PPLC filed an appeal to the state appeals court and, as expected, they lost that appeal in April 1964. In September, lawyers submitted an appeal to the U.S. Supreme Court.

The argument in this case focused on married couples and their right to privacy in the use of contraceptives. Planned Parenthood's national policy in the late 1950s and early 1960s stated that no unmarried women would knowingly be accepted as a patient at a Planned Parenthood clinic. The argument for unmarried people would have to wait until the 1970s to be fought and won in the case of *Eisenstadt v. Baird*.

Lawyers for Griswold and Buxton argued that their conviction raised three constitutional questions: whether the Connecticut law deprived Griswold and Buxton of their right to due process, violated their right to free speech, and whether the statute represented

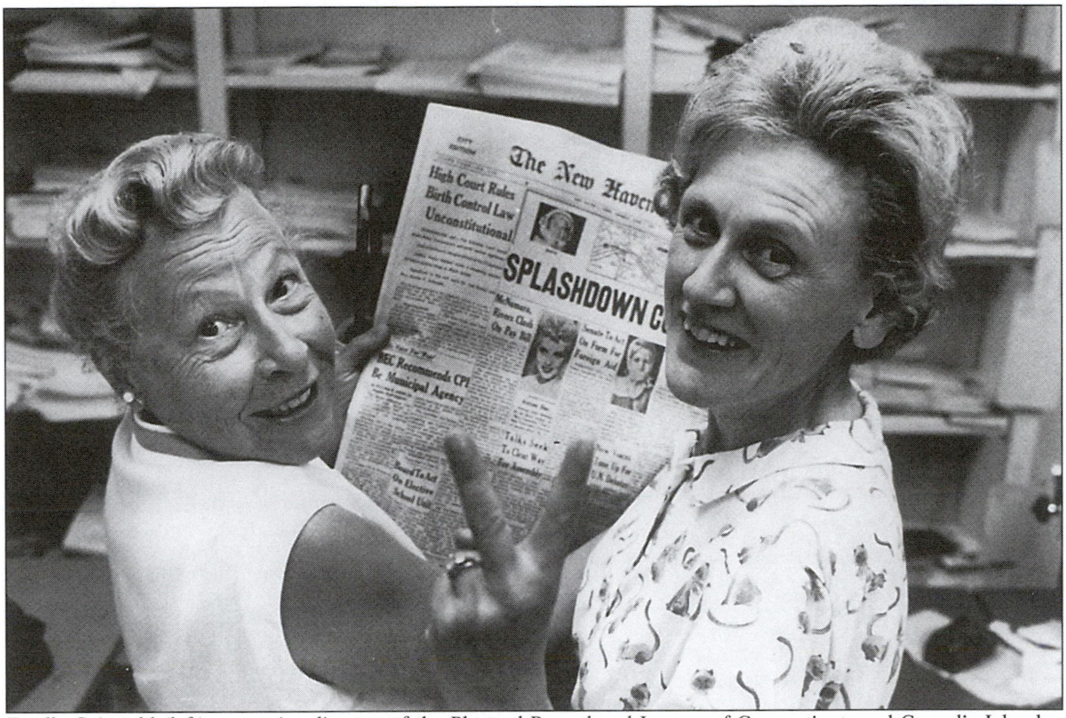
The New Haven
High Court Rules Birth Control Law Unconstitutional
SPLASHDOWN

Estelle Griswold (left), executive director of the Planned Parenthood League of Connecticut, and Cornelia Jahncke, president, celebrate the 1965 Supreme Court ruling. *Bettmann/CORBIS*

an unjustified intrusion by the state into the privacy of married couples. The court accepted the case on 7 December 1964, and heard oral arguments on 29 March 1965. In issuing its decision on 7 June, the majority argued that the right to marital privacy fell within a "penumbra" of the constitution, a hazy area of implied rather than explicit guarantees. That right, however, did exist and the state needed to prove its need to intrude into that privacy and the state of Connecticut's lawyers had not proved that point. Unable to show a compelling interest in depriving married couples of the right to contraceptives, the state lost its case.

On 20 September 1965, the PPLC opened its second clinic and those state legislatures that still prohibited the provision of contraceptives, including Connecticut, began rewriting their laws to allow for the use of contraception within marriage. *See also* *EISENSTADT V. BAIRD*; PRIVACY LAWS; *ROE V. WADE*

Further reading: Garrow, David J. *Liberty and Sexuality: The Right to Privacy and the Making of* Roe v. Wade. New York: MacMillan, 1994. Wawrose, Susan C. Griswold v. Connecticut: *Contraception and the Right of Privacy*. New York: Franklin Watts/Grolier, 1996.

Guttmacher, Alan F. (1898–1974)

Gynecologist Alan F. Guttmacher became a pioneering physician through his support of the American birth control movement and his dedication to working for the right of women to control their fertility. From the time he served as a medical intern in the 1920s to the end of his service as president of the Planned Parenthood Federation of America, a position he held until he died, Guttmacher stood out in his profession as one willing to teach people of the benefits of birth control and contraception.

Guttmacher was born 19 May 1898, in Baltimore, Maryland. He earned his medical degree from Johns Hopkins University (Baltimore) in 1923. In 1927 Guttmacher began a two-year internship and residence program in obstetrics at Johns Hopkins Hospital, then went on to complete a two-year residency at Mount Sinai Hospital in New York City.

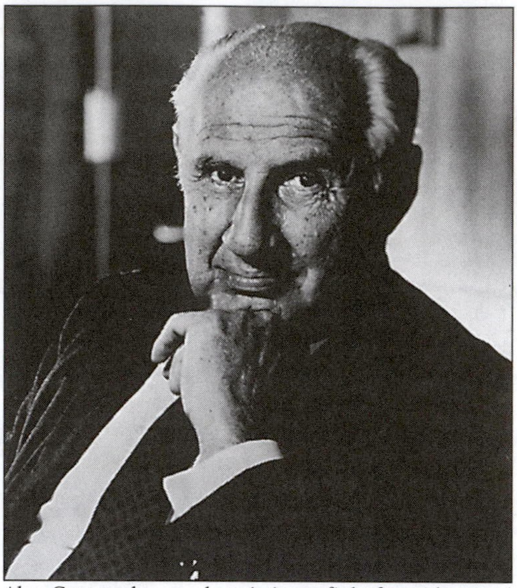

Alan Guttmacher used statistics to fight for widespread access to contraceptives. *Courtesy Alan Guttmacher Institute*

While serving as an instructor at Johns Hopkins School of Medicine from 1929 to 1952, he also maintained a private medical practice in obstetrics and gynecology.

As an intern, Guttmacher witnessed the death of a woman who had undergone a botched abortion. That experience, and his belief that the medical profession existed to serve the needs of people and to help solve the problems of society, shaped Guttmacher's strong belief in the need for birth control. Guttmacher set himself apart from the majority of the medical community when in the early 1930s he began writing, and publishing, publicly popular informational books for women on pregnancy, delivery, and postpartum care. Eventually he would write nine popular books, including *Life in the Making* (1933), *Babies by Choice or Chance* (1959), *Complete Book of Birth Control* (1961), and *Birth Control and Love* (1969).

In addition to providing women with information on sex, pregnancy, and contraception, Guttmacher sought to convince his medical colleagues to accept contraception as an important part of a woman's life and of a medical professional's service to women. In 1947, he conducted a nationwide poll of 15,000 doctors. Guttmacher found that 97.8 percent approved of birth control to protect the health of women and children, 79.4 percent favored birth control for economic reasons, and 86.5 approved of it for child spacing. He often served as liaison between members of the birth control movement and the medical profession at large. In 1947 he received the annual Lasker Award, given by the Albert and Mary Lasker Foundation for distinguished contributions to planned parenthood, for his efforts to build support for birth control by physicians, church leaders, and educators.

Since his days as an intern, Guttmacher had been an active volunteer with the Planned Parenthood affiliates in Baltimore and New York. In 1952, when he became director of obstetrics and gynecology at Mount Sinai Hospital, he began taking on more leadership positions in the national Planned Parenthood organization and eventually became the volunteer chair of Planned Parenthood's National Medical Committee. In 1962 Guttmacher was appointed president of the national organization. In the 1960s, he also became involved in the International Planned Parenthood Federation, serving as chair of its medical committee and traveled to Asia, Africa, and Latin America to support family planning efforts.

Guttmacher encouraged and fought for governmental involvement in providing contraceptive services to women and in the 1950s convinced officials in New York City to end a ban they had placed on municipal hospitals to prevent doctors there from prescribing contraceptives. By 1964, birth control services were available in that city's nine municipal hospitals as well as the 13 volunteer clinics.

Guttmacher witnessed the liberalization of U.S. contraceptive law. As an expert witness, he helped Congress in 1970 rewrite the Comstock Laws, which had hindered birth control efforts since the late 1800s. During his tenure as Planned Parenthood's president, the Supreme Court ruled that the private use of contraception was a constitutionally guaranteed right of married and unmarried Americans.

Guttmacher died 19 May 1974. In his honor that year, the Center for Family Planning Program Development, a division of Planned Parenthood, founded in 1968, was renamed the Alan Guttmacher Institute. In 1977, AGI became an independent not-for-profit corporation and is now one of the world's leading contraceptive research organizations. *See also* ALAN GUTTMACHER INSTITUTE; *EISENSTADT V. BAIRD; GRISWOLD V. CONNECTICUT*; INTERNATIONAL PLANNED PARENTHOOD FEDERATION

Further reading: Garrow, David J. *Liberty and Sexuality: The Right to Privacy and the Making of* Roe v. Wade. New York: Macmillan, 1994. "Guttmacher, Alan F(rank)." *Current Biography: 1965*. New York: H. W. Wilson, 1965. Jaffe, Frederick S. "Alan F. Guttmacher: 1898–1974." *Family Planning Perspectives* 6.1 (1974): 1–2.

Gynecology

While the roots of the word gynecology mean "woman" and "study of," this branch of medical science deals specifically with the non-pregnant aspects of the female reproductive system. Doctors who train in this speciality learn surgical and nonsurgical methods for treating women.

In the United States, gynecologists and gynecological nurses specialize in the care of the reproductive systems of women and this speciality is one of the few to include surgical practices in its training. In other countries, however, including Japan and most of Europe, much gynecological care is provided by licensed midwives.

Much of the scientific information women receive about birth control methods is obtained from their gynecologic physicians, nurses, or midwives or from a clinic staffed by these specialists. In the United States, to obtain many contraceptive devices, women need a prescription from a licensed physician or practitioner. Oral contraceptives and diaphragms and such newer contraceptives as DMPA (depot medroxyprogesterone acetate) that require injections are all made available to women through their medical professionals.

Female tubal sterilization, a surgical process in which a doctor cuts or ties a woman's fallopian tubes, is often done shortly after childbirth by a gynecologist.

Gynecology as a specialty is closely related to obstetrics, the branch of medicine that deals with childbirth and with the care of the mother before and after delivery. In current practice, the two specialties are closely related and a specialist in gynecology will also be a specialist in obstetrics.

Modern advances in the study of hormones and the endocrine system have greatly expanded the significance of this medical specialty in all of its aspects, including contraceptive methods, infertility treatment, and the treatment of the conditions of menopause. *See also* REPRODUCTIVE SYSTEM—FEMALE

Further reading: McGrew, Roderick E. *Encyclopedia of Medical History.* New York: McGraw-Hill, 1985.

H

Hispanic Americans

Hispanic people represent 10 percent of the population of the United States (about 25 million), but accounted for 18 percent of U.S. births by the middle of the 1990s. The diversity of ancestry of that group of people, who share Spanish and Portuguese origins, greatly influences the number of children to which women are likely to give birth in their lifetimes. That diversity also influences the likelihood that Hispanic women will have access to and use birth control methods.

Mexican American women had a total fertility rate of 3.3 children in 1995, while Cuban American women could expect to give birth to 1.7 children, and Puerto Rican women to 2.2 children. The greater total fertility among Mexican American women is influenced by how recently a woman or her family immigrated to the United States, her economic status, her education level, and the ease with which she can obtain information on contraception and family planning services. Hispanic women who give birth to more children are likely to be recent immigrants, living at or near poverty levels, and with little education and little access to reproductive health information and services.

A high rate of immigration to the United States from Mexico accounts for an increasing number of Mexican American women, and the cultural experiences with family size and family planning they bring with them influences their reasons for having children and the number of children they have. A traditional preference for sons among Hispanic cultures and a tradition of male dominance within Hispanic families often leads to Hispanic women giving birth to more children than women from cultures without son preferences and where male dominance is no longer the family norm.

Cuban Americans with their smaller family sizes show the influence of education and the economic transition from the poverty of early immigrants to second- and third-generation families. Increased opportunity and increased educational levels demonstrate the same influence on family size, to decrease it, that is seen among most people living in developed, industrialized nations, with universal access to education. Few immigrants from Cuba arrived in the United States in the late twentieth century. Hispanics of Cuban descent turned more frequently to contraception than Mexican Americans in part because Cuban American women had gained access to careers and social support systems for day care.

Overall, contraceptive use among Hispanics in the United States rose between 1982 and 1995, with most of the increase in use occurring later in that period. In 1995, 59 percent of sexually active Hispanic women between 15 and 44 years old used modern contraceptives. In 1982, that figure was 50.6 percent. Only 5.6 percent of sexually active

Hispanic women did not use contraceptives, a drop of 2.9 percent over 1982.

Most frequently Hispanic women relied upon female surgical sterilization to prevent pregnancy. Thirty-seven percent of Hispanic women of child-bearing age who took measures to prevent pregnancy had undergone a sterilization procedure for that purpose, an increase of 14 percent over 1982. Only 4 percent of the male partners of Hispanic women had undergone vasectomies as of 1995.

Use of contraceptive pills and intrauterine devices, however, decreased substantially within the same time period. In 1995, 23 percent of Hispanic women used contraceptive pills, compared with 30 percent in 1982. IUD use fell even more significantly, from 19 percent in 1982 to only 2 percent in 1995. That trend mirrored the nationwide decrease in use of intrauterine devices among all U.S. women.

More frequently, Hispanic women turned to the male condoms to prevent pregnancy and to protect against sexually transmitted diseases. Use of this method tripled from 1982 to 1995 when 21 percent used condoms, many in conjunction with another birth control method. This use pattern suggested that disease prevention became increasingly important to Hispanic women.

Teen pregnancy rates among Hispanics increased between 1989 and 1995, from 100.8 births for every 1,000 Hispanic teenage girls to 106.7 births in 1995. Most of those teens were married at the time of birth.

Further reading: Abma, J., A. Chandra, W. Mosher, L. Peterson, and L. Piccinino. *Fertility, Family Planning, and Women's Health: New Data from the 1995 National Survey of Family Growth*. Vital and Health Statistics 23, 19. National Center for Health Statistics, 1997. Unger, Jennifer B., and Gregory B. Molina. "Desired Family Size and Son Preference among Hispanic Women of Low Socioeconomic Status." *Family Planning Perspectives* 29 (1997): 284-287.

Hormonal Contraceptives

Artificial hormonal contraceptives mimic the functions of the three main sex hormones, estrogen, progesterone, and testosterone. As pills taken orally, injections, devices implanted under the skin, or as additions to intrauterine devices and new vaginal barriers, synthetic versions of estrogen and progesterone offer women success rates at preventing pregnancy that rival or better the success of permanent sterilization. Testosterone, the primary sex hormone in men, shows promise in intense research for aiding in the development of male hormonal contraceptives.

Early scientific research to isolate estrogens, the group of hormones that stimulate egg production and ovulation in women, and progesterones, hormones that support and maintain a pregnancy and suppress ovulation, relied on animal products, notably mare's urine, to obtain quantities for testing and drug designs. In the 1940s and 1950s, however, biochemists discovered that estrogens and progesterones that occurred in plants could be altered to more closely resemble human estrogens. Production of the first oral contraceptive pill relied on progestin, the term used for synthetic progesterones, manufactured by changing the chemicals distilled from the yam. As the manufacturing process matured, scientists learned to make the hormonal contraceptives through purely synthetic processes.

Following these discoveries came the revolution in birth control that social advocates like Margaret Sanger and Katherine McCormick hoped would provide the ideal contraceptive, a highly effective method of preventing pregnancy that would not need to be used during sexual intercourse and that gave women control over their reproductive process.

Through stages of refinement, the estrogens and progestins used in the first oral contraceptive pill, Enovid, approved by the U.S. Food and Drug Administration in 1960, have evolved into a wide range of synthetic drugs available to researchers, manufacturers, physicians, clinicians, and consumers for the prevention of pregnancy.

The estrogens, primarily ethinyl estradiol and mestranol, keep the level of estrogen in a woman's body at the elevated levels typically found after an egg has been released from an ovary during ovulation. The higher levels of estrogen in a woman's body during the second phase of her menstrual cycle, known as the luteal phase, prevent the pituitary gland from secreting the follicle-stimulating hormone (FSH), which would cause the ovaries to begin the process of maturing several egg cells on the woman's ovary. High estrogen levels also suppress the production of luteinizing hormones (LH), which trigger ovulation. The constant ingestion of the artificial estrogen tricks the woman's body, in a sense, into acting as if it is pregnant. By not allowing the levels of estrogen in the bloodstream to fall to the levels naturally found during the first phase of the menstrual cycle, the follicular phase, the synthetic hormones prevent ovulation.

Though progesterone is one hormone in the human body, unlike estrogen which is actually a class of hormones, more progestins have been manufactured than estrogens. The more common progestins include norethindrone, levonorgestrel, and norgestrel. As with estrogens, keeping the levels of progestins consistently higher than normal prevents pregnancy. The woman's body manufacturers progesterone in the second, postovulatory stage of the menstrual cycle. During this stage, the progesterone suppresses the pituitary gland's production of luteinizing hormone, a chemical required for ovulation and endometrium development. Progesterone also helps maintain the endometrium during the early stages of pregnancy.

Progestins also prevent cervical mucus from thinning and thus help block the path of sperm into the uterus. Research also shows that progestins have an effect on inhibiting sperm as they travel through the woman's body.

A variety of contraceptive products rely on estrogens and progestins for their function. The first and still the most popular form is the daily pill. Most of the more than 50 brands of combined oral contraceptives on the market combine doses of estrogens and progestins. In addition to their contraceptive functions, the two hormones working together reduce the side effects women feel from taking the pills. With a variety of progestins and quantities of estrogen and progestin to choose from, each highly effective at preventing pregnancy, women and their health care providers should be able to find a combination that works well for most women.

Several "mini-pills," which use a progestin alone to achieve their contraceptive effect, have proven extremely successful for women more than 35 years old and women who are unable to take estrogen.

Progestins have also proven to be highly effective contraceptives when used in forms other than pill. The first injectable contraceptive, depot medroxyprogesterone acetate (DMPA), relied upon a synthetic progesterone. The drug is suspended in tiny capsules which dissolve slowly over time, releasing a steady dose of progestin into the woman's body. Each shot gives the woman protection for three months. Progestins also worked well with the materials used in implantable contraceptives such as Norplant, where the hormone needs to secrete through the walls of tiny rods inserted under the woman's skin. A Norplant system of six tiny tubes can provide progestin for five years.

Generally estrogens proved less efficient at moving through the walls of these delivery devices. Research in the 1990s, however, led to the development of two combined injectable contraceptives that could reach world markets early in the twenty-first century.

Progestins, especially levonorgestrel, have been used in designs for intrauterine devices and new products such as vaginal rings. These small circles are designed to fit snugly into a woman's vagina where they will secrete the progestin over time. The woman might need to occasionally remove the ring to allow for menstruation with some models, or only to replace the ring with a new one.

Hormonal contraceptives provide near-perfect contraception when used strictly according to instructions. Pills provide the greatest opportunity for error since a woman must take a pill either every day of the month or for 21 days, followed by a week off, and then resume taking the pills. Manufacturers sell the combined pills either in packages with only three weeks of pills or in packages with three weeks of active pills and one week of inert pills. The difficulty of remembering to take the pill can decrease the effectiveness of hormonal contraceptive pills and cause a disparity between the perfect use rate and the typical use rate of oral contraceptives. Injectables offer less difficulty for women in that they must only remember to go to their clinics for shots every three months, a routine many women find much easier to meet than daily pill taking. Implants and intrauterine devices greatly ease a woman's need to remember to comply with the requirements of the contraceptives, since neither requires regular checkups once the devices are in place.

Overall, combined oral contraceptive pills (COC) provide a perfect use success rate of 99.9 percent; only one woman in every 1,000 would become pregnant during the first year of use. Progestin-only pills (POP) offer a slightly lower success rate of 99.5 percent where five of every 1,000 would become pregnant. However, the typical use for both, since they rely so heavily on a woman's memory to be successful is 95 percent effective, where 1 in 20 women are likely to become pregnant during the first year of use. Using 28-day packs of pills seems to improve the effectiveness of combined contraceptives and progestin-only pills.

Perfect and typical use rates for depot medroxyprogesterone acetate, marketed as Depo-Provera, and Norplant match and reflect the high degree of success of these two contraceptives. For Depo-Provera the success rate is 99.7 percent; three women out of every 1,000 are likely to become pregnant. Norplant, and its-two rod variant, Norplant 2, have the highest success rate of any contraceptive at 99.95 percent. Only five women in every 10,000 are likely to become pregnant with this device under their skin.

Studies show that women who have chosen hormonal contraceptive methods like the protection they receive from unwanted pregnancy. All of them have very high continuation rates after one year of use. Seventy-one percent of pill users continue to use this contraceptive after one year. Eighty-one percent of women using IUDs that contain a progestin continue with the device after the first year and Norplant has a continuation rate of 88 percent. Estimates for the number of women continuing to use Depo-Provera after one year vary, but studies show approximately 70 percent of women continue to use the injectable contraceptive after one year.

Hormonal contraceptives do cause side effects in many women, and not all women are able to use them. Progestins disrupt many women's menstrual periods. About 25 percent of women who use a progestin-only contraceptive find that after a year of use, their periods stop completely. Fifty percent show changes in their monthly patterns, including more days of lighter bleeding. The amount of disruption depends upon the progestin level and the delivery system. Norplant and Depo-Provera have significantly different effects upon the menstrual period; Norplant disrupts menstruation early in its use, whereas Depo-Provera causes less disruption early and more disruption after several years of use. Weight gain, depression, and breast tenderness also may accompany use of progestin-only contraceptives.

The presence of estrogen in combined contraceptives helps regulate menstruation. While estrogen often decreases the flow of menstrual blood, it does not interrupt a woman's hormonal balance to the point of stopping the periods. Nausea, vomiting, and headaches are also common side effects of estrogen.

Women at serious risk from oral contraceptives are regularly counseled not to use this method of pregnancy prevention. While heart disease has often been associated with combined contraceptive pills, research has established that lifestyle plays a greater role in this side effect than do the pills. Women who get little exercise and are overweight, with a high cholesterol ratio, or who smoke, are counseled not to take hormonal contraceptives containing estrogen. Estrogen also causes greater risk for women who have hypertension or a history of heart and vascular disease, are diabetic, or have a family history of diabetes.

Progestin alone seems to present few risks to a woman's health. Early tests showing a connection between DMPA and cancer in test dogs proved not to hold true for humans. Women studied experienced no increase in risk of cancer, heart disease, or bone loss from progestin-only contraceptives. These contraceptives also may decrease a woman's risk of ectopic pregnancy.

Emergency contraceptives also rely on synthetic hormones to prevent unwanted pregnancies. Since the 1970s physicians and clinicians have known that very high doses of combined contraceptives taken within 72 hours of unprotected sexual intercourse have a success rate of preventing pregnancy in more than 75 percent of the cases. While pharmacological companies in Europe began packaging combined oral contraceptives specifically for emergency situations, it was not until 1998 that the U.S. Food and Drug Administration (FDA) approved PREVEN, the first such specifically packaged product in the United States. In 1999, the FDA approved a progestin-only product, Plan B, designed specifically for emergency contraception.

Research in the 1990s also focused on melatonin, a hormone produced by the pineal gland and often studied for its role in sleeping and in controlling biological clocks, for its role in preventing pregnancy. Scientists in the United States and Europe studied the controversial hormone as a contraceptive and devised and tested the product B-Oval as a contraceptive. Combined with a progestin, the melatonin produced seems to shut down a woman's production of estrogen, which in turn prevents the development of mature eggs.

Biochemists have also created compounds that mimic the action of testosterone, which is the main male sex hormone. Research on testosterone enanthate shows that it successfully lowers the sperm rate in men by disrupting the development of sperm, which is highly influenced by testosterone. However, men involved in studies of testosterone enanthate needed months of weekly injections to reach low sperm counts. That delay between beginning the treatment and achieving the goal decreased the effectiveness of the trials as did the need for weekly shots. Research continues into the early twenty-first century on other synthetic testosterones to find a procedure that would allow men the same convenience and success rate that women have experienced using hormonal contraceptives. *See also* COMBINED ORAL CONTRACEPTIVES; ESTROGENS; FUTURE METHODS OF CONTRACEPTION; IMPLANTS; INJECTABLE CONTRACEPTIVES; MALE CONTRACEPTIVES; PROGESTIN-ONLY CONTRACEPTIVES; TESTOSTERONE

Further reading: Bennett, John P. *Chemical Contraception.* Columbia Series in Molecular Biology. New York: Columbia University Press, 1974. Fleeger, Carolyn A., ed. *United States Pharmacopeial Dictionary of United States Adopted Names and International Drug Names: 1996.* Rockville, MD: United States Pharmacopeial Convention, 1995. Guillebaud, John. *The Pill and Other Hormones for Contraception.* 5th ed. Oxford: Oxford University Press, 1997.

Hormones—Sex

The sex hormones of the human endocrine system play central roles in the development and effectiveness of modern contraceptives.

Most research and product development before the 1990s centered on the hormone system of females. Scientists working to improve people's contraceptive choices found it easier to prevent the release of one egg each month in women than they found inhibiting the production of millions of sperm each day in men. However, research efforts in the 1990s have increased in attempts to influence the male hormonal system and alter the production of sperm cells.

The hypothalamus, located near the middle of the brain on the brain stem, and the pituitary gland, located below and in front of the hypothalamus, release very similar hormones in men and women. The hypothalamus sends to the pituitary regular bursts of gonadotropin-releasing hormone (GnRH)—gonads are the primary sex organs, testicles in men, ovaries in women. GnRH signals the pituitary gland to release either follicle-stimulating hormone (FSH) or luteinizing hormone (LH)—in males, LH is also known as interstitial cell-stimulating hormones (ICSH).

In both men and women, the primary sex hormones are manufactured in the gonads. As FSH or LH works in men, it causes the male's body to produce large and steady amounts of testosterone. It also controls and regulates the production of sperm cells. As FSH or LH works in women, it causes the ovaries and the follicle surrounding the egg to produce varying levels of estrogen and progesterone.

The pituitary hormones have very different effects on men and women. In men during puberty, they signal the tissue of the testicles to continue developing and to begin producing sperm cells, the male sex cell. During adulthood, the male hypothalamus releases varying amounts of GnRH depending on the levels of testosterone in the man's blood stream. The two hormones work together to keep blood levels of the primary male sex hormone, testosterone, relatively constant.

In women, the pituitary hormones influence the monthly menstrual cycle. Each month, FSH encourages and supports the development of a number of eggs on her ovaries. LH helps develop the structure that surrounds the maturing egg. However, the levels of both FSH and LH needed to encourage this development of the egg are not adequate to cause ovulation, the eruption of a mature egg from its follicle sac and off of the ovary. Increasing levels of estrogen, the primary female sex hormone, actually prevent the pituitary from responding to signals from the hypothalamus to release the ever-increasing amounts of LH in that organ. As egg growth continues, the ovaries secrete greater amounts of progesterone and this increase finally overcomes the inhibiting effects of the estrogen and stimulates the pituitary to secrete its stored LH in a sudden and dramatic burst. The LH, then helps the mature egg erupt from the ovary.

The male system is constant and steady. The female system is cyclical, and while it varies more than the man's hormonal, reproductive system, it varies in predictable ways. That predictability of the female system, once science had discovered so many of its details, provided scientists and chemists with many opportunities to influence and alter the female sex hormone feedback loop.

As the levels of estrogen and progesterone decrease after an egg has failed to become fertilized, the hypothalamus and the pituitary resume their function and once again release those hormones that signal to ovaries to begin maturing eggs. Scientists discovered that if they mimicked the function of estrogen and progesterone and through daily pills or time-release injections and implants kept the levels of estrogen and progesterone levels high enough to suppress the actions of the pituitary gland, they could prevent eggs from maturing. This mimicry is the basis of modern hormonal contraceptives.

In men, research so far on hormones has also discovered ways in which manufactured hormones can mimic the natural hormones and alter a man's ability to make sperm without altering his sex drive or his secondary sex characteristics. However, the need for weekly shots with most such methods and side effects on cholesterol levels of many of them, a male contraceptive with as much safety, effectiveness, and convenience as the female hormonal contraceptives is still under research and development. *See also* HORMONAL CONTRACEPTIVES; HORMONES—SYNTHETIC; MALE CONTRACEPTIVES; REPRODUCTIVE SYSTEM—FEMALE; REPRODUCTIVE SYSTEM—MALE

Further reading: Carr, Bruce R., and James E. Griffin. "Fertility Control and Its Complications." In *Williams Textbook of Endocrinology,* 9th ed., edited by Jean D. Wilson and others, 901–925. Philadelphia: W. B. Saunders, 1998.

Hormones—Synthetic

Intense scientific research in the 1920s and 1930s into the biochemical processes that influence reproduction led in the 1940s to the discovery that hormones could be synthetically, or artificially, created outside of the human body and that those synthetic hormones could be used to alter the natural processes which hormones control.

Scientists first isolated estrogens and progesterone from the urine of pregnant women and horses in 1929. They isolated testosterone in 1931 from the urine of men. Finding these pure substances and the research on their chemical composition eventually lead to methods for manipulating the atomic structure of the hormones and altering the molecules to create very close alternatives which function like the natural hormones but which can be controlled from outside of the body. First with the isolation of the primary sex hormones and then with the reproduction of those hormones and close relatives of them moved the hormonal control of reproduction from nature to people.

While scientists first used humans and animals as the sources of the materials they needed to extract the hormones and create new forms of them, they found their resources very limited and very expensive. Work in the 1940s turned to the search for plant-produced hormones similar to the human hormones. Russell Marker, a blunt, stubborn biochemist who often pursued his own rather than expected directions in chemical research, believed that a variety of cholesterol, the building block of all steroid hormones, including the sex hormones, could be found in plants. These plant cholesterols could be converted in the laboratory to functional forms of progesterone, the hormone Marker was most interested in producing.

In the jungles of Mexico in 1942, Marker found the Mexican yam, a member of the *dioscorea* family and known in Spanish as *cabeza de negro*. That common root contained high levels of the molecules he needed. In his lab near Mexico City, Marker succeeded in cheaply altering the molecules and creating a synthetic version of pure progesterone.

From Marker's initial discovery science advanced to the stage where, through chemical and physical means such as treating with an acid or heat, scientists could alter a wider source of basic cholesterols to make an even wider variety of variations on the basic structure of nature's sex hormones. They could make versions of progesterone, known as progestins, that resembled the natural hormone but which could be processed outside of the body and used immediately by that body once a person ingested or injected the hormone.

Marker's basic findings also influenced the development of alternative forms of testosterone and estrogens so that by the 1950s, when researchers began working to develop an oral contraceptive pill, they had access to a variety of artificially created versions of the sex hormones they needed to achieve their goals.

Parallel courses of research led in the late 1950s to the development of the first pill to use manufactured sex hormones to alter the female reproductive cycle. A detailed understanding of the hormonal control of reproduction had developed through research in the late nineteenth and early twentieth centuries. By the time biochemists had isolated the three major hormone groups and learned how to manufacture their artificial relatives, physiologists had deciphered much of the relationship of those chemicals to the organs they influenced. Scientists knew that progesterone regulates and supports pregnancy after ovulation, that estrogen levels influence the pituitary gland, which secretes hormones that in turn lead to the development and release of mature eggs from the ovaries. They learned that testosterone, which supports the production of sperm and is manufactured primarily in the testicles, is also under the control of hormones released by the pituitary gland.

The challenge in the 1950s was to develop forms of the hormones that could be taken orally and easily used by the body. While administering progesterone throughout the reproductive cycle does inhibit ovulation, since progesterone is naturally produced by the body only after ovulation, pure progesterone is not effective when taken orally, where it must pass through the digestive process. Scientists needed to discover ways to modify the molecular structure to find a variation on the basic progesterone molecule that would be effective when taken orally. Work by Gregory Pincus and John Rock, the primary researchers on oral contraception in the 1950s, led to the discoveries that in turn developed the first hormonal oral contraceptive, Enovid, which was marketed in the United States in 1960. By the late 1960s, researchers had developed sophisticated yet less expensive means for producing the basic steroids used as the foundation for building the synthetic sex hormones.

Today, all hormonal contraceptives are made of artificial forms of sex hormones. Through many procedures, scientists add and delete atoms from the end chain of the cholesterol molecule and make the several dozen progestins on the market. Similarly, they build or alter the molecules to form the two primary synthetic estrogens—ethinyl estradiol and mestranol. Scientists have also manufactured several artificial forms of testosterone, notably testosterone enanthate and testosterone cypionate which are under investigation for their contraceptive potential.

In the late 1980s, scientists developed "third generation" progestins, synthetic forms of progesterone. Through technological means, chemists manipulate the arrangements of atoms in progestis; these new formulations cause varying reactions in humans. The new progestins have proven highly effective at preventing pregnancy as well as have decreased the incidence of androgenic effects, such as unwanted hair growth and menstrual disturbances caused by earlier progestins.

All of the synthetic hormones are also used for treating non-contraceptive conditions. Progestins can be used to treat pregnant women who are at risk of miscarriage and for anemia. Estrogens are used to treat acne and discomfort and life disruption caused by menopause. Both are used to prevent abnormal menstrual difficulties.

Testosterone is used to help boys who are late in beginning puberty and to treat certain types of breast cancer in women. *See also* COMBINED ORAL CONTRACEPTIVES; HORMONAL CONTRACEPTIVES; HORMONES—SEX

Further reading: Djerassi, Carl. *From the Lab into the World: A Pill for People, Pets, and Bugs*. Washington, DC: American Chemical Society, 1994. Lednicer, Daniel, ed. *Contraception: The Chemical Control of Fertility*. New York: Marcel Dekker, 1969. Nakajima, Steven T. "The New Progestins." *The Western Journal of Medicine* 161 (1994): 163. Oudshoorn, Nelly. *Beyond the Natural Body: An Archeology of Sex Hormones*. London: Routledge, 1994.

Hysterectomy

A hysterectomy, the surgical removal of the uterus, though primarily performed to relieve major medical problems, also leaves a woman permanently sterile. People generally do not see a hysterectomy as contraceptive method. However, if a hysterectomy is otherwise necessary for a woman, she must consider that added aspect of sterility and its impact on her life.

The need for a hysterectomy can result from a septic abortion, which is an abortion that "goes bad" and leads to complications such as infection of the uterus. Septic abortions and the hysterectomies that may be necessary to heal the woman cause serious health and reproductive concerns in countries where abortions are illegal or difficult to obtain. In this regard, hysterectomy and the jeopardizing of a woman's ability to become pregnant if she would hope to have children after an abortion, makes contraception education and availability important medical issues for health care providers in many nations world wide. *See also* ABORTION; STERILIZATION

I

Implantation (of Egg)

Within three to eight days of becoming fertilized in the fallopian tubes, an egg will move into the uterus and toward one wall, where it will sink into and become attached to the inner lining, a process known as implantation.

The complete implantation process takes about seven days and involves the division of cells into embryo and support structures, such as the placenta and amniotic fluid.

An intrauterine device (IUD) is designed to disrupt the implantation process and thus prevent pregnancy. Emergency contraceptives, extra large doses of oral contraceptives, work by preventing fertilization or implantation, depending upon the stage of the woman's menstrual cycle in which they are taken. *See also* CONTRACEPTION; EMERGENCY CONTRACEPTION; INTRAUTERINE DEVICE; REPRODUCTIVE SYSTEM—FEMALE; UTERUS

Implants

In 1966, the Population Council, a nonprofit organization located in New York, began researching the possibility of developing contraceptive implants, methods for releasing hormonal contraceptives over a long period of time directly into a woman's bloodstream. By 1974, the council began testing the first implants. Thin, flexible tubes made of silicon allow the hormones to pass slowly through the implant's walls. Eventually, researchers discovered that levonorgestrel, a synthetic form of progesterone, worked very well at moving out of the tubes and at regulating a woman's menstrual cycle to prevent ovulation. The new delivery system and synthetic hormone could provide contraception for up to five years.

By the early 1980s, Norplant, the first long-acting birth control system designed to be inserted under a woman's skin, was being tested around the world. The drug system is manufactured in Finland, which in 1983 became the first country to give regulatory approval to Norplant. Since then, Norplant has become available in more than 27 countries. The U.S. Food and Drug Administration approved Norplant for use in the United States in 1990.

Research on implants, notably by the Population Council, has continued. A two-rod variation of the Norplant system underwent testing in the late 1990s and was approved for use in the United States in 1996. This system can provide contraception for three years.

The council is also researching a one-rod implant that would be effective for two years and release Nestorone, another synthetic hormone.

Scientists expect that by 2010 researchers will have developed a biodegradable system for dispensing the hormones, one that would dissolve in the woman's arm after it had released all of the contraceptive. Such a system would remove the necessity of a woman returning to the physician's office or clinic for removal of the rods. The system also would be removable should a woman choose to stop its use. *See also* HORMONAL CONTRACEPTIVES; HORMONES—SEX; HORMONES—SYNTHETIC; NORPLANT; PROGESTERONE

Further reading: Alexander, Nancy J. "Future Contraceptives: Vaccines for Men and Women Will Eventually Join New Implants, Better Spermicides and Stronger, Thinner Condoms." *Scientific American* 273.3 (1995): 136–141.

India

India's population reached 1 billion about the year 2000. As of 1999, 16 million babies were born in India each year. Despite a steadily, but slowly, falling birth rate, projections suggest that by 2040, India will surpass China as the country in which the most people live. That size and the momentum of India's growth has created a challenge to the people and government of India, as they work to improve the quality of life for their citizens. With its tremendous variety of cultures, religions, and economic and social status, and the desperate poverty of hundred of millions of people, India struggles to find an effective blend of methods, both social and biological, for slowing its population growth.

By 1999 estimates, India's population was growing at an annual rate between 1.7 and 2.14 percent. Women could be expected to give birth to 3.5 children, a figure that represents the nation's total fertility rate. Efforts to meet a growing demand for contraceptives could decrease that total fertility rate to 2 children, where the population neither grows nor shrinks. If India is successful in that goal by 2006, the nation could reduce that growth rate to the point where its population would stabilize at 1.7 billion people. Failing in that goal, which government and nongovernment agencies have set for themselves, could result in a population of 2 billion people by 2060.

Through volunteer and governmental programs, contraceptive use increased slowly but steadily in India in the last half of the twentieth century. In 1997, 36 percent of married women used modern contraceptives; in 1970, only 13 percent of married women had used contraceptives. Women in India still rely heavily on sterilization to prevent unwanted pregnancies. In 1993, 67 percent of married women using a contraceptive had undergone

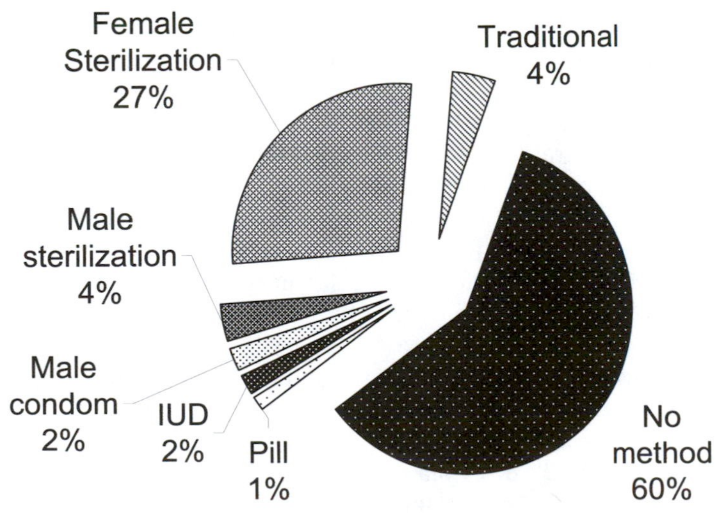

India: Contraceptive Use: 1992–1993

Source: U.S. Census Bureau Internatioal Data Base

a sterilization procedure and 9 percent of their husbands had undergone a vasectomy. While government programs have for decades focused on sterilization, by 2000, government programs changed focus to meet a wider variety of contraceptive needs.

Modern contraceptives that would offer alternatives to sterilization, provided mainly by nongovernmental agencies, have moved more slowly into India. In 1993, only 3 percent of married contracepting women used hormonal pills, 5 percent used intrauterine devices, and 6 percent used condoms. Surveys show that married women who are not using contraceptives prefer to use temporary birth control methods and that demand for alternatives to sterilization is high and increasing. Traditional methods of contraception still account for 5 percent of Indian women between the ages of 15 and 49 who said they used birth control to prevent pregnancy.

Abortion became legal in India in 1971. By the early 1990s, more than 6,900 institutions were approved to terminate pregnancies. Estimates suggest that more than 66 million abortions take place each year, though estimates are difficult since many abortions are performed in private clinics and using traditional methods.

Improved medical conditions in India dramatically increased the life expectancy rate in the twentieth century, and that increase fueled much of India's present growth. In 1947 average life expectancy in India was 32 years. By 1999 that average had risen to 63 years. The infant mortality rate decreased rapidly in India after independence in 1947. Up until then, between 200 and 225 infants out of every 1,000 born died within the first year of life. By 1999, the infant mortality rate had fallen to 73 deaths per every 1,000 births. Birth rates in the early and mid-twentieth century also remained high, with women typically having an average of 5.5 children. Now, India has a very young population with 36 percent of the nation's people under 15 years old. That bulge of children represents the focus of India's efforts to influence family size and population growth.

In 1951 India became the first government in the world to establish a national family planning program. Through a series of five-year plans, government projects worked to achieve target population goals. The total fertility rate in India fell from 5.2 in 1971 to 4.5 in 1981 to 3.3 in 1997. Governmental programs are given some credit for this decline by demographers and family planners, but those rates fell well short of ambitious government projections. For example, government population officials aimed to reduce births from 40 per 1,000 population in 1963 to 25 per 1,000 in 1973. Despite those plans and efforts, the birth rate still hovered in 1981 between 35 and 40 births per 1,000. Overzealous goals, government programs that encouraged fraudulent reporting by census takers, and accusations of regional workers who enticed citizens to undergo sterilization surgery, led to charges of unethical practices and slower than necessary decreases in population growth.

For a brief period in the 1970s India's government shifted away from population policies and worked toward improving economic development to slow population growth. That policy proved ineffective, and by the late 1980s, India officially developed a policy of supporting small family norms and legislating support for birth control efforts. The 1990s and first years of the twenty-first century have brought an emphasis to India's fertility reduction efforts that draws on the social forces of reproductive health, raising the status of women, decreasing poverty, protecting the environment, and educating youth about contraception.

The huge variety in the cultures, economics, and wealth of India's 26 states and 6 territories also tests India's efforts to slow its population growth. Generally, the four northern states are poor, have a higher fertility rate, lower life expectancy, and faster population growth than do the southern and western states. The fertility rate in northern Uttar Pradesh in 1991 was 5.2 children. In southern Kerala the fertility rate in 1991 was 1.8. Much of India's rapid growth takes place in the north where the population rate increase in 1991 was 2.33 percent. In the south, the population only increased at a rate of 1.52 percent. In Kerala, 63 percent of married women report using modern contraceptives, and less than 20 percent of married women in Uttar Pradesh do so.

Many planners believe that India's transition to a much slower population growth rate will only be achieved by improving the status of women in India—where teenage marriages have long been the norm, where boys are valued more than girls because of their socially determined ability to care for their parents in old age, and where half as many women as men learn to read. In most Indian families, women participate very little in decisions concerning finances, selection of a spouse, or most family matters. Only 38 percent of women are literate, compared to 66 percent of men. Female literacy rates have been directly linked to low fertility rates in 16 of India's states. The national average age of marriage for women now is 20 years, though in some states the average is still 16. Encouraging social change that supports an older age for marriage is also seen as a step that will help India reduce its rate of growth.

Surveys show that 59.7 percent of India's women want no more children after they have had two, yet only 41 percent of all couples practice family planning. Estimates suggest that if all couples who wanted to delay or limit their childbearing used modern birth control methods, that percentage would rise rapidly to 60 percent. This gap between desires and actions represents India's unmet need for contraception. Meeting that demand is the goal of private and governmental organizations alike.

India's social activists recognized early in the twentieth century that population growth would present serious problems for the country. In the 1930s, members of the All India Women's Conference, an association of volunteers concerned with improving women's educational and social conditions, were watching their population double, with a growth rate of 10 percent a year. Finding that growth rate alarming, the association took on family planning as one if its goals for social change. In 1935, members invited U.S. birth control activist Margaret Sanger to visit India and share her knowledge and opinions with the women of India. After this, Indian birth control activists began opening clinics and spreading knowledge of contraception.

Efforts to spread birth control knowledge progressed slowly in the pre-Independence years. Jawaharlal Nehru, who became India's first prime minister upon its gaining independence from Great Britain in 1947, recognized population growth as an important concern and expressed an interest in supporting birth control efforts. In 1949, the Family Planning Association of India (FPAI) was formed and became a founding member of the International Planned Parenthood Federation. FPAI now maintains operations in 64 locations, mostly in villages and underprivileged semirural areas and urban slums. *See also* ASIA

Further reading: Adlakha, Arjun. *Population Trends: India*. Washington, DC: U.S. Department of Commerce, Economics, and Statistics Administration, Bureau of the Census, 1997. Chandrasekhar, Sripati. *India's Abortion Experience*. Rev. ed. Philosophy and the Environment 4. Denton: University of North Texas Press, 1994. Visaria, Leela, and Pravin Visaria. "India's Population in Transition." *Population Bulletin* 50.3 (1995): 2–51.

Indonesia

The island country of Indonesia in southeast Asia shared in the economic boom that led to high prosperity and low population growth from the late 1960s to the mid-1990s, but the economic downturn at the end of the 1990s and the social turmoil in Indonesia with the breakup of several governments threatened that nation's highly successful family planning programs.

Indonesia, made up of more than 17,000 islands between the Asian mainland and Australia, is home to more than 207 million people. More than 37 percent of those people live in urban areas, including the capital city of Jakarta on the island of Java. In fact, urbanization in Indonesia is growing at a rate of more than 5 percent every five years. The remaining 63 percent of the population is unevenly distributed over 6,000 of the nation's islands.

As of 1997, Indonesia's population was growing at a rate of 1.5 percent. That rate of growth had been slowing since the 1970s. In the late 1990s, Indonesia's women could expect to give birth to 2.7 children in their lifetimes. That total fertility represents a sharp decrease from the 5.6 children per woman common in the late 1960s. Efforts to improve women's and couple's access to modern contraceptives accounted for most of that fertility decline.

More than 55 percent of the married women in Indonesia used family planning methods as of 1999. Of those women, 52 percent used modern contraceptives. That increase is the result of active government efforts to supply contraceptives to large portions of Indonesia, including hard-to-reach rural areas of the islands. Three modern birth control methods, combined oral contraceptive pills (COCs), intrauterine devices (IUDs), and injectable contraceptives, provide 80 percent of the women who used contraception with protection from unwanted pregnancy. Of all married women in Indonesia as of 1999, 17 percent used COCs, 15 percent used injectable contraceptives, and 10 percent used IUDs. Abortion is illegal in Indonesia; however, estimates suggest that unsafe abortions account for 15 to 30 percent of the deaths of women from pregnancy-related causes.

Voluntary family planning efforts began in Indonesia in 1957 when the Indonesia Planned Parenthood Association began providing information and advice to the nation's women. The organization currently maintains eight self-sustaining clinics in the islands.

The Indonesian government began its family planning program in 1968, one of the first countries in southeast Asia to take official action to influence population. Ease of access to modern contraceptives receives credit from most experts as the main reason for Indonesia's sharp fertility decline. Economic and political unrest in the late 1990s, however, threatened the success of family planning efforts. The Asian economic crisis of 1997 and 1998 led to a national depression that sharply raised prices, including contraceptive prices. Price hikes in 1998 led the Indonesia Family Planning Association to cut back severely on orders of the injectable drug Depo-Provera as prices continued to rise.

Reproductive rights activists and family planning associations worried that price alone would cause many women to stop using contraceptives, which would lead to new increase in the level of unwanted pregnancies in Indonesia and turn the annual growth rate up from its constant downward trend. They also worried that the economic decline and the rising cost of contraceptives could results in higher rates of unwanted pregnancies and would drive higher the illegal abortion rate and maternal death rates. Demographers and population analysts, however, expect fertility and population growth to continue to decrease into the twenty-first century if political and economic unrest does not weaken the convenient access to contraception that the government has helped create. *See also* ASIA

Further reading: Bureau of the Census. *Population Trends: Indonesia*. Washington, DC: U.S. Department of Commerce, Economics and Statistics Administration, Bureau of the Census, 1992. "Indonesia 1994: Results from the Demographic and Health Survey." *Studies in Family Planning* 27 (1996): 119–123. Jones, Gavin W. *Urbanization in Large Developing Countries: China, Indonesia, Brazil, and India*. New York: Oxford, 1998.

Infanticide

Infanticide was once a much-used method for limiting family size. The putting to death of a newborn child with the consent of the parents, family, or society, infanticide was permitted in ancient societies and was used as recently as the late nineteenth century to influence population size.

By the late 1800s, societies began passing laws to protect newborn children from infanticide. With the rise of modern contraceptives and with the legalization of abortion in many countries, infanticide as a form of population control faded from social acceptability and is seen now as a form of murder. Today, experts believe that the number of newborns killed by parents each year is largely underestimated and that societies still have a misunderstanding of the social and psychological forces that lead parents to kill their newborn children.

In the United States in 1991, approximately nine out of 100,000 newborn infants were killed by their parents. That figure is likely to be an underestimate since infanticide is often hidden and remains undiscovered. In Hungary, for example, official estimates suggest that 25 to 30 babies die each year from infanticide. In March 1999, Hungary raised its penalty from a maximum of two years in prison to a mandatory prison term of two to eight years for infanticide.

Psychologists and anthropologists argue that people, especially women, who murder newborns have much different motives and personality traits than women who murder older children. Woman who kill newborns, psychologists point out, deal with social and psychological pressures to deny sexual urges, deny disobedience of social norms, and doubt their ability to conceive and bear a child. The term "neonaticide" has entered popular and scholarly discussions of the crime of taking the life of a newborn child and criminal scholars have recommended changes in laws to reflect the differings motives between killing a newborn and killing an older child.

Further reading: Adshead, Gwen. "A Transient Frenzy?" *British Medical Journal* 317 (1998): 356. Hausfater, Glenn, and Sarah Blaffer Hrdy, eds. *Infanticide: Comparative and Evolutionary Perspectives*. New York: Aldine, 1984. Oberman, Michelle. "Mothers Who Kill: Coming to Terms with Modern American Infanticide." *American Criminal Law Review* 34 (1996): 1–110. Wissow, Lawrence S. "Infanticide." *The New England Journal of Medicine* 339 (1998): 1239–1241.

Infertility

Infertility is the inability of a couple to conceive a child. That inability may be a matter of choice (through contraception or sterilization) or of biological circumstances.

Several types of contraception chosen by couples or individuals effectively make them infertile. Hormonal contraceptives such as the oral contraceptive pill and Depo-Provera, which are based on manufactured versions of the hormones produced in the human body, in effect, make a person infertile and thus prevent couples from conceiving children. Voluntary sterilization through vasectomy and tubal ligation also cause, by choice, infertility.

In addition, sexually active couples who have not been using birth control devices and who have not conceived a child within one year of trying are considered medically infertile and often seek medical assistance in conceiving children. Infertility has become a growing problem for women who postpone having children until their 30s, a time when their bodies begin producing fewer healthy mature eggs. Men, too, often face fertility problems related to physiological and emotional conditions, such as disease and stress, that influence their ability to produce adequate numbers of sperm to fertilize an egg. Increases in developed countries of infertile couples led to a surge in the 1980s and 1990s in scientific ways to overcome infertility and in medical professionals who treat people with infertility problems.

As the opposite of fertility, demographers and population analysts study infertility rates, the rates at which people do not reproduce. These numbers show historical and modern trends in a society's ability to reproduce and the willingness of its people to reproduce. *See also* FERTILITY

Informed Consent. *See* ETHICS

Injectable Contraceptives

Worldwide, injectable contraceptives, made of the same forms of synthetic hormones as contraceptive pills, are growing in availability and acceptability. More than 12 million women around the world use this form of contraception, and researchers expect that number to increase rapidly as more people learn about and request injectables as their method of receiving contraceptives.

Depot medroxyprogesterone acetate (DMPA), known as Depo-Provera, is the oldest and most widely used injectable contraceptive. It is injected deep into the muscle of a woman's arm or buttock. More than 100 countries have approved and regulated the use of DMPA, a progestin that imitates the function of the natural hormone, progesterone. DMPA is effective for three months.

Another progestin-only injectable contraceptive, norethindrone enanthate (NET EN), which is sold as Noristerat, is effective for two months. As progestins, these two contraceptives work by preventing ovulation and the development of mature eggs on the woman's ovaries and by maintaining throughout her cycle the thick, dry mucus that blocks a woman's cervix when she is not ovulating.

Progestin-only injectable contraceptives have very low failure rates of between 0.1 to 0.6 percent (the percentage of women expected to become pregnant within the first year of using this method). Combined injectable contraceptives have similar low failure rates at 0.2 to 0.4 percent, during the first year of use.

In the 1980s, pharmaceutical companies developed injectable contraceptives that combine synthetic progestins with synthetic estrogens. Cyclofem (known in the United States as Cyclo-Provera) and Mesigyna have both been tested by the World Health Organization and are gaining acceptance around the world. Both require monthly injections to maintain a contraceptive level of the hormones. In clinical studies, many women found that the need for monthly shots made combined injectable contraceptives less appealing than the longer-lasting progestin-only shots. Research continues, and Pharmacia (the company formed by the merger of Pharmacia, Upjohn, and Monsanto), manufacturers of Cyclofem, awaits U.S. Food and Drug Administration approval after submitting a revised application in 1999 and renaming the device "Lunelle."

Several other monthly combination injectable contraceptives have been developed around the world, including Injectable No. 1, developed in China, though they are not readily available outside of their regions or countries of development. *See also* DEPO-PROVERA; HORMONAL CONTRACEPTIVES; PROGESTERONE

Further reading: Lande, R. E. "New Era for Injectables." *Population Reports.* Series K, no. 5. Baltimore: Johns Hopkins School of Public Health, Population Information Program, August 1995. Online: http://www.jhuccp.org/pr/k5edsum.stm, March 2000.

Insurance Coverage (for Contraceptives)

In the United States, women spend 68 percent more of their own money on health care costs than do men. Most of this imbalance results from women purchasing the contraceptives they need to prevent pregnancy. In the 1990s, when the impotency drug Viagra reached the U.S. market, people began fighting the insurance system, arguing that if insurance companies could help men pay for their ability to perform sexually, insurance should be able to help pay for women to prevent pregnancy.

In Canada and Western Europe, universal health care covers the cost of government-approved contraceptives in its provision of basic health care for the citizens of those countries. In the United States, a variety of insurance programs and government programs help people afford the rising cost of health care. The more traditional private insurance plans, known as indemnity plans, which are provided as part of an employee's benefits, offer far less coverage of contraceptives than they do of other medicines and medical devices including childbirth and abortion.

Half of all traditional fee-for-service insurance plans in the United States do not cover the contraceptives approved by the U.S. Food and Drug Administration (FDA). Only 15 percent of those insurance plans cover all approved types of contraception: contraceptive pills, intrauterine devices, prescriptive barriers, and hormonal implants and injectable contraceptives. Health maintenance organizations (HMOs) offer women the most comprehensive coverage of contraceptives. Only 7 percent of these health care providers offer no financial coverage of contraceptives.

Of the 93 percent that do offer contraceptive coverage, however, only 39 percent offer all of the FDA approved contraceptive methods. The lack of insurance support for contraceptives can be a major financial barrier to a woman's access to contraceptives. Cost can lead women to choose not to use contraceptives, especially women who live just above the poverty level and who do not qualify for government benefits programs.

In contrast, when a woman becomes pregnant, even if that pregnancy was unintended, insurance companies and HMOs in the United States cover nearly all of the costs for prenatal care and child birth. Sixty-six percent of private insurance companies and 70 percent of HMOs cover the costs of induced abortions.

Nationwide polls show that 78 percent of U.S. adults would support coverage of contraceptives even if their financial contributions to the plan increased. Eighty-eight percent of reproductive age women support expanding insurance coverage to include contraceptives and 86 percent of men support such plans. According to the cost reports of insurance companies that do cover contraceptives, that additional charge, for the contraceptives only, would be $21.40 per employee each year (in 1998 dollars). Most plans cover 80 percent of the cost of a prescription, with the employee paying 20 percent. An insurance company's costs would increase by $17.12 and the employee's cost would be $4.28. Now, most women and families pay the entire cost of the contraceptives they use. A four-week cycle of 28 contraceptive pills cost approximately $25 in 1998.

Members of the U.S. Congress introduced legislation in 1998 and 1999 to require insurance companies to begin offering policy holders help with affording contraceptives just as they help people afford other prescriptive medicines. As Congress pursued this issue, state legislatures sent forth and passed similar bills. In 1998, Maryland became the first state to pass a law requiring employers to provide full coverage of contraceptives. By the middle of 1999, 10 states had passed such laws. Only three states allowed no exceptions to this coverage; seven states allowed businesses to chose an exemption if such a policy violated religious beliefs of the organization. Proponents of religious exemptions note that not all employees will hold those religious beliefs and that those employees should not be deprived of the insurance help in affording contraception.

Experts expect the number of unplanned pregnancies to decrease significantly once insurance companies broaden their coverage of contraceptives. *See also* ACCESS (TO CONTRACEPTIVES); COSTS (OF BIRTH CONTROL)

Further reading: Dailard, Cynthia. "U.S. Policy Can Reduce Cost Barriers to Contraception." *Issues in Brief*. New York: Alan Guttmacher Institute, 1999. Online: http://www.agi-usa.org/pubs/ib_0799.html, 6 October 1999. Darroch, Jacqueline E. *Cost to Employer Health Plans of Covering Contraceptives*. New York: Alan Guttmacher Institute, 1998. Online: http://www.agi-usa.org/pubs/kaiser_0698.html, 8 October 1999.

Intercourse

The physical insertion of a man's penis into a woman's vagina during sexual arousal and stimulation is the most common meaning of the term "intercourse" when used in casual discussions of reproduction. Known scientifically as coitus, and also referred to as sexual intercourse, this physical joining provides the means for human reproduction. The desire for the physical stimulation of intercourse without the risk of conceiving children gives rise to people's need for birth control.

When a man and a woman become sexually aroused during what is often called "lovemaking," their bodies undergo physical changes that lead to increased physical and emotional pleasure. Should the drive for sexual pleasure lead to intercourse, the man's erect penis will enter the woman's vagina. The climax of this intense physical process, where muscles tense, blood pressure rises, and nerves become greatly sensitive, results in the man's body shooting sperm-filled semen into the woman's body. The sperm, the male sex cell, travels through the woman's reproductive tract where it may meet a mature egg, the female sex cell. Should intercourse result in a sperm penetrating an egg, fertilization occurs and pregnancy may follow.

The complicated emotional state of sexual arousal often leads people to forget the risks from pregnancy and sexually transmitted diseases connected to acts of intercourse. If a sexually active couple does not take measures to prevent a sperm cell from fertilizing an egg, that act of sexual intercourse has the potential to result in pregnancy. A healthy man is always fertile. He makes sperm daily, constantly; mature sperm leave the body of a healthy man with each ejaculation. A woman is fertile only during the few days after a mature egg has been ejected from one of her ovaries. Because a woman's menstrual schedule is never absolutely predictable, she is always at risk of pregnancy when she engages in sexual intercourse.

All birth control methods reduce the likelihood of the sperm reaching the egg or of a fertilized egg implanting in the wall of the woman's prepared uterus. Abstinence from intercourse is the only absolute way for a woman to assure that she does not become pregnant or for a man to assure that he does not impregnate a woman.

Sterilization of a man or a woman results in a minute chance of pregnancy resulting from intercourse. Hormonal contraceptives, if used properly, result in levels of protection close to those of sterility by altering a person's hormones. While testing is underway on male hormonal contraceptives, those on the market as of the late 1990s were based on female hormones and used by women exclusively. Barrier methods of birth control prevent ejaculated sperm from traveling through the woman's cervix. Spermicides inserted into the vagina kill the sperm.

Intense emotions also cause many couples to have difficulty remembering to use birth control methods, even if they do not wish to risk pregnancy. Barrier methods of birth control are intercourse- or coitus-related since they must be inserted or applied with each act of intercourse. These methods can require interrupting intercourse to be used, or they require a person anticipate when he or she is likely to enter a sexually stimulating situation. This interruption of intercourse often leads people to not use their chosen contraceptive method in order to increase spontaneity during intercourse and thus increase physical and emotional pleasure. Hormonal contraceptives work continuously in a woman's body and protect her from pregnancy at all times. This allows couples to maintain spontaneity in their sexual encounters but a woman, and perhaps soon a man, must remember to take the pills or receive the required shots to keep the hormones in these contraceptives at their functional levels in the blood.

Fertility awareness methods of birth control, also commonly known as natural family planning or the "rhythm" method, require that a couple have no sexual intercourse during the woman's peak fertile period which is at and for several days after she ovulates.

The spontaneity associated with intercourse and the need for planning birth control can cause conflicts. Intercourse is highly emotional and sudden. Decisions about birth control often require a long, careful decision-making process and much time spent learning and discussing options, with partners, medical professionals, and friends. Recognizing the risks of intercourse at all times will help women and men act upon their planned decisions when their emotions heighten during intercourse. *See also* BARRIER CONTRACEPTIVES; FERTILITY AWARENESS; FERTILIZATION; HORMONAL CONTRACEPTIVES; REPRODUCTIVE SYSTEM—FEMALE; REPRODUCTIVE SYSTEM—MALE; SPERMICIDES

Further reading: Hatcher, Robert, James Trussel, Felicia Stewart, and others. *Contraceptive Technology*. 16th rev. ed. New York: Irvington, 1994. Winikoff, Beverly, and Suzanne Wymelenberg. *The Whole Truth about Contraception*. Washington, DC: Joseph Henry Press, 1997.

International Planned Parenthood Federation

The International Planned Parenthood Federation, formed in 1952, today represents the world's largest volunteer family planning organization. With members and affiliates in 180 countries, IPPF relies on a global network of volunteers to bring knowledge and support for family planning services to people from the largest to the smallest countries in the world.

Each of the autonomous family planning association members sets its own goals and objectives based upon the culture and government of the country or region in which it operates. The local goals fall within the major challenges the international association sees as important for providing reproductive health care. Those international challenges include the need to meet the demand for quality family planning services, to promote sexual and reproductive health, to eliminate unsafe abortions, to empower women, to help adolescents understand their sexuality and to help them meet their own reproductive health needs, and to provide the highest possible standard of reproductive health care.

In 1952, following an international conference in Bombay, India, members of family planning organizations from countries already active in helping people prevent unwanted pregnancies agreed to come together and work as an international organization. Germany, Great Britain, Hong Kong, India, the Netherlands, Singapore, Sweden, and the United States joined together and formed IPPF. As global understanding and international spending on family planning grew over the decades, IPPF grew. In the 1990s, IPPF chapters formed in Russia, Romania, and South Africa.

In the 1990s, IPPF revised its charter to incorporate family planning into the broad range of human rights, including reproductive rights, developed by the United Nations in a series of international conferences, including the International Conference on Population and Development held in Cairo, Egypt, in 1994. Those rights, now incorporated into IPPF's charter, include a person's right to life, liberty, security, equality, privacy, access to information and education, and to decide whether or not to marry and have a family and whether or not to have children. It also includes the right to health care and protection of health.

It the early days of IPPF and the organizations that came to join it, family planning volunteers struggled to bring knowledge and methods for preventing pregnancy to poor women who had little or no access to such knowledge. Influenced by the growing birth control movements in Europe and the United States in the late 1800s and early 1900s, nations facing poverty and hardship as a result of burgeoning population, increasing birth rates, and decreasing death rates turned to founders of the international birth control movement, such as Margaret Sanger from the United States and Elise Ottesen-Jensen from Sweden, for moral and financial support. From those beginnings to help poor women around the world, IPPF worked to help and teach all people about family planning: how to have the number of children they wished in order to improve their lives and the lives of their children.

International Planned Parenthood Federation focuses its attention on preventing unwanted pregnancies and providing contraceptives to the people who want and need them. It also works to eliminate unsafe abortions. Advocates of contraception rather than abortion, the IPPF nonetheless supports a woman's right to choose an abortion. It supports efforts to legalize abortions as its members work to decrease the number of women who risk illegal abortion each year, estimated in 1999 at 20 million women. Less than one half of one percent of IPPF's annual budget funds abortion activities.

The federation works with the United Nations, serving as a consultant to that international assembly, to share concerns and actions to improve reproductive health for all people. It shares information and resources with the United Nations Fund for Population Activities, the United Nation's International Children's Emergency Fund, the World Health Organization, and the World Bank.

Funding from IPPF comes from grants from more than 20 countries, from private foundations, and from individuals. The individual family planning associations also raise funds to support their programs.

IPPF maintains a site on the World Wide Web that contains reproductive and population information on 160 nations and details the work of the members associations. *See also* PLANNED PARENTHOOD FEDERATION OF AMERICA

Further reading: Huston, Perdita. *Motherhood by Choice: Pioneers in Women's Health and Family Planning*. New York: The Feminist Press at the City University of New York, 1992. International Planned Parenthood Federation Web site: http://www.ippf.org.

Intrauterine Device

A small flexible object inserted high into the uterus, an intrauterine device (IUD) gives a woman protection against pregnancy that rivals if not surpasses the effectiveness of sterilization. Made of plastic and containing synthetic hormones or copper, modern intrauterine devices provide thorough contraception that requires little attention from the woman once it is in place.

Worldwide, approximately 100 million women use intrauterine devices to prevent pregnancy; more than half of those women are in China. In the United States, however, fewer than 1 million women use IUDs. Researchers attribute this low use to difficulties with the Dalkon Shield IUD which in the 1970s was found to contribute to toxic shock syndrome and to lack of awareness by medical professionals of the safety of new IUDs. In the mid-1970s, 10 percent of contracepting women in the United States used IUDs.

While five forms of IUDs are available outside the United States, only two, the Copper T 380 (ParaGard Cu-T 380A by Ortho-McNeil Pharmaceutical) and the Progesterone T, (Progestasert by Alza Corporation) have been approved for use by the U.S. Food and Drug Administration. Recent medical research into the safety of IUDs and education of medical professionals and women in the safety and methods of inserting IUDs may increase their use.

The first modern IUDs were developed in the 1930s in Germany and Japan; however, high incidence of pelvic inflammatory disease and other complications discouraged women and doctors from using them. In the 1950s, research sponsored by the Population Council led to new developments in IUD safety and design and thus to a high level of worldwide use of the devices.

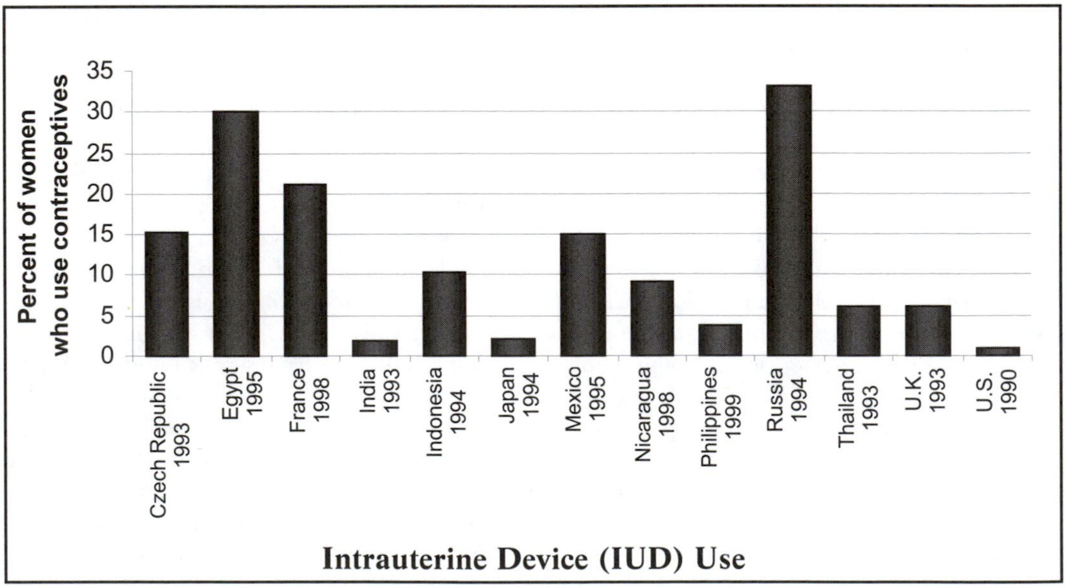

Source: U.S. Census Bureau International Data Base

IUDs are small and T-shaped; the horizontal bar fits into the wide top of the uterus. The vertical bar extends down through the uterus, though when properly placed it should not touch or extrude from the cervix. All IUDs have strings, commonly called tails, that attach to the bottom of the T and travel out the cervix and well into the vagina. A woman would be able to feel that string when the IUD is properly in place and learns to check for it after each menstrual period to make certain the flow of blood has not washed the IUD out of the uterus. Generally, with proper insertion, expulsion is not a problem; expulsion occurs most frequently in the first three months of use. Some IUDs used worldwide are unmedicated, such as the Lippes Loop, and rely on the physical presence of a foreign substance in the uterus to create their effect. The Copper T 380 uses copper as an agent to prevent conception and the Progesterone T-releasing IUD and Levonorgestrel IUD (available in Finland) use artificial hormones to add to their action and effectiveness.

Recently, scientists studying the IUD's function have shown that the device does far more than cause an irritation to the uterus, as any foreign body would, and does not merely cause a fertilized egg to fail to implant. Chemicals in the uterus, such as white blood cells that try to fight off the device and copper from the Copper T, flow to the fallopian tubes where they likely destroy eggs before they are fertilized. These same chemicals act much like spermicides and cause similar harm to the sperm cells as they enter the uterus and fallopian tubes. Studies of women who use IUDs have found very few fertilized or unfertilized ova or viable sperm in the women's fallopian tubes as compared with women who were using no contraceptives.

IUDs have very high success rates. As a group, their effectiveness ranges from 0.1 percent to 3 percent of the women using IUDs becoming pregnant in the first year of use. The Levonorgestrel IUD, which is not available in the United States, offers the lowest failure rates, where typical use and perfect use match at 0.1 percent. With typical use of the Copper T 380 IUD 0.8 percent of women become pregnant and with perfect use 0.6 percent become pregnant. Most pregnancies that occur among IUD users result from the device being expelled. On those rare occasions when the device does fail, ectopic pregnancies, or pregnancies where the zygote implants in the fallopian tube, may occur and require prompt medical attention.

The greatest advantage of the IUD is that once inserted, it requires little of the woman's attention, thus increasing the effectiveness of the devices and increasing user satisfaction. The Copper T 380 may remain in place up to 10 years according to the FDA's latest recommendations. The Progesterone T must be changed each year. Women who have used IUDs report high satisfaction with the device and many choose the device several times during their reproductive years. In the United States, 98 percent of the women who use IUDs are very happy with this birth control method and 60 percent have chosen the device more than once during their fertile years.

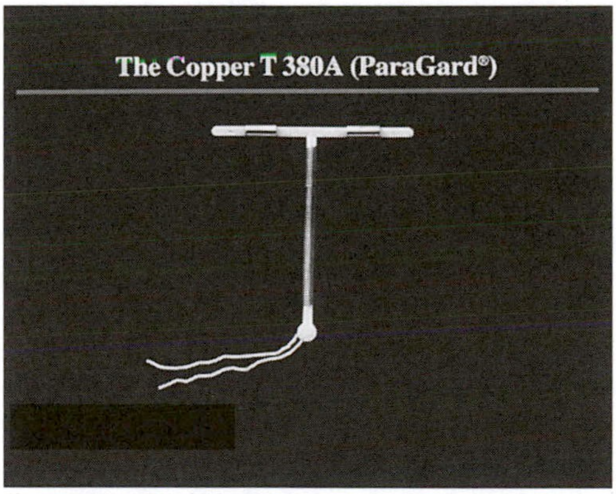

The quarter-sized plastic and copper IUD works in the uterus. *Ortho Pharmaceutical Corporation*

A woman must have a prescription to buy an IUD and a trained medical professional must insert the IUD. Insertion presents the greatest risk to IUD users, for during this procedure an untrained person or a person working too quickly could puncture the uterine muscle or fail to fully insert the device. Thorough training and slow, careful work allow the medical practitioner to feel the inside of the uterus and insure accurate placement. While a high incidence of pelvic inflammatory disease (PID) has long been associated with IUD use, recent studies have shown that a woman's greatest risk of this disease, as related to an IUD, comes at the time she first has it inserted. Studies by the World Health Organization in the mid-1990s revealed that women who have PIDs, such as vaginitis, or a history of PID, could still be successful candidates for using IUDs if their medical histories are carefully evaluated. Specialists often recommend that a woman receive antibiotics shortly before insertion to reduce the risk of infection. The "tail" of the IUD has also been blamed for causing pelvic inflammatory disease, but studies show that the tail is not a contributing factor.

Research has also verified that women who are at high risk from sexually transmitted diseases because they have several sexual partners are also at risk from pelvic inflammatory disease if they use an IUD.

Women best suited for using IUDs have had one or more children, have one steady sexual partner, and are not at risk for sexually transmitted diseases. Older women who have had children experience less trouble with expelling the IUD than do younger women.

Research is underway on new IUDs, such as a device that hangs six copper sleeves from a single thread that is anchored into the top of the uterus. Work is also underway to develop an IUD using norgestrel, a synthetic hormone that resembles progesterone, that could remain in place for three to five years.

Studies into the safety of IUDs, training of gynecologists in medical schools, and a large variety of types to choose from could make IUDs a very popular contraceptive choice for women in the U.S. as they have been in France, China, and much of the world. *See also* DALKON SHIELD; EFFECTIVENESS (OF CONTRACEPTIVES); HORMONES—SYNTHETIC

Further reading: Faundes, Anibal. "Opinion: Women Deserve Accurate Information." *Network* 16, 2 (1996). Grimes, David A., et al., eds. *Modern Contraception: Updates from The Contraception Report.* Totowa, NJ: Emron, 1997. Mishell, Daniel R., and Patricia J. Sulak. "The IUD: Dispelling the Myths and Assessing the Potential." *Dialogues in Contraception* 2nd series 2 (1997): 1–4.

Ireland

For the people of Ireland, a large island nation in northern Europe, family planning, fertility rates, and abortion remain controversial issues. In both the Republic of Ireland, an independent country that makes up most of this island, and Northern Ireland, which is part of the United Kingdom with nearby Great Britain, people's attitudes toward contraception, birth control, and abortion are changing, yet people are faced with issues of

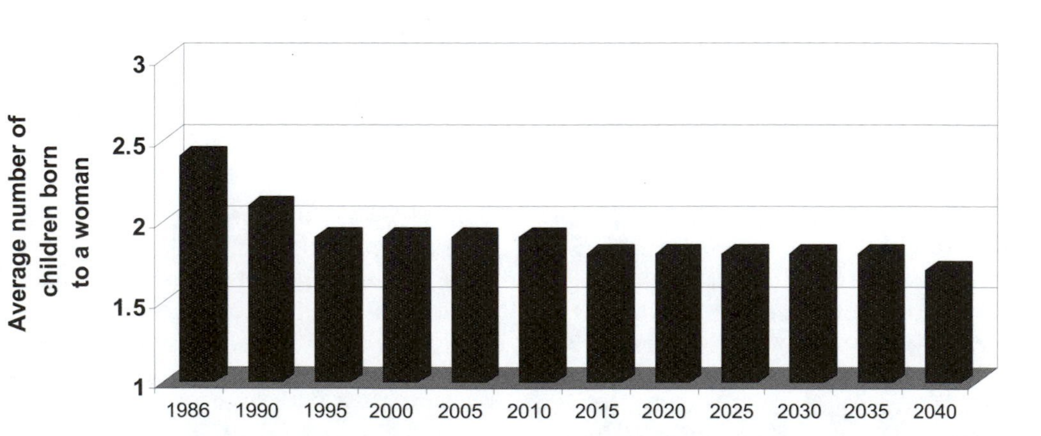

Ireland: Total Fertility Rate: Actual and Projected

Source: U.S. Census Bureau

access to contraception and abortion on a regular basis. Highly influenced by their religions—Catholics are in the majority at approximately 75 percent in the Republic, but Protestant and Catholic populations are nearly balanced in Northern Ireland—people often take stands on issues in support of the teachings of their religions.

Part of the developed world and the European Union, Ireland's total fertility rate of 1.9 was the highest of the EU member countries in 1997, though that was down from 3.96 in 1965. In religiously divided Northern Ireland, where Catholics and Protestants for decades have fought over the fate of that province, the question of which religion people belonged to and how many children those people were bearing has for several generations been a controversial issue.

Abortion remains illegal in most circumstances throughout Ireland. When Great Britain legalized abortion in 1968, ministers from Northern Ireland agreed not to oppose the law for the right to exempt that province from its requirements. Court cases have since made abortion legal in the case of protecting the woman's health or in the case of rape, but the law varies between the two governments. In 1998, more than 6,000 Irish women, from north and south, traveled to Great Britain to undergo abortions.

Public opinion in Ireland increasingly favors changes in the abortion laws. Opinion polls in Northern Ireland show that 79 percent of the people favor passing laws that make abortion legal to protect the physical and mental health of pregnant women, 72 percent in case of rape or incest, and 59 percent in case of fetal malformation. Women are increasingly willing to tell friends and family of their plans to have an abortion before leaving for England. In 1995, half of the women who left Ireland for an abortion told someone of the trip. In 1999, two-thirds of the women told someone of the trip.

Even access to contraception showed a different history between the two portions of Ireland. Northern Ireland gained access to birth control methods as Great Britain updated its laws in the 1950s and 1960s. Women in the Republic had to wait until 1980 for the official removal of the criminal charges they would face if they imported contraceptives and for birth control methods to become available in their country. In 1971, the famous "contraceptive train" returned to Dublin from Belfast, filled with more than 50 women who'd traveled north to buy contraceptives, mostly condoms. In 1973, an Irish Supreme Court case made legal importing contraceptives for personal use but not for sale or distribution to other people. Several years of high court rulings broke down the laws prohibiting the importation, manufacture, sale, and advertising of contraceptives and in 1979 parliament passed that country's first family planning legislation, the Health Act of 1979.

Modern contraceptives became legal in the Republic of Ireland but the law gave preferential status to fertility awareness methods of family planning, which are still important to Irish Catholics in limiting the sizes of their families. Overall, the use of modern contraceptives has risen steadily in both parts of Ireland. Gynecologists and family practice physicians regularly prescribe contraceptives to married and unmarried women. In Northern Ireland, all contraceptives, including condoms, are available at no cost in pharmacies through a national health care program, though most require a prescription from a doctor. Social efforts to make all contraceptives more readily available are also ongoing in both parts of the island.

Despite the official opposition of the Catholic Church to all artificial forms of contraception, almost all doctors in both parts of the country commonly prescribe contraceptives, and Catholic couples, especially women, frequently seek out their doctor's help in finding information and obtaining their method of choice. *See also* EUROPE; ROMAN CATHOLIC CHURCH

Further reading: Francome, Colin. "Attitudes of General Practitioners in Northern Ireland Toward Abortion and Family Planning." *Family Planning Perspectives* 29 (1997): 234–236. O'Grada, Cormac, and Brendan Walsh. "Fertility and Population in Ireland, North and South." *Population Studies* 49 (1995): 259–279. O'Higgins,

Kathleen. "Family Planning Services in Ireland with Particular Reference to Minors." In *The Adolescent Dilemma: International Perspectives on the Family Planning Rights of Minors,* edited by Hyman Rodman and Jan Trost. New York: Praeger, 1986.

Islam

Islam, a religion with more than 1 billion followers worldwide, stands divided on the acceptability of an individual using any means to prevent conception. That division stems from how the religious leaders and people of the Islamic faith understand and interpret the holy works of Islam, including the Qur'an, that faith's holy book, which was revealed by God to the Prophet Muhammad in the early seventh century. Muslims often disagree in their interpretations of both the writings of the prophet, the founder of the Islamic faith, and the writings of religious jurists who have studied the holy works of Islam since Muhammad died in A.D. 632.

Islam has no central hierarchy governing the church. Unlike Catholicism, which has a pope as the earthly leader and divine authority of that faith and below him an organization of lesser church authorities, Islam has no organized clergy and no central authoritative body to interpret church doctrines and laws. That decentralization in the centuries since Muhammad established the faith has led to each member of Islam being allowed to read and understand the holy works individually. Learned scholars, known as jurists, have, however, worked to interpret and understand the holy works and to pronounce rulings, known as *fatwas*, which are opinions of law delivered to individuals.

One school of modern Islam scholars, the reformists, argues that the Qur'an itself does not place a prohibition upon family planning, nor does it forbid parents from spacing pregnancies for physical, economic, or cultural reasons. Nor does the text prohibit withdrawal of the penis from a wife's vagina immediately before ejaculation, known as *al-azl*. Jurists in this school draw evidence from the writings of the prophet and early jurists approving of the use of withdrawal to prevent pregnancy and extend that evidence to include modern contraceptives. If withdrawal was allowed to maintain the health of the woman, to allow for the economic and social health of the family, then modern contraceptives that prevent the sperm from uniting with the egg are also permitted under the teachings of Islam.

The other school of scholars, the traditionalists, opposes this interpretation. They argue that the Qur'an points out that God will plant his seeds where he will and that humans cannot know God's will. In addition, the Qur'an specifically prohibits the killing of children in at least four separate sayings. This ban on infanticide extends to any act, traditionalists state, including withdrawal, that prevents pregnancy. Killing the seed, they argue, is the same as killing the child. All modern contraceptives interfere with pregnancy and would therefore fall into this category. It follows from that reasoning that any device or process that disrupts a pregnancy after fertilization, including abortion, is not permitted in Islamic law.

Reformists argue that the ban on infanticide refers only to children who have been born alive and to a fetus after the "seventh stage of creation," or 120 days after conception. They argue that withdrawal cannot be infanticide since no human being could have been created in the process and by extension they argue that modern contraceptives that work as withdrawal cannot be infanticide. Muslim teaching, according to this school of interpretation, gives reluctant approval to abortion within the first four months of pregnancy but only for valid reasons, such as a mother's inability to breastfeed a child.

According to Islamic belief, Muslims need to be open to God's will, to put their faith in Allah, and be open to the life that he sends them. Traditionalists argue that this openness must lead to accepting the possibility of pregnancy with each act of sexual intercourse. Since the early days of Islam, however, jurists have permitted the use of withdrawal to influence the outcome of intercourse to prevent a variety of problems in a person's life, arguing that the Qur'an and the prophet both describe Islam as a religion of ease and not a religion of hardship.

Marriage is strongly encouraged in the Muslim faith. Both schools agree that having children is the purpose of marriage. Though they disagree on a role that pregnancy prevention can play within that marriage, they agree that a couple cannot permanently prevent the possibility of having a child. Surgical sterilization, for either the woman or man, except for extreme reasons, is not permitted.

The two schools are also divided over the role of sexual intercourse in the lives of a husband and wife. The reformists argue that pleasure and companionship and the strengthening of the marriage is as important an outcome of sexual intercourse as are children. In fact, they argue that strengthening a marriage relationship is valuable enough reason for husband and wife to engage in sexual intercourse. The traditionalists counter that children are the only reason to engage in intercourse.

Religious leaders from many Islamic nations have issued *fatwas* in favor of family planning since the early 1990s and the development of modern contraception. They stipulate that a husband and wife, in mutual agreement, or, if necessary, without the consent of the other, may choose to block the path of sperm for economic, health, and social reasons. Family planning allows people to listen to the will of Allah in exercising prudent judgment when deciding to bring children into the world. The teachings of Islam, these leaders argue, are open to interpretation as the needs of a society and a people change over time.

Islam, as scholars point out, is as much a social system as it is a religion. How the social system of Islam expresses itself in the many governments around the world that are formed around the religion depends on a wide variety of factors other than religious interpretation of the teachings of the church. Muslims live in more than 80 countries around the world; some of them, such as Iran and Tunisia, use the religion of Islam as the central principal of the government. How these governments and the people in power choose to interpret the teachings of the Qur'an, the Prophet Muhammad, and the jurists depends on the nature of the faith among the leaders and the people living in the country. A wide variety of interpretations have influenced governments and many dominantly Muslim nations, such as Indonesia, have developed strong and influential family planning programs that rely on modern contraceptives to help their citizens plan their families. *See also* EGYPT

Further reading: Musallam, B. F. *Sex and Society in Islam: Birth Control Before the Nineteenth Century*. Cambridge, England: Cambridge University Press, 1983. Obermeyer, Carla Makhlouf. "Religious Doctrine, State Ideology, and Reproductive Options in Islam." In *Power and Decision: The Social Control of Reproduction,* edited by Gita Sen and Rachel C. Snow. Boston: Harvard University Press, 1994. Omran, Abdel Rahim. *Family Planning in the Legacy of Islam*. London: Routledge, 1992.

Israel

The citizens of Israel, a young country on the eastern shores of the Mediterranean Sea, display a wide spectrum of attitudes toward contraception and birth control, reflecting the waves of immigrants that have come to the dominantly Jewish nation since it was established in 1948, its status as a more developed nation, and the religious beliefs of its citizens.

Jews from around the world began immigrating to Israel from its formation and continued well into the 1990s with many people arriving during that decade from the states of the former Soviet Union. This immigration accounts for much of the 1.5 percent annual population growth in that nation. Israel's birth rate is high in comparison with the developed nations of Western Europe. In 1998, an Israeli woman could expect to give birth to an average of 2.9 children in her life. The total fertility rate of Israel's Jewish citizens, 82 percent of the population, was 2.6 children for every woman, while the total fertility rate for Moslems and Druze was 4.6 children. Christian citizens averaged just less than 2 children for every woman. In contrast,

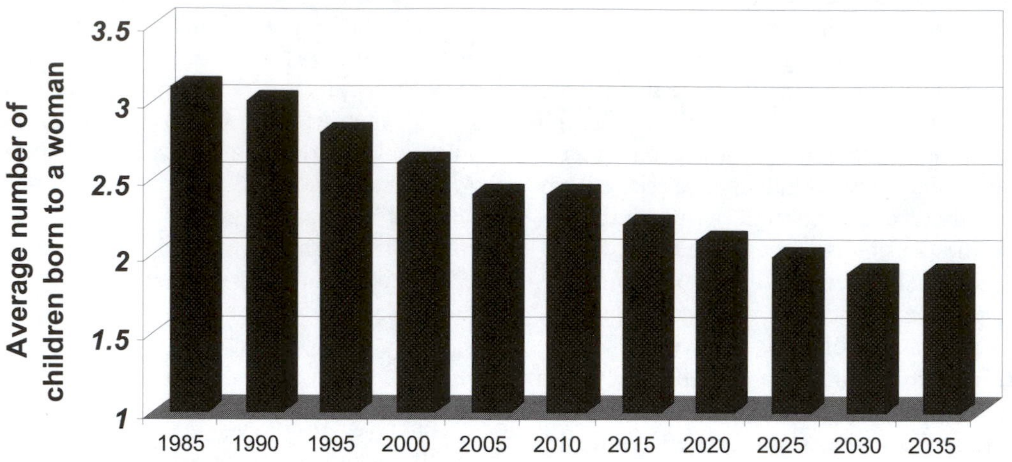

Israel: Total Fertility Rate: Actual and Projected

Source: U.S. Census Bureau

total fertility rates in Europe ranged from 1.2 in Italy to 1.9 in Ireland.

Increasingly, Israel's people were using modern contraceptives by the end of the twentieth century. Analysts expect that with that increased use the nation's growth rate and total fertility will begin to slowly decrease in the early twenty-first century. However, many forces are at work on the population growth and people's use of contraception in Israel. Countering the effect of increased contraceptive use is the fact that 40 percent of Israel's people are younger than 15 years old. As those children move into their reproductive years, fertility rates and population could increase if those children turn to the traditional Jewish law to be fruitful and multiply. Increasing economic development in Israel, on the other hand, may lead to greater participation in the work force and fewer children in each family. Confusing the predictions, Israel's government and the society's perspective on conflict in the region see larger families as a way to insure Israel's future as a nation.

As more Jews immigrate to Israel, they bring with them diverse cultural attitudes toward family and procreation. As these immigrants adjust to life in their new homes, they begin to modify those attitudes, adjusting family size and contraceptive use to meet the expectations of their new homes. As opportunities present themselves and as needs shift, they often turn acceptingly and insistently to birth control to help them meet professional and family goals. The more than 500,000 immigrants who arrived from the former Soviet Union in the early 1990s, for example, brought with them preferences for early marriage, and early and low levels of child bearing. They also brought a preference for using intrauterine devices and abortion to limit the number of children in their families. Both practices remain common in Russia and the newly independent states of Eastern Europe. These immigrants, especially the younger adults, soon adapted their contraceptive choices to include in rapidly rising numbers the use of contraceptive pills, which were not as easily obtained in Russia, but were easily available in Israel.

More than 68 percent of married women in Israel use modern contraceptives. That figure is close to the average for the more developed countries. Intrauterine devices still dominate the contraceptive use patterns in Israel as they have since the late 1970s, but more women are turning to the contraceptive pill as well. The use of withdrawal of the man's penis just before ejaculation has had a long history of use as a family planning method in Israel, particularly among immigrants from southern and eastern Europe, despite its condemnation by traditional Jewish religious law. Reliance upon this old and natural form of birth control, however, was fading as modern contraceptives became more available and accepted.

Sterilization is little used in Israel. Abortion is legal in Israel when needed to protect the health of the woman and in the cases of rape, incest, and fetal impairment. Approximately 18 of every 1,000 women in Israel have an abortion each year for a national total of more than 18,000 each year. In 1999, Israel's health ministry licensed the use of mifepristone, a chemical abortifacient.

Younger women in Israel, including those from recent immigrant groups, turn quickly to modern contraceptives to help them plan families as increasing opportunities open for them in Israel's growing economic sector. *See also* JUDAISM

Further reading: Okun, Barbara S. "Family Planning in the Jewish Population of Israel: Correlates of Withdrawal Use." *Studies in Family Planning* 28 (1997): 215–227. Remennick, Larissa I., Delila Amir, Yuval Elimelech, and Yliya Novikov. "Family Planning Practices and Attitudes Among Former Soviet New Immigrant Women in Israel." *Social Science and Medicine* 41 (1995): 569–577.

J

Jacobs, Aletta (1854–1929)

Dutch physician and feminist, Aletta Jacobs in 1882 opened Europe's first clinic to publicly provide birth control to women. This twice-weekly clinic in Amsterdam became the model for the clinics opened in the United States by Margaret Sanger in 1916 and Marie Stopes in London in 1921.

Jacobs, the daughter of a physician, was born 9 February 1854, in Sappemeer, the Netherlands. She entered the University of Groningen at 17 and became the first woman in Holland to attend university classes. She later entered medical school in Amsterdam and in 1879 became the first woman physician in Holland.

Driven by a belief that women deserved equal access to education and deserved the same social rights as men, Jacobs refused to conform to society's expectations of female behavior and was often seen walking unescorted through the streets of Amsterdam. In her studies and her career, Jacobs met many women whose health had suffered from too many pregnancies, women who could not afford to raise the large numbers of children they were bearing, and prostitutes who suffered from society's unwillingness to acknowledge their existence. This exposure to the hardships many women faced led Jacobs to devote her medical career to women. That medical work, in turn, led to her intense involvement in the international women's movements of the late nineteenth century.

Within two years of opening her medical practice in 1879, Jacobs began openly dispensing birth control devices to women. Then, in 1882, after having learned about the new "Mensinga pessary," an early form of a diaphragm, a barrier contraceptive which covers the cervix during intercourse, Jacobs dedicated two days each week to a small clinic. The "Dutch cap," as this diaphragm became known, was the same device Sanger and Stopes would provide in their controversial clinics.

Jacobs operated the clinic for 12 years. It became the model for a network of clinics in her country that remained popular with the public despite reluctance by many people, including women doctors, to disseminate and discuss birth control in public. In 1894, Jacobs ended her clinic work and her medical practice and began devoting her energies to fighting for women's rights. She remained active in fighting for women's reproductive rights, especially access to contraception, as she broadened her fight for women's suffrage and her involvement in the women's peace movement.

Jacobs believed strongly, however, that doctors should provide contraception and refused to meet with Sanger, a nurse by training, who traveled to the Netherlands in 1915 to study that country's efforts at providing birth control. Jacobs did, however, in 1925 in New York, attend an international conference on birth control organized primarily by Sanger.

Jacobs died 10 August 1929, at Baarn, the Netherlands, after helping win suffrage for Dutch women in 1919, and having seen birth control clinics spread across her country and her country become a source of knowledge for birth control activism around the world. *See also* SANGER, MARGARET HIGGINS; STOPES, MARIE C.

Further reading: "Aletta Henriette Jacobs." In *Notable Women in the Life Sciences,* edited by Benjamin F. Shearer and Barbara S. Shearer. Westport, CT: Greenwood Press, 1996. Freidenreich, Harriet Pass. "Aletta Jacobs in Historical Perspective." Afterward to *Memories: My Life as an International Leader in Health, Suffrage, and Peace,* by Aletta Jacobs. Trans. Annie Wright. New York: The Feminist Press at the City University of New York, 1996. Jacobs, Aletta. *Memories: My Life as an International Leader in Health, Suffrage, and Peace*. Trans. Annie Wright. New York: The Feminist Press at the City University of New York, 1996.

Japan

Despite figures that suggest that Japan matches the family planning use and trends of other industrialized nations, women in Japan have limited access to modern birth control methods, and Japan has a much different history in its acceptance of use of contraceptives than do other developed nations.

Before the summer of 1999, the male condom was the only modern contraceptive available in Japan and it had maintained that unique role for decades. Japan's Ministry of Health repeatedly through the 1970s, 1980s, and 1990s did not approve modern hormonal contraceptives and other female-controlled hormonal contraceptives. The nation had a highly developed market for condoms and that market, experts point out, kept other methods out of Japan. Women, then, needed to rely on a man's willingness to use a condom in order to achieve any success at preventing unwanted pregnancies.

Female barriers such as the diaphragm and cervical cap never gained acceptance by Japanese women, who shied away from visits to male gynecologists who needed to fit this birth control method. With few other options, Japanese women turned to abortion to prevent giving birth to more than the two children that had become the social and cultural norm

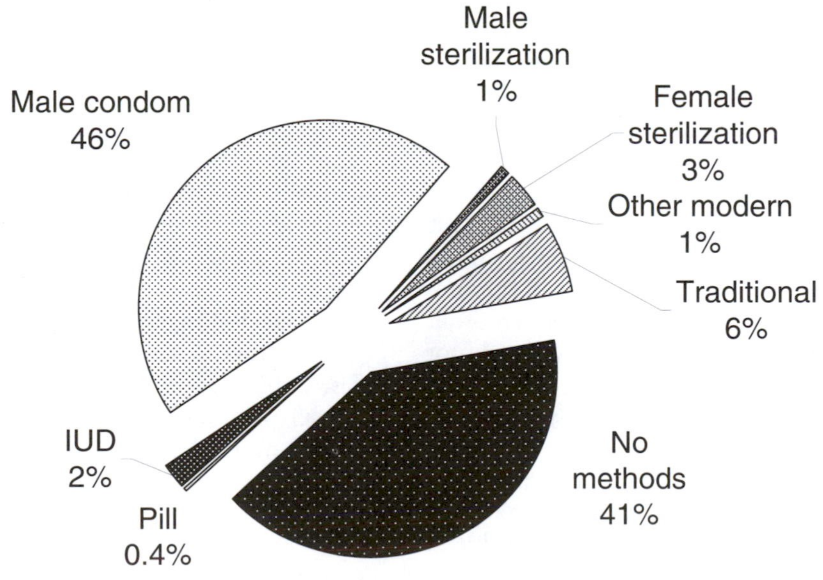

Japan: 1994 Contraceptive Use by Women Ages 15–49

Source: U.S. Census Bureau International Data Base

as Japanese total fertility rate decreased through the twentieth century.

Abortion, though technically illegal in Japan except to save the woman's life and protect her health, as well as for social and economic reasons, provided women a convenient option to giving birth to too many children. By 1999 Japanese women could expect to experience an average of two abortions in their lives. Abortion and late marriage also helped lower Japan's teen birth rate to only four for every 1,000 women between the ages of 15 and 19. Official estimates suggest that 343,000 abortions were performed in Japan in 1995. However, research suggested that at least five times more than that, nearly 1.5 million abortions, occur annually in Japan. Doctors frequently did not record information on the abortions they performed or accepted the woman's or family's fee without recording the procedure to avoid taxes on that income.

In 1999, the Health and Welfare Ministry announced it would allow the sale of the low-dose combined hormonal contraceptive pill. Available in the United States and most of the world since the 1970s, the low-dose pill contains 50 micrograms of estrogen. Japan's health ministry had argued that possible side effects and a deterioration of morals made the low-dose an unacceptable contraceptive choice for that nation. Members of Japanese women's groups and outside experts countered that argument by pointing out that the high rate of abortion and the money doctors made from the practice as well as the dominance of the condom market influenced the ministry's decisions more than the chemical nature of the pill. While higher dose combined hormonal contraceptive pills were available in Japan, they were approved only for menstrual difficulties. Interviews for research studies revealed that Japanese women who could afford them used high dose pills to prevent pregnancy. These high dose pills with 100 micrograms of estrogen were generally no longer available in other countries due to their proven health risks.

Expectations for how many women would turn to the low-dose pill varied. Some analysts believed that the private nature of the pill, that women controlled its use, and that it did not need to be used during sexual intercourse would lead women to turn enthusiastically to the pill. These experts argued that the low-dose pill would help women avoid the need for abortion and reduce in their lives a personal trauma that often sent them to Buddhist temples to perform rituals in memory of their unborn children. To the contrary, business analysts suggested that the control condom manufacturers had on the contraceptive market and the control that men had of condoms would keep women from the pill.

Other forms of modern contraceptives, such as medicated intrauterine devices or injectable and implantable hormonal contraceptives, have not yet been approved for use in Japan. While female and male sterilization are both available, people rarely use them.

Discussions of sex, contraception, and pregnancy are still considered socially unacceptable in much of Japanese society. The country provides no sex education for children within the school system, even wives and husbands seldom discuss sex within marriage, and the government itself has no official population policy. The only law governing reproductive health, the Law for the Protection of Mothers' Bodies, strictly regulates family planning workers and facilities and establishes the grounds for abortion. Most of the information on family planning comes from the Family Planning Federation of Japan, which in 1954 became an affiliate of the International Planned Parenthood Federation, only two years after that organization formed.

Women in Japan can expect to give birth to an average of 1.4 children in their lifetimes. The population of that east Asian island nation grows at only 0.2 percent each year. In Japan, more than any other nation in the world, years of low fertility rates have led to a nation facing in the early twenty-first century a time when the number of retired people equals and will soon exceed the number of workers. Known as the aging of the society, this situation challenges Japanese domestic policy and the nation now faces more concerns over caring for its senior citizens then caring for the reproductive health of younger people. *See also* ASIA

Further reading: "Bitter Pill: Japan." *The Economist,* 8 November 1997: 42–43. "The Pill, Finally." *Maclean's,* 14 June 1999: 53. Smith, Bardwell. "Buddhism and Abortion in Contemporary Japan: Mizuko Kuyo and the Confrontation with Death." In *Buddhism, Sexuality, and Gender,* edited by Jose Ignacio Cabezon. Albany: State University of New York Press, 1992.

Judaism

Approximately 12 million people worldwide are adherents of Judaism, the ancient Hebrew religion that had its origins in the lands of the Middle East. Nearly half of the Jewish people live in Israel, a country on the eastern shores of the Mediterranean Sea, which was formed in 1948 as a Jewish nation and as the homeland of the Jewish people. The remainder of the Jewish people live among cultures scattered around the world.

Followers of Judaism believe in one God as the creator and the father of humankind. They follow the teachings of the Torah, the first five books of the Hebrew Bible, and the teachings of the Talmud and the Mishnah. The teachings of the Jewish faith have been discussed over the generations and the Responsa, the collected writings of rabbis, Judaism's scholarly teachers and congregational leaders, help guide Jews in their understanding of the law. It is in those writings that the Jewish understanding of birth control and modern contraception was shaped. Orthodox and Traditional Judaism, the two older branches of this ancient religion, and the much younger Reform and Reconstruction branches within the Jewish faith base their positions on birth control upon the studies throughout history of the learned rabbis on the issues concerning family planning.

As in other faiths, each member of the Jewish faith has the responsibility to learn, understand, and interpret the teachings of Judaism according to his own conscience and according to the teachings of the religion's leaders. Some members of Judaism hold traditional views that call for a strict adherence to the laws of the Torah and the teachings of the Talmud. Other members accept great diversity in the meaning and the interpretation of the law and call for a following of the ethical principles of the law rather than a strict literal interpretation. Still others advocate compromise. How individual Jews choose to live in relation to the law becomes then a moral, ethical, and religious choice. Because Jewish people live as members of many cultures, their attitudes toward birth control and abortion are shaped by the people who surround them and the civil laws of those nations.

One of the first commands of the Hebrew God to his people calls on them to be fruitful and multiply. That *mitzvah,* or law, forms the central concept of Orthodox Judaism's attitude toward birth control. It calls upon the people to not only have children to replace themselves but to have many children to allow God's people to increase in number. As with other religions, scholars have studied and interpreted that law and the people of the Jewish faith have applied the teaching to their individual circumstances. Those circumstances include a population that has been scattered by history and conflict across the globe, a people who have learned to adapt to the societies in which they find themselves living, and who, like many others, must resolve conflicts between religious teachings and contemporary issues. In the twentieth century, the Jewish people, as did all others, faced concerns with having children, consuming the world's resources, and being faithful to the teachings of their religion.

According to traditional, Orthodox Jewish law, men, not women, have the responsibility to be fruitful. It is their charge from God. Women have the responsibility to help their husbands fulfill that calling. In their lifetimes, men cannot destroy their own ability to bear children, and they cannot remove from themselves the obligation to multiply, which means they may not be sterilized. Naturally removing their fertility is an act of God; removing it themselves violates that first mitzvah and the spirit of Judaism.

Also important to an understanding of birth control within traditional Jewish law is the concept that marital pleasure is as important a function of sexual intercourse as is procreation. Jewish law places pleasure above procreation in some instances, particularly if the man has already demonstrated a willingness to fulfill his mitzvah to have children, and if pregnancy would jeopardize the wife's health.

A third teaching of Judaism commands that the people, particularly the men, not destroy or improperly emit their seed. Confusion over the nature of the female seed, the ovum or egg, resulted in no such prohibition against women. The concept *hash hatat zera* refers most specifically to withdrawal, an attempt by the man to keep sperm out of the woman's body by removing his penis immediately before ejaculation. More generally, the term has come to include any practice that simulates withdrawal and interferes with normal heterosexual intercourse.

A final concept involving birth control, that of the *baraita* of the three women, calls into question the appropriateness of women preventing pregnancy. The story of three women seeking advice enters Jewish law through the Talmud, the teachings that expound upon and explain the Torah. In the discussions surrounding the appropriateness of pregnant women, breastfeeding women, and minor women using birth control methods to prevent pregnancy, the Jewish teachers present most of the religion's teaching on contraception.

Orthodox rabbis object to and find unacceptable devices that interfere with sperm traveling through the vagina and into the uterus unless those devices function as pregnancy would in blocking the passage of sperm. Sexual intercourse during pregnancy is permitted by Jewish law based on the principle of marital pleasure. Through an interpretation of these teachings, diaphragms and cervical caps become permissible according to law since they block the uterus as a fetus and placenta would during pregnancy. Condoms, however, are not since they interrupt the path of the sperm before it even enters the woman's body and interfere with normal intercourse. Hormonal contraceptives and intrauterine devices are also acceptable according to rabbinic interpretation since they do not interfere with natural intercourse.

In addition to determining acceptable methods for preventing pregnancy, traditional Jewish law discusses acceptable reasons for when to prevent pregnancy. Essentially, the choice to use a birth control method is a decision made by the individual, and perhaps a rabbi, on a case-by-case basis. In practice, however, protecting the health of the woman is the only generally accepted reason for a couple to use birth control methods. Abstinence is not an acceptable method of preventing harm to the woman since it interferes with married sexual pleasure.

Abortion is not a form of birth control according to the teachings of Jewish law. In determining its need, rabbis again turn to the specific case. According to traditional teachings, human life begins when the fetus exits the womb. Before then, a fetus may have life but it is not yet human in the sense that a born person is human.

The issues of birth control and abortion within Jewish life depend to a great extent on the specific beliefs of the individual. Many Jewish people practice withdrawal. Until the development of more effective contraceptives, the Jews of Israel used it regularly to prevent pregnancy. While it is fading as a practice in Israel, it was as of the end of the 1990s still an often-used option. Sterilization, however, was rare and male sterilization practically unused. In western countries, Jews often limit their children to two, as do the non-Jewish people of those nations, even though having two children contradicts the traditional law for a man to be fruitful.

Abortion divides the scholars and teachers, and the people, of the Jewish faith as it divides the leaders and followers of other religions. The majority of modern Jews accept that a silence on abortion in the traditional Jewish law with a few exceptions makes it permissible in many cases. Traditionalists argue the law allows abortions only very rarely. In the United States, a greater proportion of Jews support abortion rights than do members of other groups.

The complexity of Jewish law contrasts with the social systems in which many Jews live and makes the decision to use birth control devices and which to use, and the decision to stop a pregnancy, an issue faced by each sexually active member of that religion. According to Jewish teaching and Jewish practice, members of Judaism have choices. How they exercise those choices helps them fulfill the callings of the God of the Jewish faith. *See also* ISRAEL

Further reading: Berke, Matthew. "Jews Choosing Life." *First Things: A Monthly Journal of Religion and Public Life,* April 1999, 34. Feldman, David M. *Birth Control in Jewish Law: Marital Relations, Contraception, and Abortion As Set Forth in the Classic Texts of Jewish Law*. 2nd ed. Northvale: Jason Aronson, 1998. Levy, Sharon Joseph. "Judaism, Population, and the Environment." In *Population, Consumption, and the Environment: Religious and Secular Responses*. Albany: State University of New York Press, 1995.

L

Lactational Amenorrhea Method (LAM). *See* BREASTFEEDING

Lea Contraceptive

A new one-size-fits-all, female-controlled barrier birth control device, the Lea Contraceptive gives women an alternative to the diaphragm and cervical cap. Because it does not need fitting by a medical professional, as do the diaphragm and the cervical cap, the Lea barrier is more privately and conveniently available to women.

Once filled with a spermicide, the woman pushes the small cup gently into the top of the vagina where it falls into place. Suction keeps it securely there. The woman pulls on an attached loop to remove the device. A woman may insert the device hours before intercourse and leave it in place up to 48 hours. For fullest protection, a woman leaves the shield in place for eight hours after having intercourse.

The silicon device provides an alternative for women and men who are sensitive to latex. The Lea Contraceptive also provides a barrier for women with uteruses that tip at angles that make diaphragms difficult to affix. Lea is reusable for six months, requires careful cleaning between uses, and needs to be replaced after six months.

In tests, the Lea Contraceptive had a success rate of 92.3 percent, making it at least as effective as the diaphragm and the cervical cap.

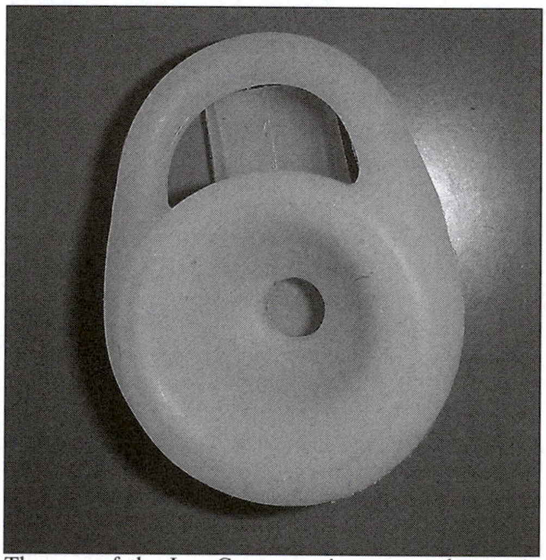

The cup of the Lea Contraceptive covers the cervix. *Courtesy Shelhigh, Inc.*

The Lea Contraceptive, originally called Lea's Shield, though available outside the United States, failed to receive approval from the U.S. Food and Drug Administration in 1996. However, Family Health International and the Contraceptive Research and Development Program are conducting long-term studies of the Lea Contraceptive that they expect will lead to FDA approval for sale in the United States. *See also* BARRIER CONTRACEPTIVES; CERVICAL CAP; DIAPHRAGM; EFFECTIVENESS (OF CONTRACEPTIVES)

Further reading: Kuo, Lena. "The Lea's Shield is Denied FDA Approval." *The Network News,* January–February, 1997, 5.

Life (Beginning of)

Science cannot answer definitively the question of when a person's life begins. In their attempts to do so, religious and non-religious groups, for moral and scientific reasons, often disagree. Also important to the discussion of family planning and fertility control is the question of which human life is of greater moral, ethical, and social importance, the life of the pregnant woman or the life of the fetus growing in her uterus.

The role of sexual intercourse in starting a new human life complicates the debate surrounding life. Some people, most predominantly the authorities in the Roman Catholic Church, believe that the only purpose of sexual intercourse is to allow the possibility of uniting sperm with eggs and creating a new human being. For these people, the emotional and physical pleasure of sexual intercourse and its role in maintaining an intimate relationship between a man and a woman is an unacceptable reason for the two people to unite sexually. Other people, including many individual members of the Catholic Church, disagree with this philosophy, and believe that creating a new life is not the primary reason for sexual intercourse. They challenge the belief that it ever was, suggesting that physical pleasure and biology, more than a moral obligation to reproduce, drives sexual intercourse.

Using any method to prevent the union of the egg and the sperm becomes morally and ethically objectionable to people who believe that each act of sexual intercourse must be open to the union of an egg and a sperm. For some who hold this belief, all forms of birth control, including the method of a man withdrawing his penis from the woman's vagina before he ejaculates his sperm, is immoral and unethical. Others argue that only natural methods of birth control are acceptable, including the recently refined and studied forms of fertility awareness that involve periodic abstinence by the woman and man. Traditionalists among the Islamic faith accept only withdrawal as an acceptable means of preventing pregnancy. Traditionalists among the Jewish faith find withdrawal abhorrent and illegal according to traditional Judaic law. For centuries the hierarchy of the Catholic Church, in fact, banned all actions that prevented conception. In the 1800s, after the discovery of the ovum and the discovery that a woman is fertile only when a mature ovum is traveling through her fallopian tubes, the church's hierarchy allowed couples to use the then poorly understood "rhythm" method to attempt to prevent pregnancy. By the middle of the twentieth century and the development of modern fertility awareness methods, the Catholic Church broadened its stance and allowed the use of all these forms of birth control, but not artificial or modern contraceptives. Reformist Islamic leaders accept most modern methods of birth control as replacements for withdrawal and permit their use, though they too argue that people must remain open to the possibility of conceiving a new human life and therefore do not allow permanent sterilization. Reform Jews, too, accept modern forms of contraception, even withdrawal under certain circumstances, as acceptable and as not interfering with the life.

The number of people who believe that all acts of sexual intercourse must be open to fertilization of an egg is rapidly declining around the world. An increasing number of people believe that the emotional expression of the already living woman and man is primary in the sexual act and that people have ethical and moral and personal reasons for choosing to prevent pregnancy. Modern birth control methods that keep sperm away from mature ovum, including barriers such as condoms and diaphragms and hormonal contraceptives, which prevent eggs from maturing on a woman's ovaries, are acceptable and do not violate their moral beliefs.

As the debate moves beyond the sexual act, it focuses on the nature of the cells that begin to form almost as soon as a male sperm penetrates the outer layer of female egg, or ovum. Here the debate is less certain for many people. Around the world members of many religious faiths and non-religious people argue that from the moment of fertilization, a human life is present in the cells that are forming. To them that new human life has the same moral and legal standing as the woman in whose body the cells replicate. In fact for many people those developing cells, often referred to as a conceptus, have even more rights because they are unable to protect themselves. These people accept only those modern birth control methods that prevent a sperm from fertilizing an egg.

Other people hold that those early cells are not yet human. A zygote, the early formed cells, are a potential human, they argue, much as an acorn is a potential oak tree. Since those early cells have the potential to divide and grow into two separate humans, twins, the early cells cannot themselves represent human life. Much has to happen in the biological process to transform those early cells into a full human entity. Included in that activity is the beginning of brain activity, which does not appear to take place until the fourth or fifth month of pregnancy.

People who hold that the early conceptus is not yet human find acceptable modern birth control methods that interfere with a pregnancy after a sperm has fertilized an egg, such as emergency contraception, which uses hormonal contraceptives to disrupt either implantation of the egg in the uterine lining or to cause the lining to dislodge. They also accept forms of menstrual regulation, processes that empty the uterus of its lining without determining first if a pregnancy has started.

Moral and ethical concerns over abortion also center on the question of life. For many of the Islamic faith, ensoulment, the arrival of the God-given soul in the conceptus, is the moment at which ethics and morals enter the discussion. According to Islamic learned opinion, that happens at about the end of the fourth month after a pregnancy has begun. In western schools of thought the issue is viability. At what point can a conceptus, if removed from the uterus, survive on its own? Brain activity and the development of the central nervous system also enter the discussion as a way of determining viability. Modern medicine has pushed the time of human viability closer and closer to the moment of fertilization. The United States Supreme Court held in its 1973 ruling in *Roe v. Wade* that viability occurred after the first trimester or after the first three months of pregnancy. That ruling has held in the United States, though medical technology is able to help babies born prematurely as young as four months.

Complicating the birth control and abortion debates is the question of the greater right of the already living woman as compared to the right of a potential human represented in either the conceptus or the as yet un-united egg and sperm. Many abortion laws, including laws in states in the United States before the *Roe v. Wade* decision, held that the life represented in the conceptus was more valuable than the woman's life and that even in the case that a pregnancy jeopardized the woman's life, the conceptus needed protecting first. In this case, laws disallowed abortions at any time. The Supreme Court in the *Roe v. Wade* ruling gave supremacy to the woman and her life.

By 1999 almost all of the world's countries allowed abortions to save a woman's life if they allowed them for no other reason. Even in the few countries that do not easily allow such abortion, legal appeals have been successful in granting an abortion in emergency cases.

Additional issues surrounding the role that life plays in birth control discussions include the right of a potential child to a valuable productive life. The tenets of Buddhism, for example, argue that human beings are entitled to lives that are neither too hard nor too easy and that people have no obligation to bring children into the world but that when they do, the parents have an obligation to provide for the quality of life of that child. Legal cases have been filed by children in developed countries arguing that their parents also had an obligation to consider the physical and emotional life that child would be able to lead in making the decision not to use birth control or not to have an abortion. *See also* ABORTIFA-

CIENT; ABORTION; ISLAM; JUDAISM; ROMAN CATHOLIC CHURCH

Further reading: Kogan, Barry S., ed. *A Time to be Born and a Time to Die: The Ethics of Choice.* New York: Aldine de Gruyter, 1991. Steinbock, Bonnie. *Life before Birth: The Moral and Legal Status of Embryos and Fetuses.* New York: Oxford University Press, 1992.

Long-Term Contraceptives

Long-term contraceptives—IUDs, implants, and injectables—are used to provide women protection against unintended pregnancy from three months to eight years. Unlike oral contraceptive pills, which a woman takes daily, and barrier contraceptives, which she must use each time she has sexual intercourse, long-term contraceptives need little attention from the woman, removing memory and a desire for spontaneity as obstacles to women who want pregnancy prevention. Long-term contraceptives also provide the greatest cost effectiveness of all current modern contraceptive methods.

Current long-term contraceptives allow a woman to return to fertility soon after she stops using them, immediately for unmedicated intrauterine devices (IUDs) and from three to six months for methods that contain synthetic hormones.

IUDs and subdermal implants prevent pregnancy for one year, and women need only make one visit to a medical professional to have the devices put in place. The Copper T 380 is effective for eight years. The Progesterone T device provides contraceptive protection for one year. Their long life makes IUDs, when left in place for years, the least expensive contraceptive choice.

Norplant, a series of tiny rods inserted under a woman's skin, lasts for up to five years. Other implant systems undergoing testing are intended to provide protection for from one to three years. Hormonal contraceptives, such as Depo-Provera, which are injected deep into a woman's muscle also provide months of contraception.

Perfect use is far easier to achieve for women who choose these long-term contraception than is perfect use with oral contraceptive pills, which they may forget to take, or with barrier methods, which many women and men feel interfere with intimacy. IUD failure rates range from 0.1 to 2.0 percent of the women using them experiencing an unintended pregnancy. Norplant's failure rate is even lower at 0.09 percent. Depo-Provera has a failure rate of 0.3 percent. *See also* HORMONAL CONTRACEPTIVES; IMPLANTS; INJECTABLE CONTRACEPTIVES; INTRAUTERINE DEVICE

Further reading: Huezo, C. M. "Current Reversible Contraceptive Methods: A Global Perspective." *International Journal of Gynecology and Obstetrics* 62, Supplement 1 (1998): S3–S15.

M

Male

Male refers to the basic designation of the members of a species that produce sperm, a cell containing one half of the genetic material necessary to reproduce that species.

In human biology, "male" refers to the members of this species for whom the major reproductive organs, the testicles and the penis, are located outside of the body below the abdomen. The word "male" distinguishes these members of a species from females, who provide the egg, a cell containing the other half of the genetic material needed to reproduce a species. The genetic material in the female egg and male sperm join to begin the process that can lead to a new individual of either sex.

Much of the biological development needed to form a male or female occurs in the very early stages of fetal development.

Because the male's sperm cell enters or penetrates the egg within the female's body, males are said to fertilize an egg and thus beget rather than bear offspring. *See also* FEMALE; REPRODUCTIVE SYSTEM—MALE

Male Contraceptives

While women have a widening range of modern contraceptive options available to them, men currently have only two, the condom and surgical sterilization. Researchers have been working for more than two decades to develop hormonal and chemical contraceptives that would allow men greater participation in the decision-making process of when and if to conceive children. Many difficulties in developing male contraceptives derive from the tremendous quantities of sperm (in the tens of millions) that healthy adult males produce each day.

The traditional means of preventing pregnancy, withdrawal and abstinence, still much in use, do not provide men with the full expression to sexual activity that modern methods such as birth control pills and long-term contraceptives like Norplant offer to women. Chemists, pharmacists, and doctors have been working to close the gap between modern contraceptive methods for men and women.

Generally, science has been better at interfering with the reproductive system of the female to provide long-term contraceptives. During fetal development, a woman's body produces all of the eggs, or sex cells, that she will have. At puberty, her body begins to release those eggs, generally one during each monthly menstrual cycle. Men are born without sperm. At puberty, they begin producing sperm constantly, between 30 and 40 million being produced each day in the young adult male. While that production rate diminishes with age, a man in his 70s and 80s still produces enough sperm to remain effectively fertile. Interfering with that constant process has caused significant difficulty for researchers.

The condom provides men and their partners with a highly effective physical barrier to the path of the sperm as it leaves the man's body. Commonly made of latex, with development underway for a thinner polyurethane sheath, the modern condom fits over the man's penis. Semen collects in the tip after ejaculation. Men have used condoms made of animal skin since ancient times. Their popular use grew rapidly in the late 1980s and 1990s as men and women realized condoms were the only birth control devices that also protected them effectively against sexually transmitted diseases. As of the end of the twentieth century, condoms were the only device to protect men and women from the human immunodeficiency virus (HIV), which causes acquired immunodeficiency syndrome (AIDS), a leading cause of death among young men and women.

Besides this easily available one-time use barrier, men may choose to have their two vas deferens, the tubes that carry sperm from the epididymides to the urethra, severed in the surgical procedure known as a vasectomy. This form of permanent sterilization was growing in popularity worldwide at the close of the twentieth century, though it was only half as popular as similar forms of female sterilization. Though scientists have developed an expensive procedure to reattach the severed ends of the vas deferens, a vasovasostomy, doctors carefully advise their male patients that vasectomies are permanent. In the 1980s, the no-scalpel method of performing vasectomies gained popularity around the world, offering men a less painful and complicated form of the sterilization procedure.

Biological contraceptives for men that would mirror the near-perfect success rates of female hormonal contraceptives gained significant research attention globally in the 1990s. Research sponsored by nonprofit organizations focused on methods for suppressing the production of sperm in the testicles and for altering the sperm themselves to make them incapable of fertilizing a female egg. All have been tested on men and all have shown serious drawbacks.

Hormonal approaches to developing long-term male contraceptives focus on the substances produced by the hypothalamus and the pituitary gland. The Population Council, a nonprofit organization based in New York City, conducted research on forcing the body to develop antibodies to gonadotropin hormone-releasing hormone (GnRH), which is secreted by the hypothalamus and which signals the pituitary gland to release luteinizing hormone (LH) and follicle-stimulating hormone (FSH). Both of these hormones influence a man's fertility although LH controls the production of testosterone in the testicles. By developing a system to inhibit GnRH production or effectiveness, researchers hope to stop or slow the development of sperm. However, without the natural production of testosterone, men begin to lose their secondary sex characteristics and their sex drive. In studies, men received synthetic forms of testosterone in addition to the GnRH inhibitor to prevent these side effects.

Scientists also have worked to suppress sperm by giving men manufactured forms of testosterone. In 1994, the World Health Organization (WHO) tested 399 men in nine countries in Asia, Australia, Europe, and North America using testosterone enanthate (TE). The men received weekly injections of the synthetic hormone. It effectively stopped or greatly lowered the sperm production rate in 98 percent of the men, reaching contraceptive effectiveness rates comparable to the high rates of female hormonal contraceptives. Men returned to natural fertility levels within two or three months of the last injection. However, the weekly shots made the approach impractical and research continued toward a more long-lasting injection. The WHO is also studying the effectiveness of two other synthetic hormones, testosterone buciclate and testosterone undecanoate.

While most of the research into male contraception focused on hormones, some scientists have been studying chemical forms of sperm suppression, most notably the study of gossypol, a cottonseed oil extract. Use of the oil in cooking in China apparently led to low fertility rates in men. Chemical research identified gossypol as the antifertility ingredient. Research then began to understand how the plant extract affected a man's reproductive system. A decade of study in China showed that the chemical lowers sperm production rates effectively after a 60 day "loading period," in which levels of the chemical built up in the man's body. Natural sperm production remained low in almost half of the men after they stopped taking gossypol. This high infertility rate lead researchers to adjust the dosage rate, and studies continue into gossypol's effectiveness as a long-term male contraceptive. However, its use as a contraceptive has also met with regulatory and research difficulties, though research into its potential as an accepted contraceptive method continues.

Other technological approaches to male contraception involve the growth of sperm and their ability to fertilize an egg and the ability of scientists to interfere with that process. Sperm-maturation inhibitors would stop the sperm from fully developing within the testicles. Sperm-altering approaches include drugs that would change sperm biology, removing enzymes the sperm needs to penetrate the outer surface of an egg, or depriving sperm of chemicals it needs to move normally and fertilize an egg. Two drugs already on the market, nifedipine, used to treat high blood pressure and migraine headaches, and mifepristone, used in chemical abortions, alter the structure of the sperm cell. Studies are underway to assess the value of these drugs as long-term male contraceptives.

Heat, too, is under study as a form of decreasing sperm counts while not altering a man's hormonal balance. Hot water, infrared heat, microwaves, and ultrasound, used to raise the temperature of the inside of the testicles, all underwent testing to determine their effectiveness at lowering sperm production. The testicles hang outside a man's abdomen in the scrotum behind his penis. This location keeps them two degrees cooler than they would be inside the abdomen. Warming the testicles that two degrees slows the sperm and prevents them from functioning normally. Men who through disease of dysfunction have had the temperatures of their testicles raised have proven to be temporarily infertile. Scientists are studying the effectiveness of heat and heat therapies as a means for giving men greater contraceptive alternatives.

Scientists and research organizations do not expect their efforts to lead to widely acceptable highly effective alternatives to the condom and sterilization until well into the twenty-first century. Social factors more than research dollars may drive the research effort into male contraceptives. Studies show that in 70 percent of the couples using contraceptives worldwide, women take charge of meeting the contraceptive needs. These women would gladly share that responsibility, the studies show, if men had greater choice in effective contraceptives with equal effectiveness and low risk of side effects. *See also* CONDOM—MALE; HORMONAL CONTRACEPTIVES; MODERN CONTRACEPTIVE METHODS; REPRODUCTIVE SYSTEM—MALE; STERILIZATION; TESTOSTERONE; TRADITIONAL METHODS OF CONTRACEPTION; VAS DEFERENS; VASECTOMY

Further reading: Alexander, Nancy J. "Beyond the Condom: The Future of Male Contraception." *Scientific American Presents: Men,* Summer 1999, 80–4. Best, Kim. "Contraceptive Update: Experimental Male Methods Inhibit Sperm." *Network* 18 (1998). Online: http://resevoir.fhi.org/en/fp/fppubs/network/v18-3/nt1835.html, 16 April 1999. Bonn, Dorothy. "Male Contraceptive Research Steps Back into Spotlight." *The Lancet* 353.99149 (1999): 302. "The Rights of Man: Contraception." *The Economist,* 16 August 1997, 63.

Maternal Mortality

Social and cultural circumstances, as well as biology, put women at serious risk from maternal mortality and morbidity, or death and illness, related to pregnancy and childbirth. Each day more than 1,600 women die during pregnancy and childbirth, 99 percent of them in developing countries. Women in developing countries, notably sub-Saharan Africa, have a 1 in 48 chance of dying from complications during pregnancy and childbirth during their 30 reproductive years, compared to a 1 in 1,800 chance of death for women in developed countries.

Hemorrhaging, the primary cause of pregnancy-related death, accounts for 25 percent of maternal deaths. Hemorrhaging can occur during delivery or be a consequences of an unsafe abortion, which alone accounts for 13 percent of the pregnant women who die in developing countries. Infections cause 15 percent and obstructed labors cause 8 percent of maternal deaths.

Lack of information about family planning and services that can provide them with that information, including post-abortion care, are one of the leading social reasons that women in developing countries are at risk from pregnancy-related death and injury. Lack of adequate health care before, during, and after delivery and undernourishment also threaten women's lives.

Providing women with information and effective family planning methods could reduce maternal deaths by 25 percent, according to estimates made by the United Nations Fund for Population Activities in the late 1990s. By giving women the opportunity to delay their first birth until they are in their 20s, to space births so they are two or more years apart, and to prevent conception in the high-risk older reproductive years, family planning means could help mothers, families, and nations decrease women's risk of death as mothers.

Contraceptive prevalence, however, is often low in the countries where pregnancy threatens the most women. In Zaire, Angola, and Somali, more than one-fifth of 15- to 19-year-old women give birth each year, and women under 20 years old have higher risks of maternal death than do women in their 20s and 30s. In those three countries, only 10 percent of women use family planning methods.

Helping a nation reduce its total fertility rate, the average number of children a woman is likely to bear during her lifetime, also helps reduce the risk of maternal death; however, social expectations, where a woman's status is determined by the number of children she bears, increases that risk.

Educating women could also help reduce the world's maternal mortality rate. Increasing a woman's ability to find and obtain information and knowledge helps her make decisions that protect her health, during pregnancy and child bearing as well as in other aspects of her life. In many developing countries, social and cultural, as well as economic forces keep women from attending school and obtaining the education that could help them protect their health.

Providing well-equipped medical facilities with well trained staff and improving a woman's access to those facilities also helps reduce a woman's risk from pregnancy-related death. Countries struggling with poverty and economic improvement may not have the resources to improve their medical facilities.

To help nations struggle to provide family planning, educate women, and improve adequate medical facilities, the World Health Organization (WHO) and its partner organizations in the United Nations, the World Bank, and the United Nations Fund for Population Activities launched in the late 1980s the worldwide Safe Motherhood Program. Now that program, part of the Maternal and Newborn Health/Safe Motherhood Unit of the WHO works to reduce the suffering women face during pregnancy and childbirth, including death and disability.

Several United Nations conferences, particularly the International Conference on Population and Development in Cairo, Egypt, in 1994, and the Fourth World Conference on Women in Beijing, China, in 1995, established through international agreements women's human and reproductive rights. Nations have pledged themselves to improve women's lives through providing greater access to family planning, education, and social status. *See also* CHILD MORTALITY

Further reading: Herz, Barbara, and Anthony R. Measham. *The Safe Motherhood Initiative: Proposals for Action*. World Bank Discussion Papers 9. Washington, DC: World Bank, 1987. Starrs, Ann. *Preventing the Tragedy of Maternal Deaths: A Report on the International Safe Motherhood Conference, Nairobi, Kenya, February 1987*. New York: World Bank, World Health Organization, United Nations Fund for Population Activities, 1987.

McCormick, Katharine Dexter (1875–1967)

Women's advocate and scientist Katharine Dexter McCormick provided much of the money needed to conduct the research that led directly to the development of the hormonal contraceptive pill. McCormick, the daughter of a wealthy Chicago lawyer, graduate of the Massachusetts Institute of Technology, and wife of an heir to the inventor of the mechanical reaper, chose to spend the fortunes she inherited in support of women's suffrage, biological research, and eventually the search for a hormonal contraceptive.

McCormick was born Katharine Dexter, 27 August 1875, in Dexter, Michigan. In 1900, after three years of study as a special student to prepare for the entrance exams, McCormick was admitted to MIT. In 1904, at the age of 29, she received her bachelor of science degree in biology and became the second woman to graduate from that school. One year later, she married Stanley McCormick, heir to the man who founded the International Harvester Company. Soon after this, Stanley McCormick began showing symptoms of mental illness. Katharine McCormick's interest in science and her husband's worsening illness led her to investigate and invest in research into the biological causes of mental illness, particularly schizophrenia, and she helped establish the Neuroendocrine Research Foundation at Harvard Medical School in 1927.

McCormick also spent time supporting women's suffrage, and after the right to vote was granted to women in 1920, helped form the League of Women Voters. Through her advocacy, McCormick became acquainted with Margaret Sanger, the founder of the American Birth Control League and a leading advocate of a woman's right to contraception.

Having maintained her keen interest in science and proving herself as an intelligent investor, and having made many connections in the biomedical research community, McCormick began in the mid-1950s to support the research of Gregory Pincus, who, with colleagues at the Worcester Foundation for Experimental Biology, was studying the chemistry of reproduction. McCormick knew of Pincus through her connections at Harvard and through her association with Sanger. Pincus's research on the hormonal control of the reproductive system in women aroused McCormick's scientific and social interest. When the Planned Parenthood Federation of America, the new name of Sanger's birth control organization, proved pessimistic about the chances of science finding a way to manipulate hormones to prevent conception, McCormick, in frustration, personally gave money to the foundation to support its work. After visiting the foundation in 1953, McCormick, then 77, pledged to spend $10,000 a year on the research. As work developed and need arose, McCormick increased her spending and became the primary source of money to support that research, eventually giving more than $2 million to fund clinical trials of Enovid, an synthetic progestin then used for treating menstrual disorders. Through her financial involvement, McCormick became what historians now refer to as one of the two mothers of the hor-

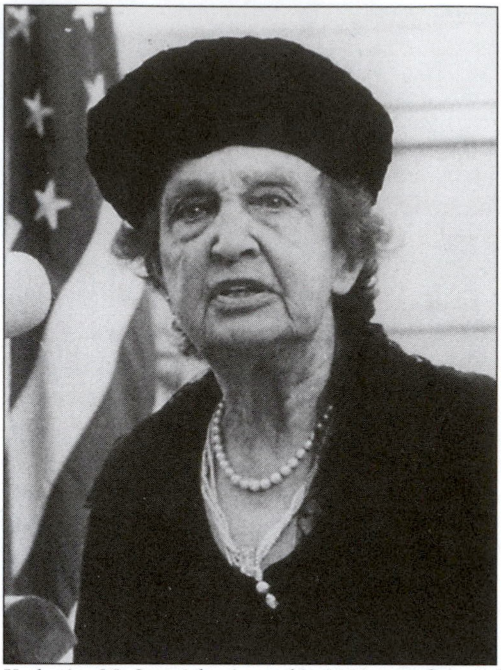

Katharine McCormick, pictured in 1963, gave financial support to the search for oral contraceptives. *The MIT Museum*

monal contraceptive pill that arrived on the U.S. market in 1960.

Katharine McCormick died 28 December 1967, in Boston. In her will she left $5 million to the Planned Parenthood Federation, which established the Katharine Dexter McCormick Library in her honor. *See also* COMBINED ORAL CONTRACEPTIVES; PINCUS, GREGORY GOODWIN; ROCK, JOHN CHARLES; SANGER, MARGARET HIGGINS

Further reading: Johnson, R. Christian. "Feminism, Philanthropy, and Science in the Development of the Oral Contraceptive Pill." *Pharmacy in History* 19 (1977): 63–78. Reynolds, Moira Davison. "Katharine McCormick." In *Women Advocates of Reproductive Rights: Eleven Who Led the Struggle in the United States and Great Britain*. Jefferson, NC: McFarland, 1994.

Melatonin

Researchers tested in Europe in the 1990s a contraceptive pill containing melatonin, a controversial hormone that appears to have a wide range of influences on the human body.

B-Oval, produced by endocrinologist Michael Cohen contained 75 milligrams of melatonin and a progesterone to create a birth control pill that, according to early reports, performed as well as combined oral contraceptive (COC) pills, which contain a progesterone and an estrogen. COCs have success rates higher than 99 percent with perfect use.

Melatonin, which humans produce in the pineal gland located near the center of the brain, became a popular food supplement and a public craze in the late 1980s after researchers discovered its relationship to sleep and discovered that it could be cheaply produced from animal and plant sources. Researchers at Yale University discovered melatonin in 1958 and while its effectiveness at resetting people's biological clocks has been firmly established, reports of its ability to lengthen human life expectancy remains unstudied. As a natural, unmodified substance rather than a drug, melatonin is not regulated by the U.S. Food and Drug Administration, as are synthetic sex hormones.

Melatonin also works to suppress the body's production of estrogen. In mammals other than humans, melatonin influences estrus, the time when they are fertile. Researchers explored the hormone's function in women in an attempt to discover dosage levels that would shut down their estrogen production as it does in females of other mammals when they are not in heat. In addition to its contraceptive influence, researchers have discovered that melatonin appears to inhibit breast cancer.

B-Oval was under study by a Dutch pharmacology company in the 1990s and tests in the United States were due to have started by 2000. *See also* HORMONAL CONTRACEPTIVES

Further reading: Cupp, Malanie Johns. "Melatonin." *American Family Physician* 56 (1997): 1421–1426. Elias, Marilyn. "The Mysteries of Melatonin." *Harvard Health Letter* 18 (1993): 6–8. Foster, Daniel. "Miraculous Melatonin." *Cosmopolitan*, July 1999, 102–103.

Menopause

For women, menopause signals the end of fertility. The term commonly refers to the time when a woman stops having menstrual periods, her menses. Scientifically, menopause refers specifically to a woman's last menstrual period, something which a woman in her 40s or 50s cannot know that she has had until she has missed several periods.

The process that leads to menopause involves the shutting down of the hormone cycle that stimulates eggs to mature and the uterine lining to thicken with blood in anticipation of receiving a fertile egg. Ovulation ceases and with the end of that process, no progesterone, a hormone created by the maturing egg follicle, is sent into her system. The absence of this one hormone triggers reactions along the hormone sequence and soon no estrogen is being produced by the ovaries. Without these two hormones, a woman's monthly reproductive cycle shuts down.

Menopause generally occurs when a woman reaches her late 40s or early 50s. About 50 percent of women reach menopause by age 50 and 85 percent reach it by age 52. *See also* MENSTRUATION; OVULATION; PERIMENOPAUSE; REPRODUCTIVE SYSTEM—FEMALE

Menstrual Cycle

During her menstrual cycle, a woman's body prepares an ovum, sometimes several, to be ready to be fertilized by a male sperm, prepares the uterus to receive a fertilized egg, and should fertilization not occur, prepares her body to produce yet another egg. On average, each menstrual period in the cycle lasts 28 days. The monthly routine begins at about age 13, with menarche, and ends at about age 52, with menopause.

The rhythm of the menstrual cycle is determined primarily by the levels of the two main female sex hormones—estrogen and progesterone—secreted by the ovaries. Estrogen production begins during puberty when the activation of some functions of the hypothalamus, which is located in the skull and is a part of the brain stem system, triggers in the nearby, tiny pituitary gland the making and releasing of two hormones important in the female reproductive cycle—follicle-stimulating hormone (FSH) and luteinizing hormone (LH). These hormones travel through the blood from the brain to the ovaries.

The first stage of the menstrual cycle, the follicular phase, begins on day one, which is considered to be the first day of blood flow from the vagina. Estrogen and progesterone levels are low, a signal to a woman's hormonal system that no egg has been fertilized, and this low level of sex hormones causes the endometrium to shed its blood-rich lining. These low levels of estrogen also allow the pituitary gland to begin releasing follicle-stimulating hormone. When this hormone reaches the ovaries, it signals them to begin maturing several of the immature eggs within small sacs, known as follicles. By about day seven, this egg growth then causes the ovaries to increase their production of estrogen. The higher estrogen levels then signal the endometrium to once again begin thickening and filling with blood.

As the level of estrogen in the woman's blood increases, it suppresses the pituitary glands ability to secrete FSH, and supply of that hormone diminishes, preventing any further eggs from developing. By the middle of the follicular phase, one egg has begun growing faster than the others and the ovaries stop the development of the other eggs, which then deteriorate. Most commonly, only one egg continues growing toward ovulation.

Also during the follicular phase of the menstrual cycle, the pituitary gland has been producing luteinizing hormone (LH), but estrogen levels have not been high enough to signal the hypothalamus to make gonadotropin-releasing hormones (GnRH) which will in its turn signal for the release of the LH, a hormone much needed to help the egg rupture from its follicular sac.

The length of the follicular phase of the menstrual cycle varies from woman to woman. On average it is 13 days long.

As an egg continues to grow, it makes ever higher levels of estrogen. By day 13 enough estrogen is circulating in the blood to trigger the hypothalamus to release GnRH. This substance then signals the pituitary gland to release, in a sudden burst, its stored supply of luteinizing hormone. This spike of LH begins the ovulatory phase of a woman's menstrual cycle.

The luteinizing hormone reacts with the follicle wall and the now large mature egg is able to erupt from the surface of the ovary. Ovulation has occurred. The egg travels quickly to the nearby fallopian tube. At this time a woman has the greatest chance of becoming pregnant, because it is when the egg is first released from the follicle that it is most fertile, most susceptible to penetration by a sperm. If sperm are present in the woman's reproductive system, if she has had sexual intercourse with a man within the last two days or so, her egg could easily be fertilized by those sperm.

The follicle on the ovary now becomes a temporary gland, the corpus luteum, and begins to secrete estrogen and large quantities of progesterone, a hormone responsible for developing and maintaining the uterine lining. High levels of estrogen and progesterone suppress the levels of FSH and LH released by the pituitary.

In the typical menstrual cycle, the egg is not fertilized and the cycle continues through the luteal phase to her next period. Soon after ovulation, the corpus luteum stops functioning, stops producing estrogen and progesterone, and fades. This decreases the amount of these hormones in the blood. Without them, the uterine lining cannot sustain the blood-filled state and the lining releases the blood in menstruation. The now decreasing estrogen and progesterone levels also allow the follicle-stimulating hormones and the luteinizing hormones to increase in quantity and begin again the process of maturing another egg and the monthly cycle begins again.

During these phases, levels of progesterone in the woman's blood influence the thickness and consistency of the mucus that plugs her cervix, the lower opening of her uterus. This mucus blocks sperm while progesterone is low and when it is thick and dry during the follicular phase. As ovulation approaches, and the follicular phase begins changes in progesterone levels causes the mucus to change consistency and become thinner and wetter and to flow from the vagina. This mucus allows the sperm to pass through and even helps support and nourish the sperm as it flows through the woman's reproductive system.

Scientific understanding of the details of the female menstrual cycle have led in the twentieth century to the development of a variety of birth control methods that alter this cycle. Most notable has been the development of hormonal contraceptives that alter the levels of the two groups of sex hormones—estrogens and progesterone. Either by pill, injection, or implants under the skin of her arm, a woman can choose to keep the level of estrogen or progesterone or both high enough to mimic the luteal phase of the menstrual cycle. These high levels of the two sex hormones suppress the pituitary gland and prevent it from secreting into the bloodstream the FSH that encourages and supports the development of egg cells. This, then, prevents ovulation.

Intrauterine devices (IUDs) inserted by a trained professional into a woman's uterus prevent fertilization and implantation and force the continuation of the luteal phase and the shedding of her thickened uterine lining. Several IUDs now contain slowly released progesterone which also inhibits ovulation.

A woman is only fertile in the days surrounding ovulation. Before an egg is released from the ovary, it cannot be fertilized. Within three days of ovulation, the egg has continued developing to a point where it can no longer be fertilized. However, the length of a woman's follicular phase can very significantly from month to month and from woman to woman. Not knowing this detail of a woman's biology led in the past to the low effectiveness of the "rhythm" method of pregnancy prevention. Understanding her cycle helps a woman use fertility awareness, or natural family planning, techniques to prevent conceiving children. Most modern methods of fertility awareness are based upon a woman's detailed knowledge of her individual menstrual cycle.

In helping her choose a hormonal contraceptive, a barrier contraceptive, or a fertility awareness method, clinicians and medical practitioners need to understand each woman's knowledge of her menstrual cycle in order to best advise her. *See also* BARRIER CONTRACEPTIVES; HORMONAL CONTRACEPTIVES; MENSTRUATION; REPRODUCTIVE SYSTEM—FEMALE

Further reading: Asso, Doreen. *The Real Menstrual Cycle.* London: John Wiley, 1983. Golub, Sharon. *Periods: From Menarche to Menopause.* Newbury Park, CA: Sage, 1992.

Menstrual Regulation

Menstrual regulation involves procedures to empty the uterus of its contents soon after a woman misses a period. These may be chemical or mechanical means and may or may not involve removal of a fertilized egg and the tissues of pregnancy.

Such procedures are generally performed to encourage menstruation after a woman has had sexual intercourse without using a birth control method or if a contraceptive fails, within days of the delay of an expected menstrual period, and before undergoing a pregnancy test. Current methods of inducing a uterus to flush its contents include chemicals such as mifepristone and suction abortion techniques.

Some nations, Vietnam, for example, and other nations of southeast Asia, allow women to undergo menstrual regulation within days of a missed period. Because these procedures are also performed without a woman first being tested to see if a pregnancy has begun, the medical professionals may not know if a conceptus (a fertilized, implanted egg) has been removed with the uterine lining. Nations where this practice is accepted as a standard part of reproductive health care do not see the procedure as being a form of abortion and do not include records of menstrual regulation procedures in abortion statistics.

Critics of the procedure see menstrual regulation as a euphemism for abortion. The procedures currently used as menstrual regulators, mifepristone, and suction, are also used to terminate known pregnancies. While missing a menstrual period may be a sign of other physical conditions, most frequently, critics argue, women seek the procedure when they suspect pregnancy and want the pregnancy stopped. These women do not seek menstrual regulation for other health reasons, they say.

Western physicians began calling in the 1990s for a more accepting attitude toward menstrual regulation. Generally, the methods used for menstrual regulation were not employed in western hospitals and clinics without first performing a pregnancy test. Advocates of the procedure argued that using menstrual regulations as did some developing nations would provide women with a private, less traumatic means of protecting themselves against unplanned or accidental pregnancy than abortion.

Abortion critics countered that such acceptance would allow people to more heavily rely upon abortion and allow them to not confront the moral questions involved in terminating a pregnancy.

Contraceptive researchers also explored the possibility of developing monthly pills that would force the uterus to shed its lining on schedule. Unlike hormonal contraceptives, these chemicals would work directly on the endometrium, the inner uterine lining.

With emergency contraceptive hormonal techniques, women take the estrogen and progestin doses within days of having unprotected intercourse. Menstrual regulation procedures are performed up to several weeks later when a woman is sure that her period is late. *See also* ABORTIFACIENT; ABORTION; EMERGENCY CONTRACEPTION

Menstruation

Menstruation refers to the three to five days during which a woman's uterus sheds its blood-rich inner lining. Blood flows out of the woman's body through the neck of the uterus, the cervix, then through the vagina.

Commonly known as her menstrual period, menstruation marks the beginning of the woman's next menstrual cycle. Generally, most women are not fertile during menstruation, since this is part of the follicular phase or pre-ovulatory phase of her cycle during which eggs begin to mature on her ovaries. However, many factors can influence fertility and women and men wishing to prevent pregnancy may choose to use a contraceptive when having intercourse during menstruation despite a low risk of fertilizing an egg.

A girl's first menstruation, known as menarche, comes at about age 13 during puberty. A woman's last period, known as menopause, occurs most commonly between ages 52 and 54. During the 40 years in between, menstruation signals the beginning of a new cycle in her reproductive process and represents, generally, that an egg has not been fertilized as a result of her sexual union with a man. Women may experience some levels of menstruation even after fertilization has occurred and until the pregnancy has firmly established itself. *See also* MENOPAUSE; MENSTRUAL CYCLE; PUBERTY; REPRODUCTIVE SYSTEM—FEMALE

Further reading: Blumberg, Joan Jacobs. *The Body Project: An Intimate History of American Girls*. New York: Random House, 1997.

Mexico

Mexico first established a national family planning program in 1973 and in 1974 family planning became a constitutional right for all Mexican citizens. At that time, the population of that country in North America on the southern boarder of the United States was growing at an annual rate of 3.1 percent. Women could expect to give birth to an average of 6.5 children in their lifetimes.

To curb that growth and the birth rate, Mexico's government worked to make contraceptives easily available to families, to educate its people, and to improve infant mortality. They set lofty goals for this achievement, hoping to reduce the annual growth rate to 1 percent by 2000.

Mexico experienced limited success in meeting those goals. By 1999 the annual growth rate had reached 2.2 percent and women were having an average of 3.1 children. Contraceptive use among middle and upper class Mexican women who lived in Mexico's cities and had at least a sixth grade education exceeded 75 percent by the end of the twentieth century. In the nation overall, where services to teens and poor women barely reached 30 percent, use of modern contraceptives had reached 63 percent.

Mexico faces many cultural and economic conditions that have led to its limited success at controlling population growth and has faced difficulties with legally and ethically persuading many of its poorer people to use

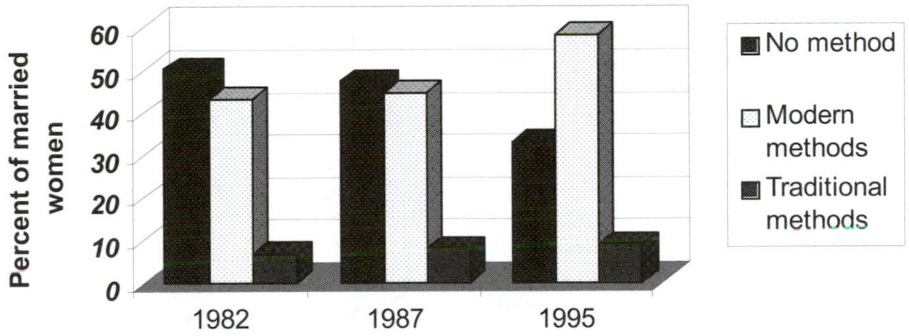

Mexico: Changes in Contraceptive Use by Married Women Ages 15–49

Source: U.S. Census Bureau International Data Base 1998

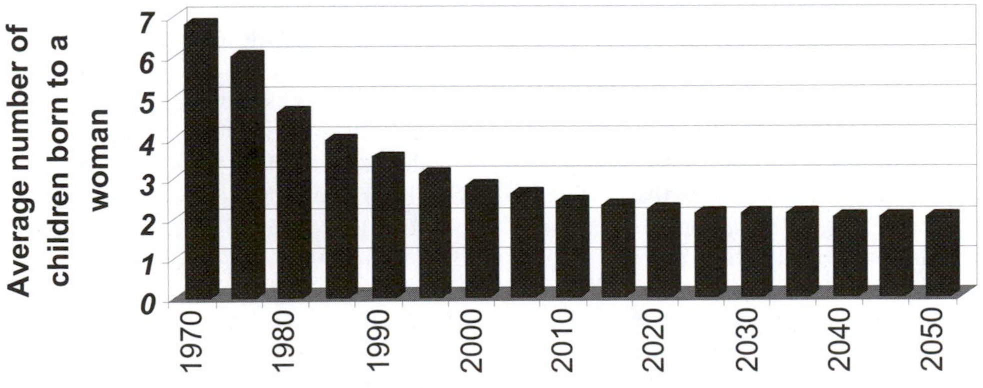

Mexico: Total Fertility Rate: Actual and Projected

Source: U.S. Census Bureau International Data Base

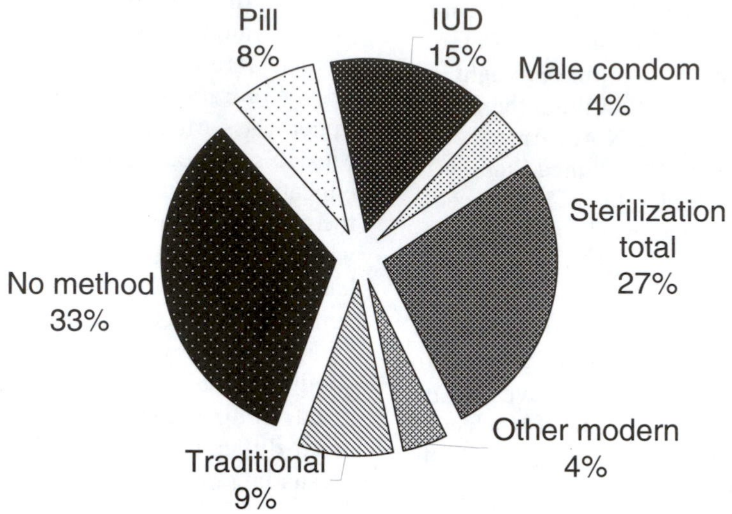

Mexico: 1995 Contraceptive Use by Married Women Ages 15–49

Source: U.S. Census Bureau International Data Base 1998

modern contraceptives. Populated by indigenous people in the southern states and by people of Spanish ancestry in the northern parts, it faces challenges from racism, poverty, and social and political unrest. All of those concerns lead to an uneven availability of contraceptives, sporadic education of the people concerning contraceptives, and difficulties in implementing the guarantees of its own constitution and of the international agreements, such as the program of action of the International Conferences on Population and Development sponsored by the United Nations and held in Cairo, Egypt, in 1994.

Nearly one-fifth of Mexico's people live at or below the poverty level. The needs of people living in poverty for reproductive health care and family planning methods goes largely unmet in Mexico. Less than 30 percent have access to information on reproductive health care. The poor have also reportedly been victims of forced sterilization and forced insertion of intrauterine devices as government workers struggle to meet unofficial quotas for population growth reduction.

Lingering social attitudes, differences between men and women, and the value the societies of Mexico place on education, also influence the still high annual growth rate and hamper efforts by the government and nongovernmental organizations to help people both gain access to family planning services and to see a value in limiting family size. An attitude that contraception, if necessary at all, is the responsibility of women, not men, decreases the choices a woman and her family have in preventing pregnancy. Though men's attitudes appear to be slowly changing, a high percentage still remain unwilling to use condoms or to take measures to assist in obtaining contraceptives. Education is free in and provided by the government in Mexico, yet the average child receives no more than five years of schooling.

As contraceptive use rose in Mexico, the incidence of abortion fell. From a rate as high as 41 for every 1,000 women in 1987, the abortion rate fell to 25 for every 1,000 women by the mid-1990s. Abortion, however, is illegal in Mexico, except in cases of rape. Most of the women who seek abortions live in poverty. With its abortions being performed illegally or with unsafe means, Mexico faces the challenge of providing health care for post-abortion complications. Most of the women who seek abortions are poor and illiterate.

Despite the social, ethical, and financial hurdles the nation faces, Mexican reproductive health professionals and policy analysts expect that nation to reduce its annual growth rate to 1.6 percent and its total fertility rate to 2.6 children per family by 2020. They will work on bringing contraceptive services to teens, primarily through education in schools, a policy strongly supported by parents, teachers, and students in Mexico. They will also work to improve reproductive health services to the nation's poor and disadvantaged. *See also* ACCESS (TO CONTRACEPTIVES); UNMET NEED (FOR CONTRACEPTION)

Further reading: Garcia, Sandra Guzman, Rachel Snow, and Iain Aitken. "Preferences for Contraceptive Attributes: Voices of Women in Ciudad Juarez, Mexico." *International Family Planning Perspectives* 23 (1997): 52-58. Kirsh, Jonathan D. "Informed Consent for Family Planning for Poor Women in Chiapas, Mexico." *The Lancet,* 31 July 1999, 419. Center for International Health Information. *Mexico: Health Statistics Report*. Washington, DC: Center for International Health Information, 1996.

Microbicides

Intense study of microbicides, chemicals designed to destroy the viruses and bacteria that cause disease, began in the late 1980s and 1990s as scientists worked to protect people from the spread of sexually transmitted diseases (STDs). Nonprofit organizations, universities, and pharmaceutical companies explored products that could work exclusively as protection from disease and products that could protect women from infection as well as from unwanted pregnancy. Researchers sought ways to combine disease-fighting agents with spermicides, commonly used with barrier contraceptives to kill sperm in a woman's vagina.

In the late 1990s, several dozen microbicides were being tested around the world by a variety of research labs. Efforts intensified as studies revealed that by 2000 women would make up nearly half of the people infected with human immunodeficiency virus (HIV) which causes acquired immunodeficiency syndrome (AIDS). Companies or nonprofit research labs hoped to introduce microbicides to the reproductive health market in the 2000s.

Researchers are attempting to develop a microbicidal product that would coat a woman's vaginal lining and cervix and prevent microorganisms from traveling through the walls of her reproductive system. The chemicals would also destroy disease organisms only without destroying or damaging the natural, beneficial microorganisms in the vagina. Complicating research into microbicides is the need to remove the product from the woman's body after intercourse. Since the vagina has natural hygienic mechanisms for cleansing and protecting the body, scientists are working on products that would themselves not breakdown and move through the vaginal tissue.

If a microbicidal product were combined with a spermicide, particularly one that did not irritate the vagina as the more popular existing spermicides do, it could provide a convenient, easy-to-use way for women to protect themselves during intercourse. Women would not have to rely on men using condoms for protection. Inconvenience, irritations, and harm to the vagina have already developed as reasons women do not use spermicides, and overcoming these preexisting obstacles would be requirements for successful microbicidal products.

In the late 1990s, the Population Council and the Contraceptive Research and Development Program reported laboratory success with potential microbicides. Scientists have discovered compounds effective at stopping in test tubes infections by chlamydia and HIV. One such product has also proven effective at preventing pregnancy in tests with rabbits.

Marketing research in the late 1990s began showing that women would be very likely to use microbicides. Research in France, Kenya, South Africa, and the United States showed a strong interest in vaginal microbicides among women. Cost for a microbicidal product appeared to be less of a concern than the cost of contraception to the women who expressed interest in protection from STDs. Cost, however, would be a factor in their using microbicides for low-income women, many of whom belong to groups at high risk from sexually transmitted diseases. Preference was high for products that would be easily available at drugstores and clinics and that would not require a prescription for their purchase. Research in the United States showed that 60 percent of women surveyed in the mid-1990s were interested in using microbicides that only protected them from diseases. Experts suspect that interest will be even higher for a product that combines contraception with disease prevention.

With HIV and chlamydia infections occurring at epidemic rates around the world, reproductive health care professionals believe that microbicides, even without contraceptive effects, are necessary in the future to protect the reproductive health of men and women. *See also* RESEARCH (CONTRACEPTIVE)

Further reading: Darroch, Jacqueline E., and Jennifer J. Frost. "Women's Interest in Vaginal Microbicides." *Family Planning Perspectives* 31.1 (1999): 16–23.

Mifepristone

Mifepristone, known originally as RU-486, stops or prevents a pregnancy by blocking the action of progesterone. When used after tests show that a pregnancy has begun, but within nine weeks of the woman's last menstrual period, after a fertilized egg has implanted in a woman's uterus, the drug causes an abortion. When used soon after unprotected intercourse, before a woman has missed a menstrual period, mifepristone prevents implantation and disrupts the earliest stages of pregnancy.

In 1980, scientists working for the French biochemical company Roussel Uclaf discovered the manufactured drug while searching for a stand-in for cortisone, a pain-relieving treatment for arthritis. Etienne-Emile Baulieu had been conducting experiments to develop an "antihormone" that would take the place of progesterone in a woman's body and block the action of that naturally occurring hormone. Researchers had discovered that chemically altered substances could attach to hormone receptors in the body and take the place of the natural hormone. The synthetic version, however, would not cause the same reaction in the receptor as would the natural hormone.

When Baulieu learned that a colleague had chemically synthesized what they originally gave the name of RU 38486, he recognized its potential as an anti-progestin and for taking progesterone's place in the biochemical cycle that supports and sustains a pregnancy. RU-486, as it soon became known, connected to the hormones to which progesterone should have connected, but RU-486 prevented, rather than allowed, the chemical reactions necessary to continue the pregnancy. With this near-identical impostor in place in the hormone cycle, the uterine lining would begin to deteriorate as if no egg had implanted and the lining, with any developing conceptus, would be washed out in menstrual blood flow.

Tests on women began in 1982 and by 1988, France had approved RU-486 as a means of chemical abortion. In 1991, Great Britain approved use of RU-486 to end a pregnancy. In 1996, after much public debate and controversy, RU-486, renamed as mifepristone, which represents its chemical structure rather than its developer, received preliminary approval from the U.S. Food and Drug Administration (FDA) for testing in the United States. Roussel Uclaf transferred the chemical's U.S. patent rights to The Population Council, a private research organization, in 1994, when the council, with financial support from the Feminist Majority Foundation, began testing the drug in 1994. Final approval of mifepristone was expected in 2000.

Medical professionals trained in its use closely supervise the use of mifepristone. It is given to the women only under medical supervision. While the procedure involves three visits to a clinic or doctor's office, it involves only one dose of this antiprogesterone chemical. On her first visit, a woman less than nine weeks pregnant, as measured from the beginning of her last menstrual period, receives 600 milligrams of mifepristone given in pill form. The mifepristone, by taking the place of progesterone in the hormonal cycle, forces the woman's body to act as if it is not pregnant and forces an eventual abortion. She leaves the clinic and returns two days later to take 400 micrograms of misoprostol, a prostaglandin that helps the uterus shed its lining.

Most commonly, the discharge of the fetus, placenta, and endometrium, occurs in the four hours the woman waits in the clinic after taking the misoprostol. Less than 5 percent experience the abortion within the two days after taking the mifepristone. In studies of its effectiveness, mifepristone has proven highly effective at ending a pregnancy with a 95 percent success rate. The earlier in the pregnancy the woman undergoes this chemical abortion, the higher the success rate. Mifepristone works most successfully within a window of progesterone levels, before the placenta takes over from the ovaries production of that hormone.

Women using mifepristone may experience painful contractions of the uterus, nausea, and vomiting. Some report diarrhea, pelvic pain, and spasm and headache. The pain of the process, about that of severe menstrual cramps according to women who have undergone medical abortions, surprised many women. These side effects also make mifepristone a less likely choice for postcoital contraception than strong combinations of hormonal contraceptives. Generally, however, women who choose this method of abortion find it less traumatic than do women who undergo surgical abortions.

Worldwide, mifepristone is gaining approval from countries for use as an early medical abortion as people seek safer, nonsurgical means of ending an unwanted pregnancy. Researchers expect its availability to all trained medical professionals will expand the availability of abortion, beyond clinics where specialists in abortion perform the more complicated methods or vacuum aspiration and dilation and evacuation. Opposition to the approval of mifepristone in the United States centers around the moral aspects of the abortion debate. As of March 2000, the FDA was awaiting answers from the U.S. manufacturer to follow-up questions.

Tests are also underway to asses mifepristone's potential as a male contraceptive and its value as a cancer treatment. *See also* ABORTIFACIENT; ABORTION; BAULIEU, ETIENNE-EMILE; PROGESTERONE

Further reading: Baulieu, Etienne-Emile. *The "Abortion Pill:" RU-486: A Woman's Choice.* New York: Simon and Schuster, 1991. Fraser, Laura. "The Abortion Pill's Grim Progress." *Mother Jones,* January 1999, 41. Winikoff, Beverly. "Acceptability and Feasibility of Early Pregnancy Termination by Mifepristone-Misaprostol: Results of a Large Multicenter Trial in the United States." *Journal of the American Medical Association* 280 (1998): 1034 (Abstract).

Mini-Pills. *See* PROGESTIN-ONLY CONTRACEPTIVES

Modern Contraceptive Methods

Barrier contraceptives, hormonal contraceptives, and intrauterine devices, all of which are manufactured, as well as surgical sterilization, represent the types of modern contraceptive methods commonly in use around the world. These products of technology provide varying degrees of success in preventing unwanted pregnancy, varying degrees of popularity of use, and widely varying costs of the method. They contrast with natural methods of contraception, such as abstinence and fertility awareness, and traditional forms of pregnancy prevention such as herbs, amulets, and even douches.

Contraceptives considered to be "modern" include hormonal contraceptives, whether pills, injectables, or implants, intrauterine devices, voluntary surgical sterilization, and recent designs of diaphragms and condoms. Spermicides and research into microbicides also fit in the modern classification of contraceptives. Recent research, however, is beginning to support the educated and diligent use of natural contraceptive methods, such as fertility awareness and abstinence, as an alternative for women and men who choose not to use modern contraceptives.

Overall, worldwide use of these modern contraceptives has been steadily increasing since the late 1970s. According to a 1999 report of the U.S. Census Bureau, married women in all regions of the world continue to turn to modern methods to help plan their families and prevent unwanted pregnancies. Trends show that the use of modern methods is more likely and common among educated women in urban areas of the world; however, the most recent studies show steady increases in modern contraceptive use among less educated, rural women as well.

As the worldwide use of modern contraceptive spread in the twentieth century, scientists and service providers came to recognize that understanding how and why people used traditional and natural methods of contraceptives needed to be studied along with modern contraceptive use to help pair a person's desire to plan a family with the method of doing so that best fit their lifestyles and preferences. Knowing which older, perhaps less safe, methods women or men would choose would allow clinicians and family planning providers to match the person with an effective modern contraceptive. Researchers also believe that more study is needed into the effectiveness of those traditional and natural methods. *See also* BIOLOGICAL METHODS OF CONTRACEPTION; CONTRACEPTIVE; RESEARCH (CONTRACEPTIVE); TRADITIONAL METHODS OF CONTRACEPTION

Further reading: Population Action International. *Contraceptive Choice: Worldwide Access to Family Planning*. Washington, DC: Population Action International, 1997. Online: http://www.populationaction.org/programs/rc97.htm, 11 October 1999. U.S. Bureau of the Census. Report WP/98. *World Population Profile: 1998*. Washington, DC: U.S. Government Printing Office, 1999.

Monthly Contraceptives

While research is underway to develop forms of hormonal contraceptives that would need to be taken or administered once a month, such a monthly contraceptive is not yet available to prevent pregnancy.

In 1999, the pharmaceutical company Pharmacia and Upjohn, now Pharmacia, conducted research on Lunelle, a monthly injection of synthetic hormones originally known as Cyclofem that caused fewer side effects than the longer acting Depo-Provera. While eliminating the need for women to remember to take a pill every day, Lunelle still presents women with the need to go to a doctor's office to receive the injection. Designers and researchers, however, believed that Lunelle, if developed and approved for such use, could become the first monthly injectable contraceptive administered by women themselves in the privacy of their homes.

Modern science also suggests that research could lead to a monthly pill based upon the synthetic hormones, estrogen and progesterone, now used in oral, injectable, and implantable contraceptives, but in much smaller doses that would target a specific moment in the reproductive process. Such a contraceptive could prevent the specific hormone sequence that triggers the process of beginning to mature eggs in the preovulatory phase of a woman's menstrual cycle.

Such monthly contraceptives would be specifically intended to be used regularly, unlike emergency contraceptive methods that are intended for a one-time use. This long-term nature would require that the monthly pills have fewer side effects than those associated with the larger-than-normal doses of hormonal contraceptives used in modern emergency contraceptives.

Some researchers suggest that women will one day have available to them a monthly contraceptive pill that would force their menstrual cycles to begin. Once referred to as "menstrual regulators," women throughout history have relied on herbs and natural substances to force menstrual flow, whether or not they had missed a period and suspected pregnancy. Such a hormone-based product would prevent pregnancy by forcing the endometrium to shed the blood-rich lining that would support a fertilized egg. Such a monthly pill that forced menstruation would likely be seen by many people as an abortifacient and the ethical equivalent to an abortion, since the woman would take the pill without knowing if an egg had been fertilized and implanted in her uterus. Such a monthly pill would not technically be seen as a contraceptive since it would not be designed to prevent the union of a female egg with a male sperm.

While research is underway to develop monthly contraceptives such as Lunelle, research into more advanced and precise monthly contraceptives is at best still in the idea stages. *See also* HORMONAL CONTRACEPTIVES; INJECTABLE CONTRACEPTIVES

Further reading: "The Morning After: Contraception." *The Economist,* 27 July 1996, 68–69. Roan, Shari. "A Shot in the Arm for Birth Control—Maybe." *Los Angeles Times,* 24 May 1999, home edition.

Morning-After Pill. *See* EMERGENCY CONTRACEPTION

Multiphasic Pills

Multiphasic pills provide women with options in finding a combined oral contraceptive formula that best suits their individual biology. As they developed their products and fine-tuned the proportions of synthetic estrogen and progestin in their pills, the more than 10 companies that sell birth control pills in the United States looked for ways to alter the proportions of hormones both to improve contraceptive effectiveness and to reduce side effects. As of the late 1990s, women could choose from monophasic, biphasic, triphasic, and even estrophasic pills to find one that worked best with their bodies.

Combined oral contraceptive (COC) pills contain doses of a synthetic estrogen, either ethinyl estradiol or mestranol, and a progestin, of which more than eight are available. The first pill, Enovid, marketed by G.D. Searle in 1960 contained 150 micrograms of estrogen and 10 milligrams of progestin with the same quantity in each of the pills in a 21-day cycle.

In 1982 multiphasic pills reached the market. These COC formulations combined a steady dose of estrogen with varying doses of progestin, which works with the estrogen to prevent ovulation and to slightly alter the reproductive system to prevent fertilization should ovulation occur. Adjusting the doses of the progestin over the days of the cycle offered women better control of side effects and better control of break-through bleeding and amenorrhea, the suppression of menstruation. By 1996, multiphasic pills accounted for more than half of the COC prescriptions written in the United States.

Biphasic pills contain two levels of progestin. In the first 10 days or so of the cycle, they contain half as much progestin as the pills the woman takes in the remainder of the cycle. The estrogen level remains constant in biphasic pills. Triphasic pills even more closely fine-tune the doses of progestin by having three separate dose levels. Triphasic formulas may also vary the amount of ethinyl estradiol in the pills. Together, these two dosing systems are referred to as multiphasic. They contrast the still common formulas, often referred to as monophasic, that maintain a steady dose of estrogen and progestin throughout the 21 days of active pills a woman takes during every 28 day cycle.

In the late 1990s, "estrophasic" pills reached the U.S. market. This new variation on the pill maintained a steady low dose of the progestin throughout the cycle but adjusted the dose of estrogen. Estrostep, manufactured by Parke-Davis, gave women and their health care providers yet another means to control fertility while minimizing the side effects and risks from the synthetic hormones. Relying on ethinyl estradiol, the most commonly used synthetic estrogen, the pills contain 20 micrograms in days one through five, 30 micrograms during days six through 12, and 35 micrograms during days 13 through 21. Each pill contains 1 milligram of norethindrone acetate as the progestin.

The estrophasic pill combines the benefits of the lowest effective doses of estrogen early in the cycle with the more certain higher doses later in the cycle. This alteration of the estrogen gives women who may be sensitive to higher doses of estrogen an option in their birth control choices that does not increase their risk from unwanted pregnancy. It meets a need among women for whom monophasic and multiphasic pills create serious unwanted side effects and for whom the very-low-dose contraceptive pills, which contain a constant 20 micrograms of estrogen throughout the cycle, prove ineffective at preventing conception.

By altering the doses of either the progestin or the estrogen in combined oral contraceptives, manufacturers and researchers give health care professionals and their clients greater choice to meet the individual needs of the women using the contraceptives. *See also* COMBINED ORAL CONTRACEPTIVES

Further reading: Rowan, Jean P. "'Estrophasic' Dosing: A New Concept in Oral Contraceptive Therapy." *American Journal of Obstetrics and Gynecology* 180, part 2 (1999): S302–S306. "Trends in Oral Contraceptive Development and Utilization: Looking to the Future." *The Contraception Report* 7.5 (1997): 4–14.

N

Native Americans

Information on the importance of birth control in the lives of Native Americans, the indigenous peoples of North America, including the Eskimos and Aleut peoples of Alaska and northern Canada, is scarce. In national record keeping in the United States, information on specific contraceptive use and sexual activity among American Indians is commonly combined for statistical reasons with information on people of Asian and Pacific island origins. This "Non-Hispanic other" race category in the 1995 National Survey of Family Growth conducted by the U.S. Centers for Disease Control and Prevention presents challenges to researchers to discover the needs and attitudes of Native Americans toward family planning, reproductive health, and birth control.

In the United States as of 1997, the 2.3 million people of Native American ancestry made up 0.9 percent of the nation's population. That represented a 38 percent increase over 1980. Native Americans are a young people. The average age is 27.2. That youth factor leads demographers to expect the Native American population to reach 4.4 million by 2050.

Native American culture plays an important role in a person's use of contraceptives, but because nearly half of all Native American people live in urban areas away from the more rural native lands, and because that shift from living as a community to living apart from the community has taken place over decades, many Native Americans are more strongly influenced by the modern culture around them than by their traditional cultures. Research into adolescent sexual behavior has shown that teen Native American women are likely to retain the influences of traditional culture, such as believing that sexual intimacy equals a permanent commitment between two people. Attitudes of Native American teen men, however, have moved away from that cultural, tribal influence. The conflict between traditional and contemporary causes conflict within relationships. Native American women who have been most strongly influenced by the modern, dominant culture are more likely to use contraceptives than are women who are strongly influenced by traditional native cultures where pregnancy is viewed as a normal part of life that should be neither sought nor avoided.

Unplanned teen pregnancy concerns adolescent and adult Native Americans. In the 1980s, about 20 percent of all births on native lands were to women under 20 years old; many of them had not finished high school. Educational efforts, however, have improved teen awareness of the risks of sexual activity and the protection from early pregnancy offered by modern contraceptives. Native American teens who use contraception most commonly choose condoms. In 1992, 49 percent of teen men and 24 percent of teen women reported using a condom with their last sexual encounter.

The history of Native Americans in light of colonization of that continent by European settlers and by the domination of non-Hispanic white peoples still influences women's access to contraceptives and their attitudes toward the provision of contraceptives by the mainstream medical and government communities. Documentation of abuse of sterilization of native women in the 1970s by mostly white medical professionals has led to significant skepticism toward medical contraceptive information by many Native American women. Then in the 1980s and 1990s, native women were encouraged by health care providers to use Norplant, a long-acting hormonal contraceptive placed under the skin, but charges soon arose of providers not adequately counseling Native American women about side effects and then being unwilling to remove the contraceptive before its five-year effectiveness span had been completed.

In 1988, the Native American Women's Health Education Resource Center opened near the Yankton Sioux Reservation in South Dakota. That organization focuses much of its attention on the reproductive health needs of Native American women and advocates for ending coercive practices by medical professionals, for improving informed consent policies, and for educating Native Americans in issues of reproductive health and fertility. The organization has also begun studies into the uses of birth control methods by Native American women and men.

Further reading: Murray, Velma McBride, and James J. Ponzetti Jr. "American Indian Female Adolescents' Sexual Behavior: A Test of the Life-Course Experience Theory." *Family and Consumer Sciences Research Journal* 26 (1997): 75–95. Smith, Andrea. "Malthusian Orthodoxy and the Myth of Zero Population Growth." In *Defending Mother Earth: Native American Perspectives on Environmental Justice,* edited by Jace Weaver. Maryknoll, NY: Orbis Books, 1996, 122–143.

Natural Contraceptive Methods. *See* BIOLOGICAL METHODS OF CONTRACEPTION; TRADITIONAL METHODS OF CONTRACEPTION

Natural Family Planning. *See* FERTILITY AWARENESS

Non-hormonal Pill

As scientists searched for new contraceptives in the late twentieth century, they looked for non-hormonal pills to help eliminate the side effects of artificial hormones that often lead women to stop using pills.

Research in India in the 1970s and 1980s lead to the discovery of the first non-hormonal pill, a colorless, crystalline hydrochloride salt. Given the name Centchroman, it prevented pregnancy when given in weekly doses. Centchroman has been marketed in India as Centron and Saheli.

Centchroman disrupts the timing of the movement of an egg through the reproductive tract, though it does not prevent ovulation. After fertilization, this chemical acts as an antagonist to estrogen and progesterone, and disrupts the functions of those natural hormones. It increases the speed at which a zygote travels through the fallopian tubes, speeds up the formation of the early cells after fertilization, and suppresses the formation of the inner wall of the endometrium. All of this disruption prevents an egg from implanting in the wall of the uterus.

Developers found that if women for the first three months took two doses of the non-hormonal contraceptive twice a week and then shifted to one pill each week they experienced a very low pregnancy rate—only 1.6 pregnancies for every 100 women using the pill during the first year of use. That compares to three pregnancies for every 100 women with typical use of hormonal pills. The only side effects noted were delayed menstruation in 10 percent of the menstrual cycles. Early testing shows rapid return to fertility when women stop using Centchroman and studies have revealed no harmful effects to children born to women who used this contraceptive. *See also* COMBINED ORAL CONTRACEPTIVES; HORMONAL CONTRACEPTIVES

Further reading: "Centchroman." In *Contraceptive Advances*. Baltimore: Johns Hopkins University,

Reproductive Health Online, 1999. http//:www.reproline.jhu.edu/english/1fp/1advances/1centch/ceorvw.htm, 22 June 2000.

Norplant

Norplant, a hormonal contraceptive that is inserted just below the skin in a woman's upper arm, provides up to five years of reversible progestin-only contraception. Once they are inserted, the Norplant rods require no attention from the woman. They offer a hormonal alternative to women who prefer their effectiveness of birth control pills but who find remembering to take a pill each day ineffective.

Norplant's six tiny silicone tubes contain levonorgestrel, a synthetic hormone that duplicates the action of progesterone, a sex hormone involved in the female reproductive system. The rods, each 2.4 millimeters (0.1 inches) in diameter and 34 millimeters (1.5 inches) long, are inserted in a fan shape just above the elbow on the inner part of either arm. The rods are only slightly noticeable once in place. Over the life of the device, the levonorgestrel secretes slowly through the walls of the tube into the woman's blood stream. The supply generally lasts up to five years.

Trained doctors surgically insert and remove the rods during an office visit. While insertion is seen as a fairly straightforward process that leads to few complications, removal has created some difficulties: the rods can move from their insertion place, complicating removal, and inserting the rods too deeply can also cause removal problems.

The Norplant progestin prevents pregnancy by interfering with egg development and preventing ovulation. The progestin also helps keep thick and dry the mucus that blocks the cervix and prevents penetration by sperm into the uterus.

Norplant rarely fails. Only 0.09 percent of the women using Norplant become pregnant during the first year of use, a result that is lower than even surgical sterilization. Over five years, only 3.7 percent of people using Norplant become pregnant.

Fertility returns quickly with Norplant. Once the device is removed, progestin levels drop rapidly and women who have the device removed before they seek to become pregnant should consider using alternative birth control devices.

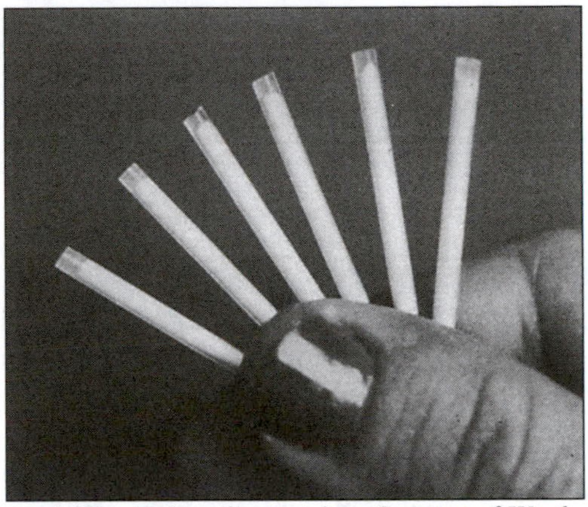

Norplant's six tiny silicone tubes. *Courtesy of Wyeth-Ayerst Laboratories*

Because Norplant relies only on a progestin, it has fewer and different side effects than contraceptive pills, most of which also contain forms of estrogen. Irregularity in menstrual bleeding is the most common side effect of Norplant. During five years of use, 45 percent of the women will experience irregular periods and 45 percent will have regular periods. The remaining 10 percent will have longer time spans with no bleeding. However, these irregularities occur most often in the early years of the implant's life and diminish with longer use. There does, however, seem to be less bleeding interference from Norplant than from Depo-Provera, a progestin-only injectable contraceptive.

Other side effects, including headache, nervousness, nausea, and skin rash are less common. More than 60 percent of the women who choose Norplant continue with the method for several years. Most who stop after one year do so because of changes in their periods.

Research by the Population Council, a nonprofit international organization, developed the subdermal (below the skin) implant system in the 1970s, and began testing it soon after internationally and in the United States. In 1983, Finland became the first country to approve public access to Norplant, a prescriptive contraceptive. Norplant now has received regulatory approval in more than 27 countries and is used by more than 15 million women.

In the United States, the Food and Drug Administration gave regulatory approval to Norplant in December 1990. While Norplant proved popular with women in its early years—800 women a day had the device inserted in 1991 and 1992—a series of product liability lawsuits filed in the mid-1990s slowed its use in the United States. Manufacturer Wyeth-Ayerst Laboratories proved successful at defending itself in the cases that went to court but in 1999 decided to settle with any woman who had filed her case before 1 March 1999. Problems with weight gain, site irritation, and difficulty removing the device led to the suits, though legal critics challenged the legal grounds of the cases and saw the complaints as a case of product liability attorneys encouraging women to sue in order to find clients. The medical community supported and continued to support the contraceptive benefits of Norplant despite the legal difficulties. By 1995, approximately 515,000 women were using Norplant, approximately 1.3 percent of women of reproductive age who were trying to prevent pregnancy.

In 1996, the FDA also approved a two-rod hormonal implant and research is currently underway by the Population Council to develop a single-rod implant. *See also* HORMONAL CONTRACEPTIVES; HORMONES—SEX; HORMONES—SYNTHETIC; IMPLANTS; INJECTABLE CONTRACEPTIVES; PROGESTERONE

Further reading: Correa, Sonia. "Norplant in the Nineties: Realities, Dilemmas, Missing Pieces." In *Power and Decision: The Social Control of Reproduction,* edited by Gita Sen and Rachel C. Snow, 287–309. Boston: Harvard University Press, 1994. "Insertion and Removal of Levonorgestrel Subdermal Implants." *The Contraception Report,* November 1994, 4–12. Segal, Marian. *Norplant: Birth Control at Arm's Reach.* Rockville, MD: Department of Health and Human Services, 1991.

O

Obscenity

By successfully classifying as an obscenity "any article or thing designed or intended for the prevention of conception or procuring of abortion," the Federal Anti-Obscenity Act of 1873, eventually known as the Comstock Postal Act or the Comstock Laws, presented a hurdle for early birth control advocates that would take until the 1960s and 1970s to overcome. That law, and the Federal Obscenity Act of 1872, which the 1873 law updated, set an example for state lawmakers to follow. State laws would also remain in effect until after World War II and prevent people from sharing birth control knowledge and devices based on their falling into the category of obscenities.

In the late 1800s, U.S. society at large seemed to share a common understanding of obscenity, though precisely defining the concept remained a difficult and elusive task. At the time, legal tests for obscenity in U.S. courts revolved around British law, which held that the concept of obscenity was based upon the intent of the material. If the intent of a painting, written words, or an object, including a condom or a diaphragm, was to deprave or corrupt the people into whose hands that object was placed, then that material was obscene. Often judges would rely on common knowledge and everyday use in instructing juries in how to define obscenity.

Birth control advocates argued that the laws were being too narrowly interpreted, and that women had the right to information that would protect them from the hardship of too many and unwanted pregnancies. Knowledge of the biology and emotion of sex and of contraception, they further stated, could also free women from restrictive social roles that prevented them from fully exercising their rights. Such knowledge could not be obscene, they argued, since it was designed to improve health and personal welfare and not debase society.

It was the common, vague, and restrictive definition of obscene of the late 1800s that Margaret Sanger and Mary Ware Dennett in the United States and Marie Stopes in Great Britain and other advocates for contraception and the sharing of sexual knowledge struggled against in the early days of the birth control movement. As those societies changed, however, the common understanding of obscenity also changed. By the 1920s, legal cases in the United States and Europe were calling into question the scope of the anti-obscenity laws and questioned who they were designed to protect. When she went to trial in 1929 for violating the Comstock Laws for distributing her pamphlet *The Sex Side of Life* through the mail, Dennett received tremendous public support for her educational efforts. Though a jury had ruled that her sex-education pamphlet aimed at adolescents was indeed obscene and a judge had imposed a $3,000 fine, Dennett received much support from observers in the courtroom gallery and via the mail. This support convinced Dennett of society's changing attitude toward sex and the lack of a common understanding of the definition of "obscene." In 1930, an appeals court found Dennett not guilty of distributing obscene material, arguing that the dominant theme of the pamphlet was to educate and not arouse sexual impulses.

Dennett's case opened the way to broader definitions of obscenity but not for more than 30 years did national law finally reflect social opinion. In 1970 Congress rewrote the Comstock Laws and removed the obscenity label from contraception. *See also* COMSTOCK LAWS; DENNETT, MARY WARE; PRIVACY LAWS

Further reading: Gurstein, Rochelle. *The Repeal of Reticence: A History of America's Cultural and Legal Struggles over Free Speech, Obscenity, Sexual Liberation, and Modern Art*. New York: Hill and Wang/Farrar, Straus, and Giroux, 1996.

Older Reproductive-Age Women

Older reproductive-age women experience natural declines in fertility as their ovaries release fewer mature eggs and as their bodies prepare for menopause and the cessation of the menstrual cycle. Concern for women in their later reproductive years grew in the 1990s among health care providers and researchers. The contraceptive needs of women over 35 apparently were going unmet as the women themselves and their physicians underestimated or misunderstood the frequency with which older women have intercourse and their risk from unwanted pregnancies.

Nearly half of all pregnancies among women older than 35 in the United States were unintended, according to a 1998 survey conducted by the Alan Guttmacher Institute, a leading reproductive research organization. Of these, half were among women who were not using contraceptives and the other half were among women whose contraceptive had failed. Abortion rates for this age group are also very high with one-third of all pregnancies for women between ages 40 and 44 ending in abortion. Women in this age group are three times more likely to choose abortion when faced with an unplanned pregnancy than are women in their 20s and 30s. Only teens have more abortions than women over 35.

While birth control use appears high among older women in the United States, their reliance on female surgical sterilization worried health care providers that many women were needlessly undergoing the risk of surgery. Approximately 72 percent of women in the United States between the ages of 35 and 44 reported using contraceptives in 1995; 40.7 percent of the 35- to 40-year-old women and 49.8 percent of the 40- to 44-year-old women relied on female surgical sterilization. Nearly 20 percent in both age groups relied on male vasectomies for birth control. That high reliance on surgery raised concerns that women were not receiving adequate or current information on their long-term contraceptive choices and their reproductive risks. Those statistics, from the 1995 National Survey of Family Growth, do not take into consideration the women over 44 who have not yet reached menopause and who might still want or need contraceptive protection.

Researchers became concerned that women chose surgery out of a mistaken belief that it was their only long-term option. This concern led to greater efforts to educate women and their health care providers on the changing biology of older women and on the methods that would appear to be most advantageous and least disruptive to older women's lives. Researchers and health care specialists began encouraging women and their doctors to discuss frequently during a woman's reproductive years her contraceptive choices.

Before menopause, which most women experience by age 52, women's bodies go through perimenopause, a biological phase in which the ovaries decrease in activity and the production of hormones decreases. Ovulation may not occur with every cycle but women in perimenopause still produce mature eggs and still run the risk of unwanted pregnancies. While their menstrual cycles are changing, women often mistakenly believe they cannot become pregnant. However, until tests confirm that hormone levels have shifted to postmenopausal levels, women can and do become pregnant.

Pregnancy itself creates greater risk for older reproductive-age women than for younger women. After 40, women experience a high rate of miscarriage or spontaneous abortion. Older women are more likely than younger women to have hypertension, diabetes, and heart disease, all of which present significant risk during pregnancy. During delivery, women over 40 are more likely to hemorrhage than younger women. Pregnancy in the late reproductive years also brings greater risk of birth defects to the fetus.

Concern among women over the side effects of combined oral contraceptive (COC) pills and worries that long-term use of COCs could negatively effect them have led women to turn away from this contraceptive choice as they grow older. In 1995, only 5.9 percent of women between the ages of 40 and 44 who were using contraceptives chose the pill to meet their needs. While that was an increase from the 3 percent reported in 1988, it was still below the level of use experts believe would be reported if women had up-to-date knowledge of the benefits of combined oral contraceptives. Most of the fears, research shows, stem from the 1970s when studies, now proven to be erroneous, suggested that older women were at greater life-threatening risk from oral contraceptives and at greater risk from side effects. Also, the formulas for combined oral contraceptives have changed significantly since the 1970s.

Doses of estrogen and progestin are much lower, scientists have identified smoking, not age, as the risk factor contributing to heart and circulatory diseases associated with COCs, and new hormone formulas have been approved and marketed from which older women may choose. Modern low-dose COCs, which contain 35 micrograms of estrogen or less and 1 milligram or less of a progestin, offer women a contraception with fewer side effects than higher, older pill formulations. Newer very low dose contraceptive pills, with 25 micrograms of estrogen and 100 micrograms of progestin provide even fewer side effects and offer women yet more contraceptive choice.

Research in the 1980s established that older women were not at greater risk from heart and circulatory disease when taking COCs as studies in the 1970s had shown. Only women over 35 who smoke 15 or more cigarettes a day or have diabetes or hypertension and who take COCs are at risk from those illnesses. With this evidence established, leading gynecological and scientific communities in the 1990s stated that older women who do not smoke or have other health complications could safely use hormonal contraceptives until they reach menopause.

Patient information distributed by the manufacturers did not reflect this new scientific understanding of the risks to older women until, in 1990, the U.S. Food and Drug Administration advised manufacturers to delete warnings for these complications for women over 40. With that change in published instructions, physicians became more comfortable in recommending COCs to their older clients. The number of women using COCs, however, grew very slowly.

Public health researchers also believe that more women will turn to combined oral contraceptives once they discover the non-contraceptive health benefits of the pill. A 1993 survey showed that between 80 and 95 percent of older women were unaware of the major non-contraceptive health benefits of combined oral contraceptives. COCs significantly lower a woman's risk from endometrial cancer, ovarian cancer, and pelvic inflammatory disease, according to extensive research conducted in developed and developing countries. They also tend to ease the disruption to menstrual flow caused by perimenopause. Studies suggest that COCs reduce the severity of rheumatoid arthritis and increase a woman's bone density, which helps fight osteoporosis.

Other birth control methods, including alternative hormonal contraceptives, provide still greater opportunity for women to find successful means of preventing pregnancy other than surgical sterilization. Progestin-only "mini-pills" use no estrogen to achieve their contraceptive effect and have proven highly effective for older women as their estrogen levels change. Norplant and Depo-Provera, an implanted and an injected form of progestin-only hormonal contraceptive, also give women long-range, low-risk alternatives to pills containing estrogen. Intrauterine devices can protect for up to 10 years and work very effectively for women in long-term monogamous relationships. However, IUDs can cause serious risk from sexually transmitted diseases for women with more than one sexual partner. With decreasing frequency of ovulation, older women might find barrier contraceptives such as diaphragms and vaginal sponges more effective than they did in their younger years. *See also* COMBINED ORAL CONTRACEPTIVES; HORMONAL CONTRACEPTIVES; MENOPAUSE

Further reading: Blaney, Carol Lynn. "Contraceptive Update: Contraceptive Needs after Age 40." *Network*. 18 (1997). Online: http://resevoir.fhi.org/en/fp/fppubs/network/v18-1/nt1811.html, 25 June 1999. Grimes, David A., et al., eds. *Modern Contraception: Updates from The Contraception Report*. Totowa, NJ: Emron, 1997. Speroff, Leon, and Patricia J. Sulak. "Contraception in the Late Reproductive Years: A Valid Aspect of Preventive Health Care." *Dialogues in Contraception* 4 (1995): 1–4.

Oral Contraceptives

Hailed by scientists, health care professionals, and birth control advocates as a contraceptive revolution, the invention of oral contraceptives in the United States in the 1950s and their first approved sales in 1960 provided women with a highly effective means of preventing pregnancy that did not require action during or immediately before sexual intercourse.

In the more than 40 years since their discovery and marketing, oral contraceptives have evolved and changed to become more effective and safer. More than 70 million women worldwide now rely on oral contraceptives to protect them from unwanted pregnancy.

Today, the more than 50 brands of oral contraceptives approved for use in the United States come in two basic forms, the more common combined oral contraceptives (COC), commonly known as "The Pill," and progestin-only pills, also known as "mini-pills." The combined pills contain doses of the synthetic or manufactured forms of progesterone and estrogen. As its name indicates, progestin-only pills rely on synthetic forms of progesterone to achieve their contraceptive effect. Synthetic estrogens and progestins mimic the function of natural hormones, maintaining throughout her cycle levels of these hormones in the woman's bloodstream similar to those found naturally only in the second half, or luteal phase, of her menstrual cycle. Levels of the two hormones, in COCs, or progestin alone in progestin-only contraceptives, prevent ovulation primarily by preventing the pituitary gland from secreting either follicle stimulating hormone (FSH) or luteinizing hormone (LH) which are necessary to begin ovulation. Synthetic hormones also alter the inner lining of the uterus to make it inhospitable to a fertilized egg, in the unlikely event that ovulation should occur and a sperm penetrate the progestin-altered cervical mucus.

Oral contraceptives are among the most highly effective products on the market for preventing unwanted pregnancy. With perfect use, when women follow package directions precisely, including when they forget to take a pill, COCs are 99.9 percent effective; only one out of every 1,000 women taking them is likely to become pregnant during the first year of use. With mini-pills, the effective rate is slightly lower at 99.5 percent; five women out of 1,000 are likely to become pregnant during the first year of progestin-only pill use. With imperfect use, where women do not follow package directions, especially when they have missed a pill, the effective rate is significantly lower at 95 percent, where one in every 20 women is likely to become pregnant in the first year of use.

All of the oral contraceptives on the market today must be taken daily, at least on each of 21 days, to maintain postovulatory levels of these two pregnancy-related hormones. In addition to 21 days of active ingredients, some products are packaged with seven pills that contain no hormones. Women may choose a product that builds the habit of taking one pill every day for as many years or months as they choose to use oral contraceptives, or they may choose a product that allows them to take pills for three weeks and then take no pills for one week.

Prior to the discovery of artificial ways to chemically manufacture forms of the sex hormones progesterone and estrogens, women and men had only barrier contraceptives, such as diaphragms and condoms, as well as spermicides, available to them should they wish to prevent pregnancy. As discoveries of the functioning of the female reproductive and hormonal systems advanced during the first half of the twentieth century, scientists learned that they could influence the hormonal system which timed and perpetuated female fertility. In the 1930s, researchers discovered that estrogens and progesterone distilled from mare's urine could alter a woman's menstrual cycle to prevent ovulation. In the 1940s, biochemists discovered several naturally occurring plant estrogens and progesterone's that, with chemical alterations, also functioned in humans to mimic reproductive hormones. The availability of these cheap and abundant plant sources eventually led to the development of pharmaceutical means of creating pills that women could take to change hormone levels and prevent pregnancy.

In 1960 G. D. Searle received approval from the U.S. Food and Drug Administration to package and sell Enovid as an oral contraceptive. The pills contained 150 micrograms of mestranol, a synthetic estrogen, and 10 milligrams of norethynodrel, a progestin. The drug was developed and approved in the early 1950s to help regulate menstrual problems, but laboratory tests and then field trials in Puerto Rico demonstrated that Enovid was highly effective at preventing ovulation.

Once publicly available, COCs became immediately popular and sought after by women in the United States and Great Britain, and proved to be highly effective at preventing pregnancy. By the late 1960s, 12 to 15 million women worldwide were using oral contraceptives to prevent pregnancy.

As the number of women who used the pill increased, health care providers began to notice a high number of women who were suffering and dying from circulatory problems, most notably blood clots that caused blockage in the blood vessels. These problems were connected to COCs. Continuing research into COCs led to decreased doses of estrogen in the contraceptives and the approval of new formulas for pills. By the late 1990s, most COCs contained only 35 micrograms of estrogen and still retained their effectiveness at preventing pregnancy. New very low dose COCs, marketed as Alesse and Estrin, contain only 20 micrograms of estrogen and very low doses of a progestin.

Early research into hormonal control of fertility had focused exclusively on progesterone since studies in the 1930s had shown that hormones' vital role in establishing a pregnancy after an egg had been fertilized. Work in the 1980s, however, showed that estrogen worked more effectively as a contraceptive and progestins reduced side effects and played a lesser role in contraception. In efforts to broaden the forms of hormonal contraception available to women, research in the 1970s refocused on progestin working alone. With minimal doses, progestins proved highly effective at interrupting a woman's ovulatory cycle. The progestin-only pills, offered women who cannot take estrogens, because of risk of circulatory problems or other health reasons, a convenient oral, daily contraceptive. Progestin-only pills do cause greater changes in the woman's menstrual cycle than do COCs, suppressing or greatly reducing the amount of monthly bleeding, and for this reason are less frequently prescribed than the contraceptives that balance the influences of estrogen and progestin.

While pills are becoming increasingly popular in developing countries, their effectiveness is hindered by ineffective education of women in how to take them and what to do should they miss a dose. As they work to improve the effectiveness of oral contraceptives, health care providers focus on educating women in face-to-face sessions so that women have the knowledge they need to achieve their reproductive goals.

Continuing scientific and technological advances led in the late 1970s and early 1980s to the development of products that allowed the synthetic hormones to remain in the woman's body for longer than one day. Injections of estrogens and progestins contained in slowly dissolving microspheres and rods containing progestins inserted into a woman's arm base their development on the scientific discoveries that lead to oral contraceptives. Even the development and study of synthetic hormones designed to work in men's bodies is based on the work in the 1950s and 1960s that lead to the "contraceptive revolution" ushered in by the pill. *See also* COMBINED ORAL CONTRACEPTIVES; HORMONAL CONTRACEPTIVES; MALE CONTRACEPTIVES; PROGESTIN-ONLY CONTRACEPTIVES

Further reading: Hatcher, Robert A., and John Guillebaud. "The Pill: Combined Oral Contraceptives." In *Contraceptive Technology,* 17th rev. ed, edited by Robert Hatcher, James Trussel, Felicia Stewart, and others, 405–466. New York: Ardent Media, 1998. Mishell, Daniel R. "Evolution of Oral Contraception: 1960–1985." *Dialogues in Contraception* (1985): 1–6.

Ovaries. *See* OVUM AND OVARIES

Ovulation

Ovulation is the erupting of a ripe egg from the follicle on a woman's ovary in which it has been maturing. From that moment until the egg passes well into the uterus some days later, the woman is fertile and any normal, mature male sex cell, or sperm, that enters her body through sexual intercourse can fertilize that egg.

One egg erupts from a follicle, on average, once every 28 days. Most often, a woman's body releases one egg during each ovulation and either of her two ovaries may release that egg.

The timing of ovulation and the length of the menstrual cycle vary from woman to woman and women rarely maintain absolutely regular cycles; therefore predicting the exact day of a woman's ovulation is very difficult. Chemical methods of birth control, the pill and implants, use synthetically created hormones to upset the woman's hormonal cycle and prevent ovulation. Determining when ovulation is likely to have occurred by using changes in a woman's body, most notably body temperature and the secretion of cervical mucus, is the primary process involved in natural family planning methods of trying to prevent or plan a pregnancy. *See also* BIOLOGICAL METHODS OF CONTRACEPTION; ORAL CONTRACEPTIVES; OVUM AND OVARIES; REPRODUCTIVE SYSTEM—FEMALE

Ovum and Ovaries

The ovum, or female sex cell or gamete, is known commonly as the egg. This one cell provides the female half of the chromosomes needed to begin a new human life.

Ovum are produced by the ovaries, the two almond-sized and -shaped sex organs nestled on either side of a woman's pelvic cavity. The ovaries prepare female reproductive cells, ova or eggs, for the journey through the body, and they produce the two major female sex hormones, estrogen and progesterone.

As a female fetus develops in the womb, the ovaries first grow near the kidneys then descend to their location in the pelvic cavity. They are attached to the pelvic muscles but not to the rest of the reproductive system. During prenatal development, several million egg cells begin to form on the outer layer of each ovary. By birth, most of these cells have died, leaving an estimated 1 million immature eggs on the ovaries. These early cells continue dying during childhood, and by puberty about 400,000 remain. During a woman's reproductive years, her ovaries will release only about 400 mature eggs.

At about age 13, a girl's body begins the process that each month results in one of these eggs growing to maturity and being released from the ovary. Each month, hormones trigger the ovaries to continue the development of 12 immature eggs. Generally, one of these 12 cells matures faster than the others and grows until it is ejected from the ovary into the nearby fallopian tube. The other eggs stop growing, and deteriorate.

Typically, one ovum is released from an ovary during each female menstrual cycle. After ovulation, the ovum travels through the fallopian tube and into the uterus. If on this journey, a male sperm cell penetrates the ovum, the egg becomes fertilized and begins the cell combination and division that can lead to the forming of a new human being. If this fertilized egg implants in the lining of the waiting uterus, pregnancy begins.

The ovaries also produce sex hormones, chemicals that trigger and control the development of unfertilized eggs and either the continued development of a fertilized egg or the expulsion from the body of an unfertilized egg.

The hormonal function of the ovaries plays an important role in birth control. These small oblong organs produce two important groups of hormones: estrogen and progesterone. Most modern hormonal birth control methods, such as the pill and implants, are based on manufactured versions of these hormone groups and are aimed at preventing ovulation or at stopping the production of mature eggs. *See also* HORMONAL CONTRACEPTIVES; MENSTRUAL CYCLE; OVULATION; REPRODUCTIVE SYSTEM—FEMALE

P

Patch (Contraceptive)

A contraceptive patch, currently in research and development, is a hormonal contraceptive device that would be worn like an adhesive bandage on a woman's arm, buttock, abdomen, or upper chest. The new patch method of delivering synthetic hormones to the bloodstream is based upon "transdermal" therapies used to administer other medications such as testosterone and estrogen for non-contraceptive uses.

Ortho-McNeil, a subsidiary of Johnson and Johnson, an American pharmaceutical company, announced in the summer of 1999 that it was in the final stages of testing a transdermal patch that women would wear on their skin. The patch, which the company named "Evra," is the size of a half dollar and can easily be hidden. The Population Council, a nonprofit organization devoted to contraceptive research, was also developing a patch delivery system.

Each patch would last one week and move the estrogen and progestin used in combined oral contraceptives through the skin. The patch would have the benefits of eliminating a woman's need to remember to take a daily pill, being simpler to use than injected or implanted hormonal contraceptives, and providing a steadier dose of the hormones than do injections or implants. In testing, the patch decreased common side effects such as nausea and vomiting.

Women in the Johnson and Johnson study appreciated the convenience and privacy of wearing the patch. They found the patch easier to remember to use and more successful at contraception. Others found that the adhesive did not stick well to their skin, a problem for women who sweat excessively or who participate in athletics. As of October 1999, the company had not yet submitted Evra for United States Food and Drug Administration approval. *See also* FUTURE METHODS OF CONTRACEPTION; HORMONAL CONTRACEPTIVES

Further reading: "Another Option: Contraceptive Patches are Now Under Research." *Contraceptive Technology Update* 20 (1999): 113. "Johnson & Johnson Patch." *Wall Street Journal,* 21 July 1999, B4.

Penis

The penis, an external part of the male reproductive and urinary systems, is essentially a transportation device. This cylinder-shaped organ is located below a man's pubic bone and protrudes at its root from a man's lower abdomen. The urethra, a thin tube, runs through the penis and carries, under different circumstances, urine and semen out of the body.

When a man becomes sexually aroused, three large areas of tissue in the penis that surround the urethra fill with blood, enlarge the penis, and cause it to become rigid and erect. This rigidity allows a man to insert his penis into a woman's vagina, the canal that leads from the outside to the woman's internal reproductive organs.

As sexual arousal begins, sperm cells travel from the testicles, where these male reproductive cells are formed, through the vas deferens into the urethra. In that process, the sperm combine with semen, a whitish substance that contains hormones and proteins that aid the sperm in surviving in the woman's vagina. When a man reaches the climax of sexual arousal, his body ejects semen through the urethra and into the woman's vagina.

The penis is the location for the application of the condom, one of the most commonly used forms of birth control. A condom is a manufactured sheath, often of latex or rubber, that covers the penis and captures the semen once it is ejected from the man's body.

Many people mistakenly believe that the penis must be inserted into the woman in order for fertilization of an egg cell to take place. However, the pre-ejaculatory fluid that rinses urine from the urethra may contain a small amount of sperm. Research suggests that sperm in this fluid may be left in the penis from a previous, recent ejaculation. In heavy petting which does not include insertion of the penis into the vagina but which does result in pre-ejaculatory fluid coming in contact with a woman's genitals, sperm can enter the vagina and survive long enough to fertilize an egg and cause pregnancy. Researchers still do not agree on the risk of pregnancy from contact with pre-ejaculatory fluid. *See also* CONDOM—MALE; EJACULATION; PRE-EJACULATORY FLUID; REPRODUCTIVE SYSTEM—MALE

Perimenopause

As the worldwide population of women who have experienced menopause increases, scientists have turned their attention to studying the perimenopause, the period of time that precedes a woman's last menstrual period.

The eggs a female needs for reproduction are formed in her own early fetal stages, and a girl is born with approximately 1 million immature eggs. By puberty she may have 400,000 remaining immature eggs, and by about age 37, only several hundred to a thousand follicles may remain on the ovaries and many of these are incapable of maturing to the stage of ovulation. The depletion of the egg supply on her ovaries decreases a woman's fertility, the actual physiological means of reproducing. Estimates suggest that by their mid-40s women are 50 percent less fertile than they are in their early 20s.

By the time of perimenopause, generally women will begin ovulating less frequently and may experience changes in their menstrual cycles, sleep disturbances, and psychological and cognitive changes. These symptoms affect women differently; some women may experience none of them. The woman in perimenopause is still capable of becoming pregnant, but the decline in the number of egg follicles has brought about significant changes in her ovaries, and these changes can cause confusion over the need for contraception and her ability to conceive. Doctors and public health professionals increasingly recommend that women seeking to prevent unwanted pregnancies use contraception until menopause has been confirmed through tests of estrogen levels. *See also* MENOPAUSE; OLDER REPRODUCTIVE-AGE WOMEN; REPRODUCTIVE SYSTEM—FEMALE

Further reading: Alexander, Ivy M. "Contraceptive Options for Perimenopausal Women." *Contraceptive Technology Update* 20 (1999): 122. Lobo, Rogerio A. "The Perimenopause." *Clinical Obstetrics and Gynecology* 41.4 (1998): 895–897.

Pessary

The general term "pessary" refers to a device inserted into a woman's vagina.

Until the early twentieth century "pessary" commonly referred to removable devices that couples used to prevent conception. In ancient and medieval times these were often made of bundles of herbs or concoctions of oils and tars.

Until the 1920s, "pessary" referred generally to early forms of the modern diaphragm and the cervical cap, and more precise terms replaced this older, generic term in discussions of birth control. By the late twentieth century, the term almost exclusively came to mean a medical device used to ease symptoms from uterine dysfunction. The term "pessary" is still used, however, in historical discussions of birth control devices. *See also* TRADITIONAL METHODS OF CONTRACEPTION

Further reading: Riddle, John M. *Eve's Herbs: A History of Contraception and Abortion in the West*. Cambridge, MA: Harvard University Press, 1997. Robertson, William H. *An Illustrated History of Contraception: A Concise Account of the Quest for Fertility Control*. Park Ridge, NJ: Parthenon, 1990.

Philippines

As a southeast Asian country, the Philippines shared in the economic boom of the 1980s and 1990s that led to prosperity for that region of the world. However, its share of that prosperity was not as great as that of other nations, limited in part by the Philippine's inability to decrease population growth and the fertility rate as significantly as its neighbors had.

The Philippines covers 7,100 islands that separate the South China Sea from the Pacific Ocean. Of those islands, people live on 880. They speak more than 50 languages and mix a wide variety of religious influences. Much of that diversity, however, is diminishing as the Philippines, like most nations, is evolving to a country where more and more people live in cities. In 1999, 47 percent of Filipinos lived in urban areas. More than 75 percent of Filipinos also follow the Roman Catholic religion.

The impact of the island geography, the dominance of the Catholic Church, and political change in the nation has made introducing family planning measures difficult in the Philippines, despite the availability of modern contraceptives in some areas since the early 1970s. In 1999, the Philippine population was growing at a high yearly rate of 2.3 percent, a much faster growth rate than neighboring Indonesia, which grew at 1.5 percent a year, and Thailand, which grew at 0.9 percent a year. Women in the Philippines could expect to give birth to an average of 3.5 children in their lifetimes in 1999. Despite that decrease in fertility, demographers expect no further drop in that rate into the middle of the twenty-first century. Without further decreasing fertility levels, the

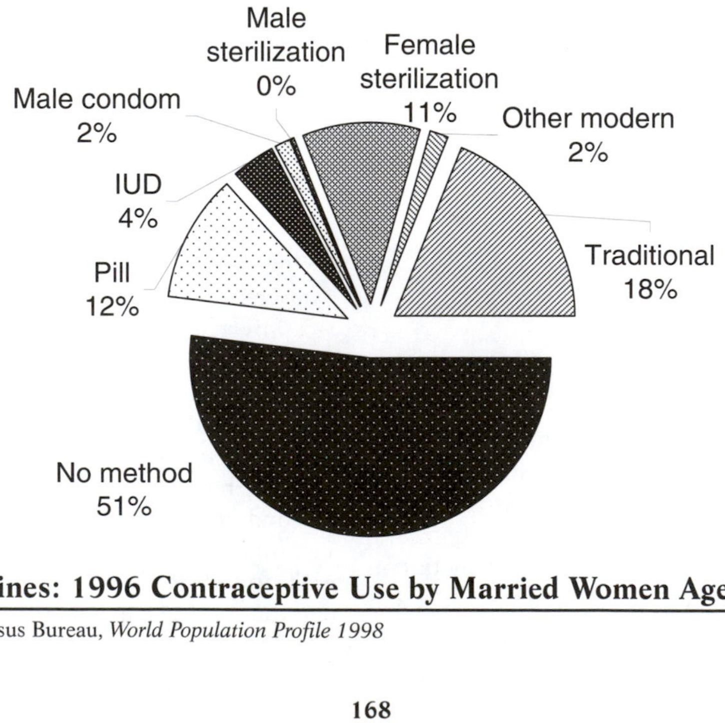

Philippines: 1996 Contraceptive Use by Married Women Ages 15–49

Source: U.S. Census Bureau, *World Population Profile 1998*

Philippines's high rate of growth will continue and its 1999 population of 75 million people could easily reach 112 million by 2020.

Fewer than 30 percent of women of childbearing age in the Philippines use modern contraceptives. Efforts to bring greater use to the Philippines have been hampered by getting supplies to people in their rural communities. Typically, women can gain access to only a six-month supply of their choice at one time. In some provinces, as many as 60 percent of the women who had begun using a method quit within a year of beginning that method. Women who had intrauterine devices inserted were least likely to discontinue that method. Side effects most often caused women to reject a method, most frequently the pill. Men's complaints about condoms, that the latex covering interfered with the sensations of intercourse, irritated the penis, or didn't fit, also caused women to stop using that method. Use rates and drop-out rates prompted the Philippine government in 1999 to renew efforts to promote birth control and family planning. Health officials increased efforts to encourage people to use modern methods of contraception, including condoms, hormonal pills, and IUDs, despite political opposition from the Catholic Church.

Abortion is illegal in the Philippines, though rare exceptions are made to save a woman's life. Despite this restriction, admissions to hospitals of women suffering from complications from abortions suggest that 25 women out of every 1,000 have an abortion each year, a rate close to that of the United States where abortion is legal. At that rate 16 percent of pregnancies in the Philippines each year end in abortion. Another 37 percent of pregnancies are unwanted, according to estimates. That level, in addition to the high growth rate, shows that the Philippines has a high level of unmet need for effective birth control methods.

In recent years, the Catholic Church has worked to introduce fertility awareness to the people of the Philippines. That method, however, has proven unsuccessful there, despite limited success in some regions. The influence of their religion on people's lives, however, seems as variable in the Philippines as it does in other parts of the world with a slowly growing number of Catholic women expressing greater interest in using modern birth control methods and a growing number turning to abortion to end unwanted pregnancies. *See also* ROMAN CATHOLIC CHURCH

Further reading: Biddlecom, Ann E., John B. Casterline, and Aurora E. Perez. "Spouses' Views of Contraception in the Philippines." *International Family Planning Perspectives* 23 (1997): 108–115. *Center for International Health Information Health Statistics Report: Philippines*. Center for International Health Information, 29 October 1999. Online: http://www.cihi.com/PHANstat/PHILIPPINES.html, 12 November 1999.

The Pill. *See* COMBINED ORAL CONTRACEPTIVES; ORAL CONTRACEPTIVES

Pincus, Gregory Goodwin (1903–1967)

Biologist and physiologist Gregory Goodwin Pincus had spent more than two decades studying reproduction in mammals, when in 1951 American birth control activist Margaret Sanger met with him and encouraged him to begin work on developing a simple, foolproof method of preventing conception.

Born in Woodbine, New Jersey, 9 April 1903, Pincus, received his Bachelor of Science degree at Cornell in 1924 and his Doctor of Science degree from Harvard in 1927. He focused his studies exclusively on the mechanisms of reproduction and developed a distinguished reputation in reproductive biology. Pincus was the first in 1934 to unite the sperm and egg cells of rabbits in a laboratory dish.

After having been a research professor of biology in Cambridge, England, and Clark University in Worcester, Massachusetts, Pincus became in 1944 director of laboratories at the Worcester Foundation for Experimental Biology in Shrewsbury, Massachusetts. There he conducted experiments with progesterone, a hormone made by the ovaries that helps sustain a pregnancy. His research focus remained on deciphering the reproductive process until Sanger invited him to dinner in 1951. His growing concerns with world population, combined with Sanger's ability to find money to fund birth control research, persuaded Pincus to begin intensive work toward inventing a chemical means of preventing pregnancy.

Research since 1942 and work by pharmaceutical companies, notably G.D. Searle, to develop and market progestins, synthetic progesterones, gave Pincus a starting place for his contraceptive research. With the intense scrutiny of detail and methodology he was known for, Pincus directed M. C. Chang, his assistant, to begin tests on rabbits of the progestins.

In 1952, Pincus renewed an acquaintance with John Rock, a Boston gynecologist who had been using progesterone to try to help infertile women become pregnant. Eventually, Pincus persuaded Rock, a Roman Catholic with serious misgivings about his church's prohibition on contraception, to begin testing progesterone on volunteers who wanted not to become pregnant.

In 1956, Pincus and his team began tests with the progestin in Puerto Rico. During those experiments, they first used only a progestin. However, a laboratory error at G.D. Searle led to the inclusion of a synthetic estrogen in a batch of Enovid, the specific pill they were testing. The estrogen prevented the break-through bleeding that women experienced and made the pill much more affective and convenient. After that discovery, G.D. Searle redesigned Enovid to contain both a progestin and an estrogen and the first combined oral contraceptive pill became an effective tool for contraception. In 1960, Pincus and his team, working with G.D. Searle, received U.S. Food and Drug Administration approval to market the estrogen-progestin version of Enovid as the first contraceptive pill.

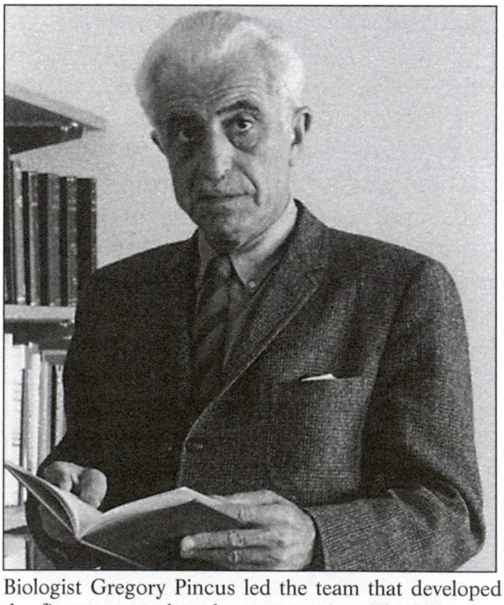

Biologist Gregory Pincus led the team that developed the first approved oral contraceptive. *The Worcester Foundation for Biomedical Research*

Pincus sought to increase scientific research into chemical contraception and tried during the research years to report on his team's successes with progestins but others were unwilling to believe that people would accept the manipulation of the reproductive system and refused to pay much attention to Pincus's discoveries until after Enovid had been marketed. With the huge and rapid social acceptance of the pill, Pincus felt somewhat vindicated in his strong belief that scientific research needed to produce social benefits and argued fervently for the responsibility of scientists, including biologists and physiologists, to apply the results of scientific research to helping solve society's problems.

Pincus also believed in informing the public of the work scientists engaged in and wrote in 1965 *The Control of Fertility* to explain to people, and not only scientists, exactly what he and other researchers understood of the biology of the hormonal contraception.

Pincus died 22 August 1967, in Boston. It was not until 1973 that scientists themselves, through a study by the National Science Foundation, were able to acknowledge that Pincus, a "technical entrepreneur," had changed the world in a way basic science could not have. *See also* HORMONES—SYNTHETIC; MCCORMICK, KATHARINE DEXTER; ROCK, JOHN CHARLES; SANGER, MARGARET HIGGINS

Further reading: Asbell, Bernard. *The Pill: A Biography of the Drug that Changed the World*. New

York: Random House, 1995. Johnson, R. Christian. "Feminism, Philanthropy, and Science in the Development of the Oral Contraceptive Pill." *Pharmacy in History* 19 (1977): 63–78. Pincus, Gregory. *The Control of Fertility*. New York: Academic Press, 1965.

Planned Parenthood Federation of America

The Planned Parenthood Federation of America, a national and international advocate for reproductive rights and provider of reproductive health care, is the world's oldest and largest volunteer organization supporting access to contraception and reproductive health. Through its clinics, this nonprofit organization provides women and men with reproductive health care, with family planning counseling and birth control methods, sex education resources, abortions and abortion referrals, and adoption referrals, and screens and treats people for reproductive diseases.

From headquarters in New York City and regional offices in Chicago, San Francisco, and Washington, DC, the staff of Planned Parenthood coordinates the efforts of 17,000 staff members and volunteers in 900 health care centers. They provide health care and sexual health information to more than 5 million people each year.

In addition to providing medical services, Planned Parenthood's 132 affiliate chapters work to educate people concerning their reproductive rights and choices. The organization's advocacy efforts include going to court to defend reproductive freedom, informing the public when people who oppose individual reproductive rights take action to limit choice, improve access to reproductive health services, and provide information on reproductive issues.

In the 1960s, Planned Parenthood began advocating for the legalization of abortion. As an advocate and an organization that provides abortions in the United States, where abortion is now legal, Planned Parenthood also comes into conflict with individuals and organizations that oppose abortion. A mission of Planned Parenthood is to support the legal standing of abortion, and contraception, in the United States.

Planned Parenthood had its organizational beginnings in the twentieth-century birth control movement. In 1916, Margaret Sanger, an early and powerful advocate for the legalization of birth control, though herself an opponent of abortion, founded in New York City the first birth control clinic in the United States. In 1921, following the first American birth control conference, Sanger formed the American Birth Control League. Under her direct control, the league fought state and national laws that prohibited the discussion of contraception and the showing, spreading, and mailing of contraceptive devices. By 1942, the league had opened 218 birth control clinics across the country. In an effort to better describe its purposes, the leaders of the league, including Sanger, who agreed with reservations, changed the organization's name to the Planned Parenthood Federation of America.

Planned Parenthood has long been active in supporting contraceptive development and helped fund the research that led to the development of the first combined oral contraceptive (COC) pill in the 1950s. Planned Parenthood clinics have often been sites for clinical tests of new contraceptives, including spermicide foams, intrauterine devices, and COCs.

See also INTERNATIONAL PLANNED PARENTHOOD FEDERATION; SANGER, MARGARET HIGGINS

Further reading: Brown, Cecelia. "In Memory of Mary Steichen Calderone." *The Journal of Sex Research* 36 (1999): 218–219. Planned Parenthood Federation of America Web site. http://www.plannedparenthood.org. Tell, David. "'Responsible Adults' and Abortion." *The Human Life Review* 24.4 (1998): 99–101.

Population Council

The Population Council, when it was formed and funded by John D. Rockefeller III in 1952, became the first foundation to focus its attention exclusively on concern for the world's rapidly increasing population. Arising out of a series of private conferences sponsored by Rockefeller in 1952 and 1953, the council aimed its activities at foreign and worldwide problems arising from population size and distribution. After World War II, many nations became aware of the rapidly growing world population, which doubled between the late 1950s and 1999, and the demands of that population on the world's resources. The Population Council worked to study and understand population growth, and encourage change that would influence that growth. Supporting access to family planning and contraceptives became one of the ways the council hoped to achieve its goals.

Two divisions, biomedical and demographic, formed the original council. The first focused on issues of individual contraception. The second focused on collecting data on population and promotion of family planning efforts. Today, three divisions make up the Population Council: the Center for Biomedical Research, the International Programs Division, and the Policy Research Division. Staff in those divisions conduct research into reproductive physiology and the development of new contraceptives for men and women, study economic development issues and personal decision making as it relates to population, and work to incorporate reproductive health services into programs to improve the quality of reproductive care and contraceptive choice around the world.

As of 1999, 480 employees from 65 countries worked for the council, more than half of them in developing countries. From headquarters in Washington, DC, the council directed the work of regional offices in Cairo (Egypt), Nairobi (Kenya), New Delhi (India), Dakar (Senegal), and Mexico City (Mexico), and 13 country offices. In 1999, the council was supported by grants and private donations and had as its budget $69 million, a 65 percent increase since 1993.

Vaginal rings, implants, intrauterine devices, transdermal patches, and chemical abortion methods were all under development in the 1990s by the Population Council. Research in contraceptives for men focused on implants and immunization-like contraceptives. The council also conducted research into microbicides, methods for killing or preventing the spread of sexually transmitted diseases.

Social issues of concern to the council included adolescent reproductive behavior, including the transition to adulthood, managing unwanted pregnancies and preventing unsafe abortions, women's economic contributions to family life, men's partnerships in women's reproductive health, and the consequences of urbanization, poverty, and child survival on population.

The council shares its research with professionals and the public through several publications including the peer-reviewed international quarterly journal *Studies in Family Planning.* This journal contains research articles, reports, and commentary, and statistical data for individual countries. Other publications include *Population and Development Review* and the working papers of the Policy Research Division. The council also maintains a site on the World Wide Web, where many of its publications are accessible to the public.

In 1994, the Population Council received the U.S. patent rights to mifepristone, the controversial chemical abortion pill known originally as RU-486. Developers of mifepristone, Roussel-Uclaf, a French pharmaceutical company, made the arrangement to remove itself from the conflict surrounding the drug's testing and approval in the United States. By 1996, after testing on more than 2,100 women, the U.S. Food and Drug Administration Advisory Committee recommended approval of the drug. In 1997, the Population Council formed with its project partners Advances for Choice, a new company to oversee the completion of the approval process, which is expected to be completed sometime in 2000. *See also* MIFEPRISTONE; RESEARCH (CONTRACEPTIVE)

Further reading: Back, Kurt W. *Family Planning and Population Control: The Challenges of a Successful Movement.* Boston: Twayne, 1989. Population Council. *Annual Report: 1998.* Online: http://www.popcouncil.org/about/ar/default.html, 6 March 2000. Population Council Web site. http://www.popcouncil.org.

Population Growth

In 1999, the size of the human population reached 6 billion. With 77 million babies born each year, the world population growth rate in 1999 was 1.33 percent annually. Demographers, environmentalists, religious leaders, ethicists, feminists, and world leaders, among many others, worried that that level of human habitation had already neared the maximum that the world's resources and human ingenuity could support. With more than 30 percent of the human race living in extreme poverty and another 40 percent living only slightly above that level, continued human growth would endanger too many people, threaten the health of the globe, and lead to global strife and social stress.

An overwhelming consensus of world opinion held in the year 2000 that nations needed to spend even more resources to influence in a downward direction that population growth. The manner of that influence, however, evolved during the last half of the twentieth century. It changed from population control efforts, where the wealthy nations of the world donated money to help supply modern birth control methods to poorer countries, to reproductive health efforts, where the nations of the world worked to ensure those 6 billion people their reproductive rights. Through several international agreements, nations agreed upon methods to improve individuals' lives that would have the residual effect of also lowering their dependence upon more children for their welfare. Improved living standards and economic opportunity, they believed, would lead people to want and need fewer children, a trend seen in all of the developed nations of the world and in many of the developing nations, particularly east Asia and Latin America.

At the beginning of 2000, the United Nations stated that the world population could rise at three different rates—low, medium, and high—depending on the actions nations took to slow their population growth. In the low scenario, population growth rates could continue to decline as they have since reaching a peak at 2 percent each year in the 1960s. The population would reach 7 billion by about 2020 and level off, beginning a slight decline by the year 2050. In the medium scenario, growth rates would decline more slowly and the population would reach 8 billion by 2030 and 9 billion by 2050 before eventually leveling off. In the high scenario, the current growth rate would continue, even increase slightly, and the population would climb steadily to 10.5 billion by 2050. United Nations Department of Economic and Social Affairs experts believe the medium scenario is most likely. United States Census Bureau predictions found the high scenario more likely.

In the mid-1950s, a woman on average across the world could expect to give birth to 5.1 children. In that decade Europe had the lowest regional total fertility rate at 2.6 children; north Africa and western Asia had the highest at 6.6 children. Across the world, due in large part to the invention and development of modern contraceptives, the total fertility rate declined steadily and in many cases rapidly during that decade. By the mid 1990s, Europe's total fertility rate stood at 1.4 children and the world's high was sub-Saharan Africa at 5.5 children. In north Africa and western Asia women could expect to give birth to 3.5 children in mid-1990.

Much of the fertility rate decline of the developed nations of Europe and North America took place in the late 1800s, with increasingly rapid declines occurring after the development of the modern birth control methods of oral contraceptive pills and intrauterine devices in the twentieth century. In those wealthy, highly urbanized nations, economic and industrial development preceded decreases in the sizes of families people were having. However, even in those nations fertility decrease occurred first in wealthy families, then middle class families. The increasing availability of modern contraceptives in the twentieth century allowed poorer families to choose the number of children they raised. In the developed nations, economic change and family planning changes occurred at the same time and worked together to improve the quality of life and to lower population growth rates.

In the 123 years from 1804 to 1927, the world's population doubled from 1 billion to 2 billion. It reached 3 billion by 1960 and reached 6 billion in 1999. World population growth reached its peak at 2.3 percent in the mid 1960s. The scientific advances of the late nineteenth and early twentieth century accounted for most of the rapid population growth. Discoveries of immunizations to prevent diseases that had plagued nations and contributed to slow population growth meant more children survived infancy. In the United States in 1920, nearly 85 of every 1,000 infants born, died each year. By 1990, fewer than 10 infants died each year out of every 1,000 born. The infant death rates in many of the world's poorer countries decreased as rapidly in the latter half of the twentieth century, though by 2000, the poorer nations of Asia and north Africa had infant mortality rates of between 50 and 60 for every 1,000 births. In the nations of sub-Saharan Africa more than 90 infants for every 1,000 children born died before the age of 1.

Around the world, people in 2000 lived an average of 20 years longer than they did in 1950. In developed countries, people lived an average of 79 years. In less developed countries, their life expectancy rose to 67 years. That increase in the chances of a child surviving infancy and people dying at older ages, known as the gap between birth and death rates, contributed to a great extent to the rapid increase in population seen in the twentieth century.

Observing those trends led to concern by many people around the world, both in developing and developed nations. At issue was the ability of nations to grow economically and provide quality of life for its citizens. By 1 January 2000, nearly 90 percent of the people in the world lived in countries considered less developed, and less able to provide their citizens with a quality of life common to more developed countries.

Modern contraceptives played an important role since the 1960s in lowering the population growth rate. Estimates in Asia alone suggest that modern contraceptives accounted for between 48 and 64 percent of those nations' dramatic fertility declines. Some population experts calculate that without the international action beginning in the 1960s to lower worldwide the number of children to which women typically gave birth and to help nations achieve higher rates of economic success, world population could have reached 7 billion by 2000. Chinese demographers estimate that without that nation's population measures, the "one-child" program, 1996 would have been the year in which the 6 billionth baby was born. Instead, the world's population reached 6 billion in 1999.

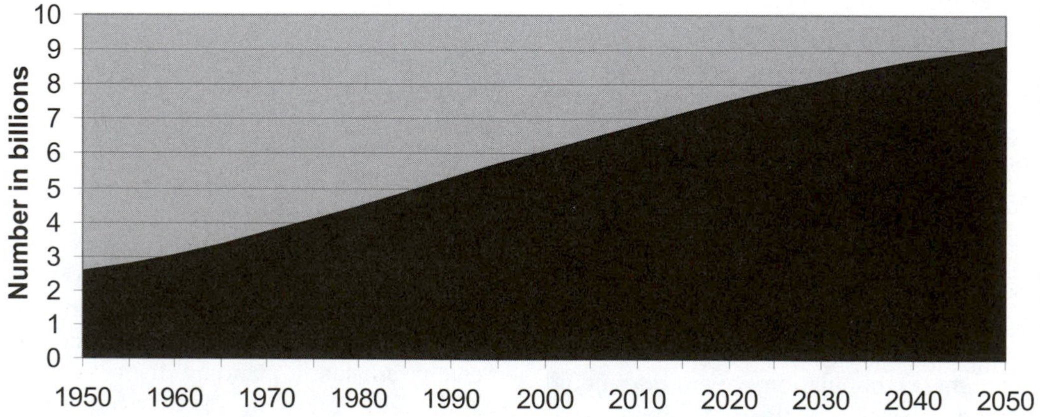

World Population Annual Growth Rate: Actual and Projected

Source: U.S. Census Bureau

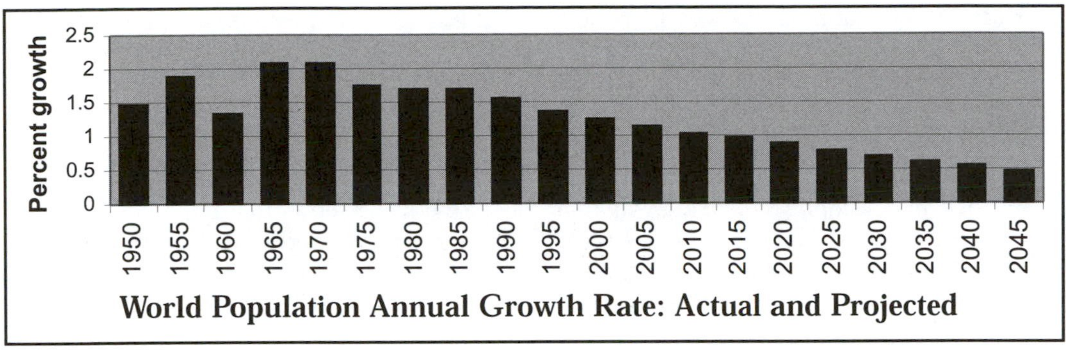

Source: U.S. Census Bureau

As nations developed, they came to rely on contraceptives with greater frequency both to meet individual personal family planning needs and to meet nations' efforts to influence population growth. In developed nations, contraceptive use reached 90 percent of sexually active women in the mid-1990s. Developing nations showed steady increases in the use of contraceptives, with Latin America and the Caribbean rising above an average of 50 percent. In Asia, demand also rose above 50 percent in most countries by 2000. Only in sub-Saharan Africa did contraceptive use remain well below 50 percent by 2000.

Demand for contraceptives rose as they became more socially acceptable around the world. It rose still higher as the children born in the 1960s and 1970s reached reproductive age. Not only did greater percentages of people seek contraceptives, but those percentages represented larger and larger numbers of individuals. Experts predict that other factors, such as the rate at which cities are growing and the increasing levels of education of women, will also increase the demand for contraceptives, since urbanization and education both influence the number of children people choose to have. People between the ages of 15 and 24 years made up more than one-fifth of the world's population in 2000. Estimates suggest that these people want far fewer children than did their parents. Levels of education have been rising steadily around the world as has the population, and those educated children are delaying childbearing in greater numbers as they enter adulthood.

While demographers, scientists who study human populations, are not in complete agreement, the majority opinion by the year 2000 was that the world was close to holding as many people as it could without causing irreversible damage to the ecosystem and without causing greater hardship to the world's poor. Continuing the steady decreases in the annual population growth will depend to a large degree on increasing people's interest in using contraceptives to plan their families, on people wanting fewer children than their parents had, and on manufacturers and nations being able to produce and purchase the contraceptives the people need.

Further reading: Cohen, Joel E. *How Many People Can the Earth Support?* New York: W.W. Norton, 1995. Ravenholt, R. T. "Taking Contraceptives to the World's Poor." *Free Inquiry* 14.2 (1994): 1–6. Rostow, W.W. *The Great Population Spike and After: Reflections on the 21st Century*. New York: Oxford University Press, 1998.

Poverty

The plight of large families living in poverty stirred early birth control advocates to work for making contraceptives easily available to all people. Wealthy people, at the beginning of the century, had access to means of limiting family size unknown to poor women. Even today, people with greater financial means have easier access to family planning than do poorer families. Discrepancies between the resources of wealthier urban populations and poorer rural populations, and people living in crowded slums challenge societies to ease the hardships of poverty and provide family planning services to people who want them.

Measured by income levels, between 20 and 25 percent of the world's people live in absolute poverty, earning less than US$400 each year. More than 90 percent of those people live in developing countries, which in turn experience 90 percent of the world's population growth. When poverty is defined in terms of income, scientific studies have not shown that large families are the result of poverty or that large families cause poverty. Neither has science established that family planning methods directly lead to the elimination of poverty, within a family or within a society.

When scientists and social advocates broaden the definition of poverty to include poor access to education and health care and the inability of people to lead creative and productive lives, then the impact of large families on poverty is clearer and the impact of family planning methods to influence quality of life is clearer.

In families with many children, resources are stretched so that older children often receive greater personal attention, greater access to education, and greater access to health care than younger children. Older children, however, may have to cut short their schooling to help support the family, either by caring for the younger siblings or by working to bring money into the family.

Where infant mortality is still high, or in countries where diseases such as acquired immunodeficiency syndrome (AIDS) increase the mortality rate of younger adults, parents may be likely to give birth to more children to insure their own care in old age. Growing families and limited financial resources can force parents to choose between which children will receive the benefits of what income they have to spend on children. This can leave some children, especially girls, disadvantaged. Girls may be expected to stay home to care for the family when sons are allowed to go to school. Son preference in many cultures may also lead parents to have more children than family resources might comfortably support, in hopes of producing at least one son. In this case, the extra girls may not receive the attention and education their brothers receive and may themselves then have few options other than to enter into marriage and have more children to support them.

Evidence shows that large families experience greater deprivation in societies and groups already at risk from economic poverty. Societies then, according to international agreements and changes in social attitudes, have an obligation to help families gain the knowledge and access to family planning that will help them use family resources to benefit their children. Societies also have been called upon to create social security systems to help support parents in their old age so that parents can limit their family size and allow children to achieve levels of education that will allow them to earn wages higher than the poverty level.

Family studies show that worldwide, if not in every culture, women want fewer children than their mothers wanted. Those studies also show that parents will voluntarily limit their size when given adequate means to control their fertility and adequate means to support their children and themselves. *See also* FAMILY PLANNING; FAMILY SIZE; REPRODUCTIVE RIGHTS

Further reading: Cassen, Robert, ed. *Population and Development: Old Debates, New Conclusions*. New Brunswick, NJ: Transaction, 1994. Population Action International. *Why Population Matters*. Washington, DC: Population Action International, 1996.

Pre-Ejaculatory Fluid

Part of the biological process that prepares a man's reproductive system to expel semen and sperm from his penis during sexual intercourse involves the creation and emission of pre-ejaculatory fluid, which neutralizes any urine that may remain in the urethra. The fluid also provides some lubrication to the end of the penis to aid in inserting that organ into a woman's vagina.

The man's body produces this fluid in the bulbourethral or Cowper's glands that surround the upper portion of the urethra. The glands secrete the fluid into the urethra before ejaculation. The Cowper's glands also produce small amounts of sperm, though the numbers are still in the millions, that could impregnate a woman even if the man's penis only touches her external sex organs.

Studies conducted in the mid-1990s, however, are leading to some rethinking of this biological process. These studies have found no sperm in the pre-ejaculatory fluid and have lead some scientists to argue that pre-ejaculatory fluid itself does not contain sperm. Rather, the sperm found in this fluid remains in the urethra after an ejaculation. If men urinate after one ejaculation and before again having sexual intercourse, they will wash any remaining semen from their urethras.

This scientific difference over the fertility level of pre-ejaculatory fluid is not yet resolved, and most contraceptive and fertility experts recommend that men and women who engage in heavy petting in which the man's penis comes in contact with the woman's genitals use birth control methods if they wish to prevent pregnancy. *See also* EJACULATION; PENIS; REPRODUCTIVE SYSTEM—MALE; SEMEN; SPERM

Further reading: Hatcher, Robert, James Trussel, Felicia Stewart, and others. *Contraceptive Technology*. 16th rev. ed. New York: Irvington, 1994.

Pregnancy

Pregnancy describes the time during which an offspring is growing within a woman's uterus. Also known as the gestational period, pregnancy is seen by most people as beginning at or near the time a sperm fertilizes an egg and ends when a child is delivered into the world.

Most contraceptives work by preventing the union of the sperm and egg and thus preventing pregnancy. However, several birth control mechanisms, most notably the intrauterine device and emergency contraception, function by preventing a fertilized egg from implanting in the uterine wall. These are seen as interrupting pregnancy, and considered by some as abortifacients.

The complex process of early cell development often is disrupted by nature. Fertilization does not guarantee that the zygote will develop into a human embryo. The fertilized cells must evolve through many precisely timed and coordinated biochemical steps for the growing zygote to implant in the uterus.

Scientists estimate that 50 percent of all embryos do not survive. Most are lost during the first two weeks after ovulation, while the fertilized egg travels through the fallopian tube or while it floats within the uterus. Once the egg implants spontaneous loss is less common. Only approximately 15 percent of established pregnancies end in loss of the embryo.

With implantation, the embryo begins secreting human chorionic gonadotropin (hCG), a hormone that maintains the uterine lining. This hormone provides a clear signal that a pregnancy is underway.

Scientific, moral, ethical, and religious debate surrounds those days between fertilization and implantation. The high rate of natural loss of eggs leads many people to believe that pregnancy does not commence until implantation. Likewise, individuals and groups hold different opinions on whether devices that interrupt pregnancies are contraceptives or abortion devices. *See also* ABORTION; CONCEPTION; FERTILIZATION; REPRODUCTIVE SYSTEM—FEMALE

Further reading: McBride, Wayne Z. "Spontaneous Abortion." *American Family Physician* 43 (1991): 175–182. Rothman, Barbara Katz, ed. *Encyclopedia of Childbearing: Critical Perspectives.* Phoenix, AZ: Oryx Press, 1993.

PREVEN

The first oral contraceptives specifically packaged to serve as emergency contraceptives, PREVEN, manufactured by Gynétics, a privately held women's health care company in New Jersey, reached the U.S. market in September 1998. PREVEN provides doctors and women with a method of preventing unintended pregnancy in the event of unprotected sexual intercourse.

PREVEN uses oral contraceptives according to the procedure first described by Canadian Albert Yuzpe in 1974. The PREVEN kit, currently obtainable only by subscription in the United States, contains four combined oral contraceptive pills, each containing ethinyl estradiol, a synthetic estrogen, and levonorgestrel, a synthetic progestin.

PREVEN works to prevent a pregnancy by disrupting the woman's hormonal balance, as do oral contraceptives taken daily. The higher doses of estrogen and progestin mimic the hormonal balance that naturally occurs during the second half of her menstrual cycle and prevent the hormonal changes that would lead to the eruption of a mature egg from a woman's ovary. By preventing ovulation and disrupting the lining of the uterus, PREVEN works like regular contraceptive pills to protect a woman against unwanted pregnancy. PREVEN, like "off-label" uses of oral contraceptives for emergency contraceptive purposes, does not stop a pregnancy once it has begun. Package instructions advise women not to use the product if the pregnancy testing kit included shows she is pregnant. When used correctly, PREVEN has proven successful in preventing six of the eight pregnancies that would be expected if 100 women had unprotected intercourse during any one menstrual cycle. This 75 percent success rate, while effective for an emergency contraceptive, makes PREVEN and other emergency contraceptive pills far less effective than the 99.9 percent effective rate for daily combined oral contraceptive pills.

The most common side effects of PREVEN include nausea or vomiting that may last for a few hours or one to two days. As with oral contraceptives, women with existing medical conditions that create greater risk from estrogen and progestins, such as smoking, would be advised not to use emergency oral contraceptives.

The FDA's approval of PREVEN was based upon 10 studies of emergency contraceptive pills conducted since 1977. Those studies were based upon research conducted during the approval process for similar specific packaging and marketing of emergency contraceptive pills in Europe and New Zealand. The studies verified that the higher doses are highly effective, though not as effective as oral contraceptives taken on a daily basis, at preventing unwanted pregnancy. *See also* EMERGENCY CONTRACEPTION

Further reading: "Emergency Contraception Kit Approved." *Journal of the American Medical Association* 280 (1998): 1472. Food and Drug Administration. "FDA Approves Application for PREVEN Emergency Contraceptive Kit." FDA Talk Paper. 2 September 1998. Online: http://www.fda.gov/bbs/topics/ANSWERS/ANS00892.html, 9 June 1999. Gynétics, Inc. "PREVEN Emergency Contraceptive Kit: The First and Only Emergency Contraceptive Product: Approved by The FDA." Press Release, 2 September 1998. Online: http://www.gynetics.com/gynetics/news/releases/pr199809021.html, 9 June 1999.

Privacy Laws

Arguing that the state and nation had the right to protect the morals of society, and to protect virginity and chastity until marriage, national and state legislators passed laws in the late 1800s in the United States that prohibited the distribution and use of contraceptives even in the privacy of a person's home and within the privacy of marriage.

During the early 1900s, birth control activists fought against these laws, and by the mid- to late twentieth century, legal cases concerning the private use of contraception began arriving in the U.S. Supreme Court. In a series of three specific cases, as well as rulings in aspects of privacy other than regulating fertility, the court established a couple's right to privacy within marriage, an adult's right to privacy in the decision to have children, and expanded the individual right to privacy to include the choice to have an abortion. Before these rulings, many states had already revised existing or written new legislation making legal the use and dissemination of contraceptives and legalizing abortion. The U.S. Supreme Court rulings resulted in all states adjusting their laws to fit the constitutional interpretations of the courts' decisions.

Married couples gained the right to privacy within their legal union when in 1965 the Supreme Court, in a seven-to-two vote in *Griswold v. Connecticut*, struck down an 1879 Connecticut law prohibiting the use of contraceptives, even within marriage. The 1972 six-to-one ruling in *Eisenstadt v. Baird* extended that right to all individuals, whether inside or outside of marriage. Finally, in the *Roe v. Wade* (1973) decision, the justices continued the reasoning that made bearing and begetting children a private matter. Recognizing the conflict between the woman's right to private decisions over her body and the potential rights of the fetus and its potential as a human being, the court limited the right to privacy in the case of abortion to the point of "viability," where the fetus could survive as an individual person outside of the womb.

Nations around the world have had or still have similar restrictive laws concerning the sharing of information and methods and using that information on contraception and abortion.

An individual's right to private decisions in childbearing comes into conflict with state policies and concerns when the health and strength of a nation are determined by the size and health of its population. Charges of coercion have been made against China in enforcing its "one-child" policy, against Peru in forcing sterilization on poor indigenous women, and in India where governmental policies in the 1970s enticed men to have vasectomies without full and knowledgeable consent. In many nations, abortion has put the state in conflict with individuals, both with people who want to terminate pregnancies and with people who want to prevent what they see as the death of a human being in the destruction of a conceptus at any point after fertilization.

International efforts, including the 1994 International Conference on Population and Development in Cairo, Egypt, have worked in the 1990s to increase people's rights to reproductive health, including the private decision to use contraceptives. An agreement adopted by 184 nations during the Cairo conference specifically holds privacy as a specific reproductive right and set goals for countries to meet in ensuring that its citizens have the ability to exercise that right to privacy. *See also* EISENSTADT V. BAIRD; GRISWOLD V. CONNECTICUT; OBSCENITY; REPRODUCTIVE RIGHTS; ROE V. WADE

Further reading: Goldstein, Leslie Friedman. *Contemporary Cases in Women's Rights*. Madison: University of Wisconsin Press, 1994. Strossen, Nadine. "The Right to Be Let Alone: Constitutional Privacy in *Griswold, Roe*, and *Bowers*." In *Benchmarks: Great Constitutional Controversies in the Supreme Court,* edited by Terry Eastland. Grand Rapids, MI: William B. Eerdmans, 1995.

Progesterone

Progesterone, a major female sex hormone, works with estrogen during a woman's menstrual cycle to prepare her reproductive organs to receive a fertilized ovum.

Small amounts of this hormone are made and secreted from a woman's ovaries during the first half of her menstrual cycle, while an egg is still maturing in a follicle on one of her ovaries. After that egg erupts from the pouch of cells during ovulation and begins to travel toward the nearby fallopian tube, the wall that protected it as it grew collapses onto the ovary. Now called the corpus luteum, this convoluted structure begins manufacturing large amounts of progesterone and estrogen. During this, the second half of the woman's cycle, the progesterone prepares her uterus to receive a fertilized egg. At the same time, progesterone changes the consistency of the mucus that plugs the cervix of the uterus, transforming it from a thick plug that sperm cannot penetrate to a thin, slippery substance that actually helps sperm cells travel into the uterus.

Significantly increased levels of progesterone in the blood provide a noticeable signal that ovulation has occurred. These levels remain high until the uterine lining begins to shed during the onset of menstruation when the corpus luteum fades. As the level of progesterone drops, this hormone's influence on the pituitary gland diminishes, allowing the pituitary to once again release follicle stimulating hormone (FSH) and begin again the cycle of maturing eggs on the ovary. Should a fertilized egg implant in the uterine lining, the corpus luteum would continue to produce high levels of progesterone, which in turn would continue to prevent the pituitary gland from releasing the FSH.

Artificial forms of progesterone work alone or with artificial estrogens in oral contraceptives to create the biochemical effect of preventing the pituitary gland from releasing FSH and thus preventing eggs from maturing. Maintaining the levels of progesterone and estrogen in the blood that match the levels found after ovulation in essence prevents the pituitary gland from functioning as it would if a woman were not pregnant.

The ability of chemists developed in the 1940s and 1950s to create sex hormones from the chemical compounds found in certain varieties of plants led to the inexpensive production of synthetic progesterones known as progestins. These manufactured hormones form the basis of modern hormonal contraceptives. *See also* ESTROGEN; HORMONAL CONTRACEPTIVES; HORMONES—SEX; HORMONES—SYNTHETIC; MENSTRUAL CYCLE; REPRODUCTIVE SYSTEM—FEMALE

Further reading: Austin, C. R., and R. V. Short, eds. *Hormonal Control of Reproduction*. Reproduction in Mammals 3. 2nd ed. Cambridge, UK.: Cambridge University Press, 1984. Jones, Richard, E. *Human Reproductive Biology*. San Diego, CA: Academic Press–Harcourt Brace Jovanovich, 1991.

Progestin-Only Contraceptives

Progestin-only contraceptives contain doses of a synthetic, or artificial, version of progesterone, the hormone that supports and maintains a pregnancy. Many hormonal contraceptives contain both a progestin and a synthetic estrogen which work together to prevent pregnancy. The progestin-only contraceptives, such as the "mini-pill," several injectable contraceptives, and devices implanted under a woman's skin, contain only forms of progestins.

Alone, this manufactured hormone, a chemical compound that resembles but is slightly different from naturally occurring progesterone, performs three main contraceptive functions. First, progestins act upon the mucus that plugs the neck of the uterus, the cervix. They help keep that mucus dry, as it is when it blocks the cervix before ovulation. Sperm cannot penetrate this thick cervical plug and by keeping the cervical mucus dry, progestins prevent sperm from entering the woman's uterus.

Second, progestins impair ovulation. Because a woman's natural levels of progesterone are high after ovulation and during pregnancy, her taking progestins keeps her blood levels of the hormone high enough to prevent her hypothalamus and pituitary gland from recognizing a need to secrete the hormones that will begin her menstrual and ovulatory cycle. In essence, her body always thinks it is ovulating or has ovulated and therefore does not mature more eggs toward ovulation.

Third, progestins cause the endometrium to become unreceptive to a fertilized egg. Should ovulation occur, an extremely unlikely event, given the effectiveness of a progestin's first two effects, and the egg become fertilized, the woman's endometrium would not support the growth of the developing egg and menstruation would begin on time despite fertilization.

Over time, progestins commonly lead to amenorrhea, the complete stopping of menstruation. They also cause longer stretches of time between periods of menstrual bleeding. Many women report bleeding in the middays of their cycles early in their use of progestin-only contraceptives, but this generally fades with continued use.

Each of the progestin-only contraceptive methods has its potential drawbacks, including missed pills, difficulty in removing the implants, and the length of time before fertility returns after a woman discontinues use of injected progestins. However, progestin-only contraceptives provide some valuable benefits for some women. Progestins work more effectively than synthetic estrogens in implantable and injectable contraceptives. Women who for reasons such as uterine fibroids should not take estrogens find that they can use progestin-only contraceptives. Women who have had strong reactions to combined contraceptives, such as nausea, severe headaches, or hypertension rarely suffer those side effects with the progestin only products. A woman would be advised not to choose a progestin-only method if she were pregnant or had breast cancer; doctors recommend caution because studies have not completely ruled out risks from the interaction of progestins with hormone changes involved in pregnancy and cancer.

The first-year failure rates of progestin-only contraceptives are among the lowest for all forms of contraception, including sterilization. Norplant, an implant which contains levonorgestrel, prevents pregnancy 99.95 percent of the time, failing only 0.05 of the time. Because it is implanted, a woman choosing this method would not have to worry about remembering to use the method. Depo-Provera, or depot medroxyprogesterone acetate, another progestin, is given as a shot every three months and only requires that a woman choosing this method keep her quarterly appointment with a doctor or clinic. Its perfect use is slightly less easy to achieve than for Norplant, and fails only 0.3 percent of the time. "Mini-pills," which the woman must remember to take daily, have a perfect use failure rate of 0.5 percent, though forgetfulness makes their typical use failure rate 5 percent.

These success rates make progestin-only contraceptives very appealing to many women, despite alterations in their menstrual cycles. They provide easy use options for teenagers and also allow older women to avoid estrogen. *See also* DEPO-PROVERA; HORMONES—SYNTHETIC; NORPLANT; ORAL CONTRACEPTIVES; PROGESTERONE

Further reading: "International Medical Advisory Panel Statement on Steroidal Oral Contraception." *International Planned Parenthood Federation Medical Bulletin* 32.6 (1998): 1–6. Rebar, Robert W., and Leon Speroff. "The New Progestins: Pharmacologic and Clinical Perspectives" *Dialogues in Contraception* 4.1 (1993): 1–10.

Prostate Gland

A man's prostate gland produces fluids that nourish sperm, the male sex cell, and that improve the ability of the sperm to move through the female reproductive system.

This chestnut-sized organ rests below a man's bladder and surrounds the top of the urethra. It is a major producer of semen, the white fluid that carries the mature sperm out of a man's body. The seminal vesicles, attached to the prostate by small ducts, and located just above the prostate, also produce some of the semen. *See also* REPRODUCTIVE SYSTEM—MALE; SEMEN; SPERM

Protestantism

The official churches of the Protestant faiths have supported birth control within marriage since the days of the Reformation in the sixteenth century. In 1520, three years after posting his 95 theses on the church door at Wittenberg, Germany, reform leader and namesake of the Lutheran faith, Martin Luther held that love, not procreation, was the essence of marriage. John Calvin, also a reformist leader, also argued that love was the primary force in a marriage and argued that interpretation of the Bible was open for further study. From those beginnings the non-Catholic Christian faiths primarily have been open to men and women choosing when intercourse would be solely for expressing love and when they would be open to the possibility of conceiving a child.

Protestant faiths generally hold that the individual can understand God's teaching by personal study of the Bible. During the late 1600s and early 1700s in the American colonies and western Europe, people accepted birth control as an individual decision within marriage. Relying then on the natural forms of birth control of abstinence and withdrawal, and perhaps early forms of condoms and vaginal plugs, people began exerting their own influence over conception and childbearing.

With the development in the 1800s of the first modern condoms, made of vulcanized rubber, the debate amongst Protestant church members centered on the specific methods of birth control, rather than the practice of pregnancy prevention itself. Concerned with a society's morals and values, people challenged through their churches the harm that condoms, diaphragms, and spermicides would inflict on the people's morals if they could prevent the outward sign of sexual indiscretions. To protect morals, the major Protestant religions withheld their approval of modern contraceptive methods until well into the middle of the twentieth century.

The scientific understanding of reproduction grew steadily from the mid-1800s on. With the discovery of the ovum and the sperm and of the process by which a sperm fertilizes an ovum, and with the description of the female menstrual cycle and a man's constant fertility, science came to understand better the role people could play in preventing pregnancy and with interfering with the reproductive process. This scientific development led to a new general acceptance of birth control, including among the members of the Protestant faiths, who often saw science as providing them with more effective means to answer the calling for children within their lives. Rather than corrupting morals, birth control allowed people, so the churches came to believe, to further their search for God's calling in their family lives.

Beginning with the Anglican Church in England in 1930, non-Catholic Christian churches began publicly endorsing modern birth control methods. At the Lambeth Conference of the church's bishops in London, the Anglican Church officially approved of the use of artificial forms of birth control. Protestant churches throughout Europe approved modern methods during the next 25 years. In 1956 the General Conference of the Methodist Church and the United Lutheran Church both approved the use of modern contraceptives. That same year The National Council of the Reformed Churches of France and the Church of Finland, a Lutheran denomination, took a public stand approving modern birth control methods.

By the 1960s, Protestant opposition to modern birth control had faded to the degree that contraception was seen as being of no real consequence to the churches or their members. The Protestant faiths worldwide had become so accepting of modern birth control that the topic was no longer an issue. People accepted the presence of birth control in choosing when to have children as they accepted the possibility of having children.

Abortion, however, presented greater conflict among the members of the Protestant faiths. In this religion, as in Catholicism, Judaism, and Islam, more traditional Protestants and individual churches often stood adamantly against interference with reproduction once a sperm had fertilized an egg. From the moment of conception, they argued, human life began, and it was immoral and a violation of Christ's church to stop that pregnancy. More permissive Protestants did not accept that life begins at fertilization but argued that life begins at ensoulment, a moment not yet known to humankind. For these members of Protestant faiths, abortion was a regrettable but acceptable act when sought after careful thought and prayer on the part of the pregnant woman. Protestants remain divided, on a personal and organizational level, over the role of abortion in a person's life. Some argue that abortion is never right. Others argue that abortion can be the lesser of two wrongs and in those circumstances it may be permissible.

Questions of abortion for Protestant faiths also enter into the methodology of modern contraceptives. Those that prevent pregnancy, such as barrier methods and hormonal contraceptive pills which prevent ovulation, are universally acceptable in the Protestant faiths, which generally include Anglican/Episcopalian, Baptist, Congregational, Lutheran, Methodist, Presbyterian, and Quaker denominations. Those methods that interfere with pregnancy after ovulation, an important though not exclusive function of intrauterine devices, are seen as abortifacients and are unacceptable to those Protestants who hold that life begins at fertilization.

The stand on birth control of the Protestant faiths is in conflict with that of the Roman Catholic Church, which argues that the primary reason for marriage is the begetting of children and that each act of sexual intercourse must be open to the possibility of conceiving children. Some see the conflict over birth control as a major obstacle for the Christian faiths as they continue efforts toward reconciliation begun in the late 1900s. *See also* ISLAM; JUDAISM; ROMAN CATHOLIC CHURCH

Further reading: Nuechterlein, James. "Catholics, Protestants, and Contraception." *First Things: A Monthly Journal of Religion and Public Life,* April 1999, 10. Spitzer, Walter O., and Carlyle L. Saylor. *Birth Control and the Christian: A Protestant Symposium on the Control of Human Reproduction*. Wheaton, IL: Tyndale House, 1969.

Puberty

Puberty is the stage in life during which the immature body of a young human grows into the body of a sexually functional adult; the reproductive organs in girls and boys complete the growth process begun during their prenatal development.

For a girl, puberty generally begins between the ages of 9 and 13. For a boy, puberty generally begins between 10 and 14. The first sign of puberty in a girl is usually the development of breast buds, for boys it is the enlargement of the testicles and penis.

The changes of puberty in the bodies of girls and boys are signaled outwardly by rapid growth spurts and internally by dramatic increases in hormonal secretions. A biological mechanism that scientists still do not understand well causes the hypothalamus, an organ in the brain, to signal the pituitary gland, located in the brain just below the hypothalamus, to begin secreting gonadotropins which then signal the gonads, or primary sex organs, to begin secreting greatly increased amounts of estrogen and testosterone. These two primary sex hormones will trigger the final growth of the sex organs.

In girls, those pituitary hormones cause the immature ovaries to begin secreting estrogen. This increase in estrogen first causes the development of secondary sex characteristics, the development of breasts, the growth of pubic and underarm hair, and depositing of fat in a mature female pattern of rounder hips and buttocks and filling out of the breasts. Estrogen also triggers the first build up of blood in the inner lining of a girl's uterus. That first discharge, known as menarche, signals the onset of a girls menstrual cycle though not necessarily of ovulation. Girls experience the beginning of menstruation generally by age 13. Athletically active girls with low body fat percentages may see a significant delay in the onset of menstruation.

Ovulation is the final stage of puberty for a girl. The increases in estrogen will finally trigger follicles on her mature ovaries to begin growing. In those follicles, immature gametes, or ova, begin to mature. Only one egg eventually continues growing to maturing when it ruptures from the follicle and moves toward the waiting fallopian tube. If the egg does not fertilize, it passes through the uterus without implanting and that organ sheds its blood-rich lining. A girl's uterus may shed its lining for several months before the first egg is discharged from the ovary. Her growing body may be secreting enough hormones to cause the uterine lining to thicken before her pituitary gland begins secreting the hormones which trigger the development of the follicles on her ovaries. Within a year or two of her first period, a girl will generally be ovulating regularly. From that point through the onset of menopause in her early 50s, a woman will, for the days the mature egg travels through her system, be fertile.

In boys, the pituitary hormones signal the renewed and increased development of testosterone, the male sex hormone produced in the testicles. That production system has remained dormant since shutting down shortly after birth. At the beginning of puberty, under the influence of increased testosterone levels, a boy's testicles grow larger, his penis grows longer, and his external sex organs finish growing. A boy also grows greater muscle mass in the shoulders, arms, chest, and legs. His larynx enlarges and his voice drops in pitch. He also begins growing facial hair. During the first two years of puberty, boys experience noticeable growth spurts.

The increased levels of testosterone trigger the production of sperm, the male reproductive cells, also in the testicles. From this stage through most of the rest of his life, a man constantly produces sperm, which is stored and finishes maturing in the epididymides where it awaits ejaculation when his body abruptly expels the sperm, in semen, through his urethra. A boy may have his first ejaculation between ages 11 and 15, though any time between 8 and 21 is normal. This may occur in his sleep, in response to masturbation, or during sexual intercourse.

Puberty, the physical maturing of the human body, often takes less time than adolescence, the stage in life where social and psychological development continues. Both puberty and adolescence takes place during the second decade of a person's life, but both do not necessarily occur at the same pace. *See also* ADOLESCENTS; SEX EDUCATION

Further reading: Sapolsky, Robert. "Growing Up in a Hurry." *Discover* 13 (1992): 40–42. "When Your Child Is Close to Puberty." *American Family Physician* 60 (1999).

Q

Quinacrine

Quinacrine, an effective anti-malarial drug taken orally and used effectively since the 1920s, became the center of a contraceptive research controversy in the 1990s.

In the late 1970s, Dr. Jaime Zipper of Santiago, Chile, developed a method of non-surgical female sterilization that involved placing pellets of quinacrine in a woman's uterus, very close to the opening to her fallopian tubes. As the pellets dissolved, the chemical burned the fallopian tube tissue enough to cause scarring. The scarring in turn blocked the fallopian tubes, preventing sperm from entering the tubes and eggs from leaving the tubes. Since that discovery, medical professionals in many countries have used quinacrine pellets to sterilize more than 100,000 women.

Trials of the procedure in China, India, Indonesia, the Philippines, and Vietnam in the 1980s established that quinacrine provided an inexpensive, effective method of permanent contraception. Safer than surgical sterilization, the most commonly used form of contraception worldwide, quinacrine provided an option for permanent sterilization in countries with few and distant necessary medical facilities. The effectiveness of the quinacrine procedure improved with experience and refinement and by the early 1990s was reported to be between 80 and 90 percent effective at preventing pregnancy, resulting in one or two pregnancies within a year. Studies conducted in Iran from 1990 to 1994 suggested that success rates might be even higher, at 98 percent or better.

By 1994, however, a conflict between those concerned with dangers of population growth and those concerned with women's rights and acceptable ways to research, develop, and provide contraceptives slowed quinacrine's use as a sterilization method and created a battleground between some feminist organizations and population organizations. At the center of the controversy lay questions of the appropriateness of testing contraceptives, a preventive use of medicine and technology, on people in developing countries. Quinacrine, though approved by the U.S. Food and Drug Administration for its use against malaria, has not been approved by the United States as a contraceptive. The FDA requires that contraceptives undergo separate testing. Tests on animals to prove quinacrine safety in the doses used in contraception had not been completed before doctors with access to the medicine began sharing it in study programs with doctors in other countries.

Those doctors have argued that to bar quinacrine's use goes against FDA policy of allowing doctors to use approved medicines for other medical procedures. The World Health Organization also holds different and conflicting standards for development and testing of medicines for contraceptives than for tropical disease treatment and prevention. The doctors who support quinacrine's use for sterilization also argue that all modern contraceptives, most notably the oral contraceptive pill, relied upon tests in developing countries to establish their effectiveness and safety before they were approved in the United States and other developed countries. Further, advocates of quinacrine argue that this method provides a less expensive, safer alternative for women who would otherwise seek surgical sterilization as their contraceptive choice.

Feminists argue that the use of quinacrine in developing countries without the testing that would lead to approval in developed countries amounts to experimentation on women. They worry that side effects, such as risks of ectopic pregnancy and cancer, are too great to risk learning of them from women who have undergone the sterilization procedure. Feminists have called for a ban on the use of quinacrine, unless it undergoes the necessary FDA laboratory testing to establish its safety.

The controversy over the use of quinacrine continues, with the FDA banning in 1999 its sale by two American doctors who had been involved in its use worldwide. The World Health Organization has taken a stand against the chemical sterilization; however, advocates for its safety and its necessity for many women work to keep the method available and to encourage its testing and continued development. *See also* RESEARCH (CONTRACEPTIVE); STERILIZATION

Further reading: Bhatia, Rajani, and Anne Hendrixson. "The Quinacrine Controversy." *The Network News,* May 1999, 3. Kessel, Elton. "Quinacrine Sterilization Revisited." Commentary. *The Lancet,* 10 September 1994, 698–700. Lisheron, Mark. "Embracing the Complexities." *American Journalism Review,* June 1999, 40.

R

Reproductive Equality

The relative ease of interrupting a woman's reproductive cycle led in the twentieth century to a far greater number of female birth control methods than of male birth control methods. This biological, technical, and social trend, added to the gender discrimination against women within families and societies, led to concerns over a lack of reproductive equality by health advocates and women's advocates.

As of 1999, women had access to a variety of birth control methods, ranging from one-time-use vaginal spermicides with low effectiveness at preventing pregnancy to the almost perfect reversible pregnancy prevention of injectable and implantable hormonal contraceptives to permanent sterilization through surgery. Men had two contraceptives available to them—the condom, a latex barrier placed over the penis, and vasectomy, surgery to block the vas deferens, which carry sperm from the testicles into the reproductive system.

To help eliminate that imbalance, and with encouragement from women's groups and population experts, scientists began intensely studying in the 1980s and 1990s alternative forms of male contraceptives that would allow men to share more equally in family planning efforts and pregnancy prevention. As of 1999, researchers were studying and testing more than 10 methods of long-term reversible male contraception. Research into men's attitudes indicated their willingness to share more equitably in personally using contraception to prevent unwanted pregnancies.

The different actions women and men take in discussing and deciding upon whether to use a birth control method and which method to use also received close study in the 1990s as people from different aspects of the reproductive health initiatives worked to understand how couples decided to use contraception. The more equality a woman feels she has in a relationship with a man, they found, the greater her ability to discuss family planning and contraception. That half of the equation had been long understood by family planning program developers, but in the 1990s research also revealed that men were willing, even eager, to participate more fully in family planning discussions and choices. However, research also showed that clinic services directed mostly at women often shut men out of the family planning process. Growing awareness of this inequality led program developers to begin working by the late 1990s to redesign programs to be more inclusive of men. By involving men in clinic appointments and by aiming reproductive health care information at men, public health workers aimed to increase overall knowledge of family planning, to create a balance between women and men, and to raise understanding of contraception.

Earlier efforts by reproductive health care providers and family planning program developers focused almost exclusively on the use of condoms. That focus led to the dichotomy that said men were responsible for disease protection and women were responsible for pregnancy prevention. Such segregation led to stereotypes and miscommunication that family planning specialists hoped to change with a gender-balanced approach to education about contraception.

Survey findings from around the world demonstrated that men generally approve of family planning. Researchers began discovering that men, overall, wanted to be involved in the family planning decisions. Studies also revealed that men and women had different reasons for understanding, choosing, and approving of the different contraceptives available to them. This awareness of men's views and of gender differences in the family planning decisions encouraged family planning providers and contraceptive researchers to be more inclusive of men in their programs and to create reproductive equality in all aspects of family planning. *See also* FEMINISM; MALE CONTRACEPTIVES

Further reading: Brooks, Marlies. "Men's Views on Male Hormonal Contraception: A Survey of the Views of Attenders at a Fitness Centre in Bristol, UK." *British Journal of Family Planning* 24 (1998): 7–17. Drennan, Megan. "New Perspectives on Men's Participation." *Population Reports* 26.2 (1998). Grady, William R., Daniel H. Klepinger, and Anjanette Nelson-Wally. "Contraceptive Characteristics: The Perceptions and Priorities of Men and Women." *Family Planning Perspectives* 31 (1999): 168.

Reproductive Health

Toward the end of the twentieth century, focus of international health care and social justice advocates shifted from examining issues of population only as they relate to pregnancy and child mortality to a broader view of considering a person, a community, a nation, and a world's total reproductive health. This shift in attention, which was specifically written into the international agreement that arose from the 1994 International Conference on Population and Development (ICPD) in Cairo, Egypt, looks at the total health of a person, woman, man, and child, as it relates to his or her ability to reproduce and to enjoy a healthy sex life.

The ICPD's program of action specifically aims to reach the "highest attainable standard of physical and mental health," and includes providing all people with access to reproductive care, family planning, and sexual health information and services. This broadening of focus puts reproductive health above population concerns while anticipating that improved reproductive health will curb practices that threaten individual health and that encourage population growth.

This approach places an emphasis on providing information, counseling, medical services, and resources for people to use in learning about and protecting their reproductive well-being. Family planning and contraception for women and men forms one aspect of reproductive health.

Preventing, treating, and curing reproductive tract infections and sexually transmitted diseases also concerns reproductive health professionals and public health workers. Sexually transmitted diseases threaten people's lives and reproductive health. Reproductive tract infections, if undetected and untreated, often lead to ectopic pregnancies, which occur outside of the uterus, usually in the fallopian tube, and often lead to rupturing of the fallopian tube or damage to the woman's reproductive system. Sexually transmitted diseases and reproductive tract infections cause most of the world's cases of involuntary infertility.

The international effort to improve reproductive health has focused sharp attention on the health of adolescent girls, who experience a variety of early threats to their reproductive health. For many social reasons, including early marriage, girls from puberty at age 12 to about age 19 face significant risk to their reproductive health, including early pregnancy, early exposure to reproductive infections, and early threat of death from high-risk pregnancies. Efforts to protect the health of adolescent girls undertaken by nations as a result of the Cairo agreement include working for social change, developing strategies to delay the age of marriage and the age of childbearing, protecting girls from unsafe abortions, and changing customs, such as female genital mutilation, that threaten a girl's long-term reproductive well-being.

This broadening of perspective that came out of the ICPD includes men's reproductive health. Research into male contraceptives intensified in the 1980s and 1990s. Attention to the health needs of both men and women has put even more attention on work to develop contraceptives that would allow men to protect themselves and their partners from unwanted pregnancies. Protection from sexually transmitted diseases and infertility in men have received greater attention as a result of an international broadening of the understanding of reproductive and sexual health. *See also* REPRODUCTIVE RIGHTS

Further reading: Larkin, Marilynn. "Male Reproductive Health: A Hotbed of Research." *The Lancet,* 15 August 1988, 552. Mitchell, Marc D., Joan Littlefield, and Suzanne Gutter. "Costing of Reproductive Health Services." *International Family Planning Perspectives* 29 (1999): S17–S29. Population Action International. *Fact Sheet No. 9: How are Nations Responding to the Call for Increased Funding for Reproductive Health?* Washington, DC: Population Action International, 1999.

Reproductive Rights

The reproductive rights of women have been a focus of the international birth control movement since its beginnings in the late nineteenth and early twentieth century. Fundamentally, people like Margaret Sanger, in the United States, and Aletta Jacobs, in the Netherlands, believed that a woman had a right to control her own body, including when and if to have children. Images of women dying in childbirth during their eleventh or twelfth pregnancy in as many years with worn, tired bodies, or bleeding to death from botched illegal and often self-induced abortions, led crusaders to fight to develop the means by which women could protect their health and their lives as they maintained their health and expressed their sexuality.

By the end of the twentieth century, after decades of focusing international aid and fertility control efforts on world population issues, reproductive health advocates, international aid workers, and feminists worked to return the focus of family planning to the rights of women—and men—to determine for themselves when to have children. By 2000, international agreements and global efforts were working to provide people with this human right and to assure that each man, woman, and child had the means to protect and even regulate their reproductive health.

Advocates state that reproductive rights include the right to reproductive health—a persons' physical, mental, and social well-being as it relates to her or his reproductive system. Within that right women and men need to be able to have a satisfying sex life, to choose if and when to have children, and to be safe from reproductive diseases. For women, this also means to be protected against the risk of death from pregnancy and abortion due to failures by the society to provide adequate and safe means for those processes.

Implied within the right to choose if and when to have children is a person's right to the information and methods she or he needs to prevent pregnancy. Contraception and family planning, in this shift of focus in global efforts from population concerns to individual rights, became ways through which people could exercise their reproductive rights. This right requires that nations work to provide contraceptives and family planning methods to people to help individuals meet their own needs rather than to help the governments meet population control needs.

Advocates argue that a woman's right to an education is part of her reproductive rights. Through an education, a woman develops the ability to learn about and understand how to achieve her right to choose if and when to have children. They suggest that reproductive rights include the right to choose if and when to marry as well as if and when to have children. By extension, women and men should be free from coercion, by individuals or governments, in the expression of their reproductive rights. This includes the right not to be misled and coerced into undergoing contraceptive techniques such as sterilization or insertion of an intrauterine device.

Recognizing reproductive rights as part of the larger category of human rights allowed advocates to argue for the support of reproductive rights from nations through their agreements on human rights documents. According to international agreements, governments must provide adequate access to family planning and to health care, and nations must provide laws that protect people's reproductive rights as they protect their overall human rights.

In Teheran, Iran, in 1968, at the International Conference on Human Rights convened by the United Nations, participants agreed that "parents have a basic human right to determine freely and responsibly the number and spacing of their children." Since then, through succeeding international conferences on human rights, population and development, and women's rights, UN member nations and nongovernmental organizations have expanded the meaning of that statement and clarified the details of a person's reproductive rights.

In Cairo, Egypt, in 1994, nations adopted a program of action that defines reproductive rights and specifies actions nations need to take to ensure and improve access to those rights by their citizens. These rights were repeated and emphasized during the Fourth World Conference on Women held in 1995 in Beijing, China. The Cairo program of action specified measures that nations would be required to take to bring family planning into the perspective of a person's overall health and also provided actions nations could follow to provide women with the social as well as biological tools they would need to achieve their reproductive rights.

Concern among reproductive health professionals in the years following the Cairo program of action focused on the limited resources nations had to bring about such sweeping changes in their societies. Within the context of providing education and broader health services, nations would fall short of needed money for supplying contraceptives and funding specific family planning programs. International health professionals worried that less spending, not more, would be devoted to providing contraception. Reproductive rights advocates, however, contend that educating women and building social structures around the world that support women's access to the means of achieving their reproductive rights will help them fight for and achieve access to the family planning methods they need.

The United Nations reconvened in 1999 to assess the progress member nations had achieved in reaching the reproductive rights goals set in Cairo. While nations had moved steadily toward broadening their focus from supporting family planning services to supporting reproductive health services, funding to meet the goals of the 1994 conferences fell behind. Calls to action in 1999 included emphasizing the need for donor organizations and communities to meet their obligations to fund changes in reproductive rights practices around the world. *See also* FEMINISM; REPRODUCTIVE HEALTH

Further reading: Dixon-Mueller, Ruth. *Population Policy & Women's Rights: Transforming Reproductive Choice*. Westport, CT: Praeger, 1993. Packer, Corinne A. A. *The Right to Reproductive Choice*. Abo, Finland: Abo Akademi University/ Institute for Human Rights, 1996. United Nations Population Fund (UNFPA). *The State of World Population 1999: 6 Billion: A Time for Choices*. New York: United Nations Population Fund Information and External Relations Division, 1999. Online: http://www.unfpa.org/swp/ 1999, 7 March 2000.

Reproductive System—Female

Before she is born, nature provides a woman with all of the sex cells, ovum or eggs, that she will need and places them at the beginning of her reproductive system. The immature eggs grow in the female fetus and gravitate to the surface of the ovaries where, late in prenatal development, they stop developing and await the girl's birth and entering into puberty at about age 13.

The adult woman's reproductive system, in an ebb-and-tide cycle of two main sex hormones, regularly matures one egg at a time and prepares it to travel through these organs where it may or may not be fertilized by a male sperm. The female system is episodic, made up of phases of development, maturity, transportation, and either implantation or deterioration of that egg cell. From beginning to end, this cycle takes approximately 28 days. That time span is a species average and the cycle varies enough from woman to woman, and even from month to month for any one woman, to make predicting the exact stage of each monthly cycle very difficult.

However, that same episodic nature of her system has provided scientists with ample opportunities to develop methods for interrupting and even stopping the cycle. Therefore, birth control research has centered first on the female reproductive system for developing reliable accessible contraceptive methods.

A woman's two ovaries, her primary sex organs, rest on either side of her abdomen, near but not attached to the fallopian tubes. Hormones from her pituitary gland trigger one dormant egg to resume growing toward maturity. As the egg grows, the ovary produces estrogen, the primary female hormone. This hormone then triggers changes in the woman's uterine lining. It also signals the pituitary to stop sending the hormones that encourage more eggs to begin growing.

Once mature, the egg erupts from its follicle on the ovary during ovulation. It soon moves into the nearby fallopian tube and begins its journey toward the uterus. Fertilization most frequently occurs in whichever of these tubes the egg is descending if sperm are present and penetrate the surface of the egg. Whether fertilized or not, each egg takes about three days to move through the fallopian tubes.

Meanwhile, after the egg leaves the follicle on the ovary, that follicle begins secreting progesterone, as well as estrogen. Progesterone also influences the uterine lining, preparing it should the need to support a fertilized egg arise.

At the other end of the fallopian tube, the egg enters the uterus. This muscular organ has been undergoing changes as the egg has matured on the ovary and descended through the fallopian tube. The inner lining of the uterus, the endometrium, under the influence of estrogen and progesterone, has thickened with blood to prepare a rich, cushioned resting place for a fertilized egg. In the very common event that an egg has not been fertilized, the uterus sheds during menstruation this nutrient-rich lining and the bloody discharge passes out of the woman's body through the neck of the uterus, the cervix, and the vagina.

The first day of this shedding of the lining marks the end of one 28-day reproductive cycle and the beginning of the next. As women and medical professionals time the cycle, "Day 1" is counted as the first day of the menstrual period.

The vagina, as the canal that connects the outside world with the inner female reproductive organs, provides the place in which a man deposits his sperm-filled semen in the woman's body. It also provides a relatively easy and effective place to insert a barrier to the movement of that sperm further into the woman's body. The diaphragm and cervical cap cover the cervix, or neck of the uterus, which protrudes slightly into the top of the vagina. When fitted and worn properly and inserted into the vagina by a woman before she has intercourse, they offer strong protection against pregnancy.

However, interrupting the hormone-controlled cycle that matures an egg and prepares the uterus to receive a fertilized egg has given scientists the means of effectively causing temporary infertility and preventing a mature egg from leaving the ovary and in preventing a fertilized egg from implanting in the uterine lining. By manufacturing in a laboratory forms of natural hormones, science has developed highly effective contraceptives that alter the hormonal controls of her reproductive system.

These contraceptives do not alter the organs themselves and provide rates of pregnancy prevention, when used properly according to package directions, that comes very close to the pregnancy prevention of surgical sterilization. Physically altering a woman's fallopian tubes by severing them and closing the ends or by placing bands around them causes sterility. Also, removing a woman's uterus in a surgical procedure known as hysterectomy also causes sterility. In some instances fallopian tubes have been reconnected after tubal sterilization, but the process is seen as a permanent form of sterility. Hysterectomies do permanently remove a woman's ability to bear offspring.

Both the physical nature of the reproductive tract and the hormonal system involved in the female reproductive system have provided many opportunities for interfering with this biological process and preventing the union of the mature egg and the male sperm cell. *See also* CERVIX; FALLOPIAN TUBES; HORMONAL CONTRACEPTIVES; HYSTERECTOMY; MENSTRUAL CYCLE; MENSTRUATION; OVULATION; OVUM AND OVARIES; TUBAL STERILIZATION; UTERUS; VAGINA

Further reading: McKerns, Kenneth W., ed. *Reproductive Processes and Contraception*. New York: Plenum, 1981.

Reproductive System—Male

The reproductive system of a healthy, fertile male constantly produces sperm by the millions. These tiny sex cells are always available to impregnate a woman should that man reach sexual climax during intercourse and ejaculate his sperm into her vagina. The constant production of sperm in the testicles has proven a challenge to scientists in developing a chemical form of birth control, one a man could use constantly to decrease his fertility level as many women use birth control pills to decrease their fertility levels.

Modern birth control devices and techniques for men put up physical barriers to prevent the sperm from reaching a mature ovum in the woman's body. Those physical barriers, however, either result in sterility as does a vasectomy, or require the interruption of intercourse to apply them, as does the condom. However, researchers are at work on developing birth control methods that allow men to take more long-term actions to temporarily alter their fertility. Researchers are studying ways to alter sperm themselves, to change how they react when they reach the mature egg, and are studying how levels of male sex hormones influence a man's fertility. Scientists are, however, challenged by difficulties in decreasing fertility without decreasing the man's sexual desires or his physical characteristics.

Fertility for a man begins in his two testicles, small oval-shaped organs that hang in the scrotum, a small sack-like structure that

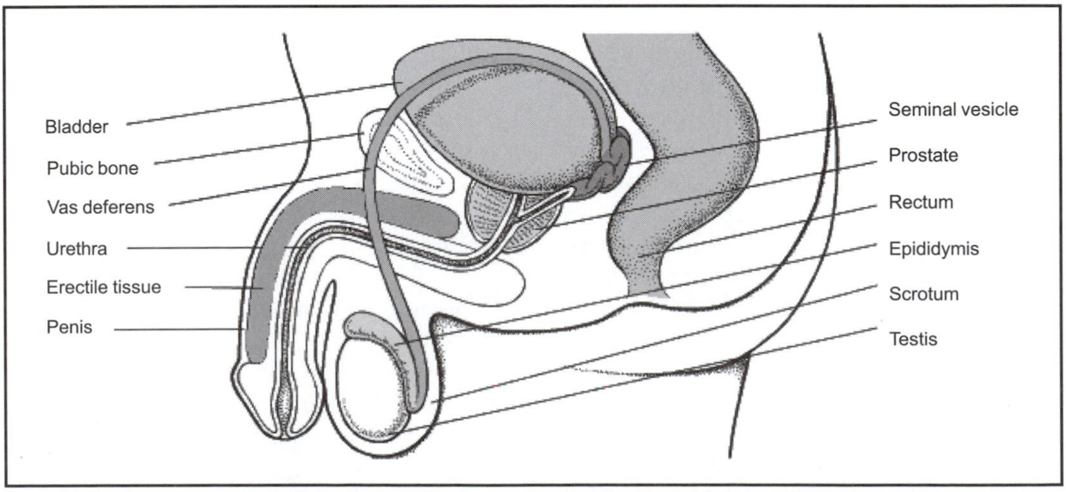

The male body makes sperm cells in the testicles then stores them in the epididymus. During ejaculation, the sperm travels through the system and out the tip of the penis. From the *Merck Manual of Medical Information, Home Edition*, p. 1056; edited by Mark H. Beers and Robert Berkow, © 1997 by Merck & Co., Inc., Whitehouse Station, NJ.

is suspended outside of his body below and in the front of his pelvis and behind his penis. A healthy man has two testicles, one on each side of his body, each having an identical biological structure. Both sides of the system produce sperm and function in the same manner.

Here in the cool temperature of the seminiferous tubules of the testicles, a man's body produces the tiny sperm cells. If the testicles were located inside of the man's body, his warm internal temperature would kill the newly made sperm and he would be infertile. In the cooler outer temperature, sex cells are produced steadily. They are stored in the epididymis, a long tube connected to and resting on the testicle. In this duct, the sperm mature and await the process that will send them through the remainder of the reproductive system.

Before the sperm travel from the epididymis, a man must become sexually aroused. Stimulation of the penis during sexual intercourse then moves the sperm cells out of the epididymis and into the vas deferens, two more long ducts that travel up through the pelvis wall and into the man's lower abdomen. They travel behind the man's ureters and in front of the bladder and connect to the seminal vesicles and finally to the prostate gland where the two halves of the reproductive system finally come together.

Semen, the fluid that carries the sperm out of the man's body, is manufactured in the prostate gland, a bulb-like organ below the bladder, and the seminal vesicles, which lie above the prostate and behind the bladder. At the lower end of the prostate, the reproductive tract connects to the urethra. In a man, this tube serves as a path out of the body for sperm as well as for urine. The urethra travels from inside the man's lower abdomen and into his penis.

During the early stages of sexual arousal, tissue in a man's penis fills with blood, causing that external organ to become large and quite stiff. Further stimulation of the tissue of the penis causes physical reactions in the nerves of the spine which signal the muscles in the testicles, the epididymides, the vas deferens, and the prostate to rhythmically contract and release. These contractions force the sperm along the reproductive tract to the internal opening of the urethra.

The much stronger contractions caused by the physical intensity of intercourse cause muscles at the base of the penis to begin contracting and eventually, in the abrupt explosive contraction of ejaculation, to shoot the sperm-filled semen out through the tip of the man's penis.

Testosterone stimulates the production of sperm in the testicles; it, too, is produced in those two external organs. Testosterone is the main male sex hormone and is responsible, at puberty, about 13 to 15 years of age, for causing the enlargement of the testicles, the production of sperm, and the development of secondary sexual characteristics in a male.

The Cowper's or bulbourethral gland, a tiny gland located below the prostate and connected to the urethra, produces the fluid that precedes the semen on its journey out of the man's body and that neutralizes any urine that may remain in this tube. Recent scientific study challenges the belief that the Cowper's gland manufactures a small amount of sperm. While sperm is often found in the cleansing fluid this gland produces, studies in the 1990s suggest that any sperm in this pre-ejaculatory fluid comes from a previous ejaculation. Still, family planning counselors and doctors warn people that pre-ejaculatory fluid may impregnate a woman if it comes in contact with her external genitalia, even if the man's penis is not inserted into her vagina. Some scientists advise men to urinate after an ejaculation to flush remaining sperm from the urethra, thus making the fluid from the Cowper's devoid of sperm.

Primarily because a man's body constantly produces sperm, scientists have turned to the woman's reproductive system, a more episodic process, to discover methods of preventing sperm from reaching mature eggs. Also, because the sperm leave the man's body and the eggs do not, scientists have found it more effective to put up barriers to sperm outside of the man's reproductive system. For those reasons, most birth control devices that have been developed to this point have had more to do with female physiology than with male physiology. *See also* EJACULATION; MALE CONTRACEPTIVES; PENIS; PRE-EJACULATORY FLUID; PROSTATE GLAND; REPRODUCTIVE SYSTEM—FEMALE; SEMEN; SPERM; TESTICLES; TESTOSTERONE; VAS DEFERENS

Further reading: McKerns, Kenneth W., ed. *Reproductive Processes and Contraception*. New York: Plenum, 1981.

Research (Contraceptive)

Reproductive choice, population demands, and epidemics of sexually transmitted and reproductive tract diseases are pushing forward research into new methods of contraception and fertility control. At the same time feminist and antiabortion social movements and the threat of lawsuits in product liability cases are opposing work to develop new contraceptives.

Science, critics and researchers believe, has the capacity to develop a "second contraceptive revolution," similar to the revolution of the 1960s that made available to women hormonal contraceptives like the birth control pill. This revolution could take advantage of recent discoveries in molecular and cellular biology to bring to women—and men—a variety of products that would prevent fertilization by focusing on precise functions of specific aspects of either sperm or egg cells. Nonprofit organizations in the late 1990s were investing in research that would alter the outer layer of the sperm cell to prevent it from penetrating the female egg. Other research explored ways to alter the egg itself to make it impenetrable. Such cell manipulations, researchers believe, will provide contraceptive benefits without the side effects associated with contraceptives that manipulate hormone levels.

This "revolution" remains in the future in part because pharmaceutical companies have been reluctant to conduct research into new products. Faced with the incidence of product liability lawsuits in the 1970s cases of the Dalkon Shield, an intrauterine device, and the 1990s cases of Norplant, an implantable hormonal contraceptive, companies veered from researching new contraceptives to researching drugs to protect people from or cure reproductive diseases.

New birth control products developed in the 1980s and 1990s refined old products. Very low dose contraceptive pills entered the market; "mini-pills" that contained only a progesterone also became available. Even the emergency contraceptive, PREVEN, that reached the U.S. market in 1998 relied on a special combination of combined oral contraceptive pills in high doses. In 1999 Barr Laboratories announced it was developing a new packaging of hormonal contraceptive pills that would prevent menstruation for three months, leaving a woman to have four periods each year.

The World Health Organization, nonprofit organizations such as Family Health International and the Population Council, and research universities, such as Johns Hopkins University, conducted most of the contraceptive research at the end of the twentieth century. With financial resources more limited than those of the business community, these groups developed new barrier contraceptives, new methods of administering hormonal contraceptives such as transdermal patches, and researched immunocontraceptives, also known as anti-fertility vaccines. While these organizations actively pursued research, their low level of funding, some suggest, prevented them from producing marketable products by the end of the twentieth century.

The development of mifepristone, originally known as RU–486, demonstrates the movement of pharmaceutical companies away from research and development and the need for nonprofit organizations to take up the task. Available in Europe since the late 1970s and early 1980s, mifepristone was undergoing testing to lead to U.S. Food and Drug Administration approval in the late 1990s. This drug, known as an abortion pill, was seen by reproductive health advocates as the most innovative product to reach the market after the hormonal pill. The French pharmaceutical company that developed mifepristone almost stopped research under protests from antiabortion activists and finally turned over rights to the Population Council in the United States to develop the product in that country.

International public health needs, including efforts to reduce unplanned pregnancies worldwide, reduce legal and illegal abortions, and help nations reach their population goals, gave rise to great concern among human rights activists and policy advisers that not enough scientific effort and money was being spent on contraceptive research. They recommended that research focus on cellular approaches to contraceptives. New products need to take into consideration the feature of current contraceptives that prevent people from using them as widely as their developers expected. Side effects, the need to remember the product daily, or to use it with each act of sexual intercourse often keep people from using the current mix of contraceptives. New contraceptive research hopes to produce contraceptives that avoid or work around these aversions. *See also* FAMILY HEALTH INTERNATIONAL; FUTURE METHODS OF CONTRACEPTION; MIFEPRISTONE; POPULATION COUNCIL; WORLD HEALTH ORGANIZATION

Further reading: Fishel, Joy. "Contraceptive Technologies: How Much Choice Do We Really Have?" *The Zero Population Growth Reporter,* March/April, 1997. Online: http://www.zpg.org/Reports_Publications/Reports/report40.html, 6 March 2000. Harrison, Polly F., and Allan Rosenfield, eds. *Contraceptive Research and Development: Looking to the Future.* Washington, DC: National Academy Press, 1996. Houppert, Karen. "The Politics of Birth Control: How Prolife Forces Strangle Research." *Village Voice,* October 1996, 23–30.

Rhythm Method. *See* FERTILITY AWARENESS

Risk

Risk from a birth control method involves the potential for a person to develop a life-threatening condition as a result of using that method. All modern contraceptive methods carry a risk for some people. With careful screening, physicians and health care professionals can help women and men avoid that risk. In some instances, contraceptive methods have been shown to protect people from the risk of developing life-threatening conditions.

In general, the medical risks women face in using modern contraceptive methods, most of which work with a woman's body, are very small. Many of those risks are more closely related to non-contraceptive aspects of a woman's health or lifestyle than to the device itself. While using combined oral contraceptives (COCs), for example, a woman's risk of heart attack was 1 in 100,000 in 1991. Her risk of stroke while using COCs was 3 in 100,000. Health care practitioners suggest that even that slight risk could be decreased with effective screening by medical professionals as they advise women concerning their contraceptive choices.

Scientific study of contraceptives continues to asses the medical risks of the methods on modern use. The results of that study can lead to even safer use for the women who choose those devices. Some people argue though that no device should be issued until all hazards have been well studied, confirmed, or refuted. To learn more about their risks, women can and are advised to carefully read package materials and consult in detail with their health care providers.

COCs have undergone intense study and modification to understand and reduce the risks to women who take them. As the only prescription drug given to people to prevent a healthy process, hormonal contraceptive pills have received intense scrutiny since they were first made publicly available in 1960. The doses of estrogen and progestin in early contraceptives, hindsight demonstrated, were much higher than necessary to prevent pregnancy. Those high doses increased the chances that women would develop blood clots deep in their veins, most frequently their legs, a condition known as deep vein thrombosis. As researchers studied this risk they discovered that doses of estrogen over 100 micrograms were a major cause of this problem. By the mid-1960s the doses of estrogen in commonly prescribed pills began falling until in the 1990s the doses were well below

35 micrograms and some very low dose pills were as low as 20 micrograms. That reduction in dose led to significantly fewer reports of circulatory risks from COCs.

This research into contraceptive doses also revealed that women who smoke are at particular risk from COCs for developing circulatory problems and accounted for a significant number of women who developed the life-threatening circulatory problem. Women who smoke are strongly discouraged, by physicians and manufacturers, from using hormonal contraceptives.

The risk of women developing cancer from hormonal contraceptives has also proven to be very slight if any risk exists at all. While studies from the 1980s suggested an increase in a woman's risk of breast cancer, when scientists reexamined those studies in the 1990s they found little or no actual risk. Further studies are ongoing. Studies have found a slight but unclear relationship between COCs and cervical cancer. In fact, COCs are known to protect women from endometrial and ovarian cancer.

The vast majority of women have no conditions that indicate a high risk of health problems from COCs. Most women can successfully use hormonal contraceptives with very low chance of health hazard or death.

Spermicides also bring with them the risk of damaging, when used in too strong doses, the the naturally protective organisms that exist in a woman's vagina. Spermicides can also cause irritation and burning.

Life circumstances can increase the risk women, and men, face from a specific contraceptive. For example, women who might choose an intrauterine device (IUD) to prevent pregnancy but who have more than one sexual partner would be at significant risk of contracting a sexually transmitted disease and developing pelvic inflammatory disease. Women who smoke, particularly those who are more than 35 years old, have a significant risk of developing circulatory problems if they take hormonal contraceptives.

The role contraceptives play in helping people plan their reproductive lives brings with it a connection to sexually transmitted disease (STD) and the risks people face from this health aspect of their reproductive lives. No contraceptive completely prevents the risk of partners passing to each other an STD. The male latex condom and the female polyurethane condom greatly reduce a person's risk of contracting STDs, such as human immunodeficiency virus (HIV), hepatitis B, and herpes genitalis (genital warts), that are transmitted primarily through vaginal-penile intercourse. Some spermicides have proven effective in the lab at destroying many STD organisms; tests are still underway to establish their effectiveness in actual use. Vaginal barriers, such as diaphragms, sponges, and cervical caps, work in conjunction with spermicides and offer people similar risk reduction to spermicides used alone. Hormonal contraceptives offer little protection against the risk of contracting most STDs though evidence suggests that they have a protective effect against pelvic inflammatory disease (PID).

To minimize the risk women face from any contraceptives, physicians and manufacturers work carefully to identify women with preexisting medical conditions that would jeopardize their health while using a specific pregnancy prevention method. Taking careful health histories and developing clear communication with a client can help a health care provider detect problems before they occur. This knowledge can help professionals direct women away from potentially harmful products to products that pose very little risk. Women who might be at risk from the estrogen component of COCs could possibly take progestin-only pills or injectable hormones or they might consider using an IUD, most of which contain no hormones. Women at risk for pelvic inflammatory disease from an IUD or a barrier contraceptive may be advised to consider hormonal contraceptives.

Inaccurate or improper use of a contraceptive also increases a person's risk of medical complications from that device. Female barrier contraceptives, such as the vaginal sponge and cervical cap, if left in too long or used during menstruation, increase a woman's chances of experiencing toxic shock.

Natural forms of pregnancy prevention, such as fertility awareness methods and withdrawal, appear to present no life-threatening physical risk to the people who use them.

Rumors and myths concerning the risks of contraceptives methods, most publicly the contraceptive pill, have led women to temporarily reject a method that they had already found effective. When reports reached the press of scientific studies of "third-generation progestins," those developed in the 1980s and 1990s from progestins already in use and well known, indicated that these newer progestins caused a greater risk of blood clots, circulatory problems, and heart attack, women stopped using their pills. Follow-up studies, however, demonstrated that the risk of circulatory problems for women taking the new progestins is no greater than the risk for other women. Medical advisory boards returned the products to the market after short moratoriums on their sales.

The scientific study and analysis of medical risks take time and often produce contradictory results that require further study. Some people argue that no contraceptive should be made publicly available until all or most of these conflicts have been resolved. Inadequate testing, they argue, puts women at greater risk from the products. The risks to women from vaccines designed to treat a fertilized egg as an invading substances led in India to the suspension of tests on those vaccines. Others, however, believe that the risk from pregnancy and abortion caused by the scare over contraceptive risks is greater than the problem credited to the contraceptive.

As women and men weigh their choice to use contraception, they consider the impact of an unwanted pregnancy against the possibility of that contraceptive causing medical complications. They weigh the risk of pregnancy against the risk of the birth control method. Since the pill reached the market, marketing efforts and governmental requirements have made significant information available to people for them to consider as they make their choices. *See also* CANCER; CERVICAL CAP; COMBINED ORAL CONTRACEPTIVES; PROGESTIN-ONLY CONTRACEPTIVES; TOXIC SHOCK SYNDROME; VAGINAL SPONGE

Further reading: Hatcher, Robert, James Trussel, Felicia Stewart, and others. *Contraceptive Technology*. 17th rev. ed. New York: Ardent Media, 1998. Hicks, D. A. "What Risk of Infection with IUD Use?" *The Lancet* 351 (1998): 1222–1223. Sadovsky, Robert. "Oral Contraceptive Use and Risk of Cardiovascular Disease." *American Family Physician* 58 (1998): 561–562.

Rock, John Charles (1890–1984)

Gynecologist John Rock, a noted researcher into the biology of reproduction, worked on the team that developed the first hormonal contraceptive pill. During the mid-1950s, Rock conducted experiments with progesterone to help infertile patients conceive. He discovered that progesterone, a naturally occurring hormone made after a mature egg leaves the ovary and that supports a pregnancy once an egg has been fertilized, actually prevents ovulation if it is ingested throughout the menstrual cycle. These preliminary discoveries combined with the research of Dr. Gregory Pincus at the Worcester Foundation for Experimental Biology, and in 1952 the two Harvard graduates began an informal sharing of information which led in 1954 to the formal collaboration that developed and tested what some expected to be the perfect contraceptive.

On 24 March 1890, John Charles Rock was born in Marlborough, Massachusetts. Raised a devout Catholic, Rock worked before attending college in Guatemala, where he saw, firsthand, deprivation to men and women caused by poverty, early marriage, and large families. Rock returned to the United States and graduated from Harvard in 1912, going on to receive his medical degree from Harvard Medical School in 1918.

As an intern in obstetrical care at the Lying-In Maternity Hospital in Boston, Rock learned of the prevalent ignorance of sexuality and reproduction, including the consequences of sexual intercourse, and the dangers women often face during pregnancy and childbirth.

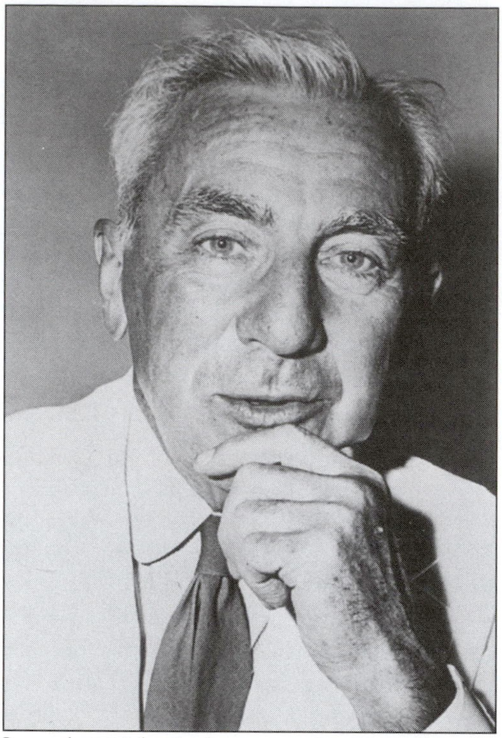

Gynecologist John Rock was one of two scientists who developed the first approved oral contraceptive. *AP/Wide World Photos*

In 1924, Rock established the Fertility and Endocrine Clinic, the first infertility clinic, at the Free Hospital for Women in Brookline, Massachusetts. He soon began offering classes on reproduction, including to medical students, where he included discussions of contraception, despite Massachusetts law that made it illegal to disseminate information on that topic. When researchers discovered in the mid-1920s that women are only fertile near the midpoint of their menstrual cycles, the "rhythm" method of avoiding conception developed. An inexact method that required close record keeping and periodic abstinence, rhythm offered some opportunity for birth control to the world's Catholics whose church prohibited contraception. In 1936, Rock opened the first clinic to teach the rhythm method. While he found the method to be chancy as a contraceptive, it worked well to help his infertile patients conceive.

In the 1930s and 1940s, Rock combined his interests in practicing gynecology with conducting research. In 1938, while working with Arthur Hertig, Rock became the first person to find and observe an intact early human ovum—a 12-day-old conceptus. He had obtained the uterus lining that contained the egg from a woman who had undergone a hysterectomy. In August of 1944, a team of researchers working with Rock succeeded in fertilizing a human egg in vitro, in a dish in a laboratory.

In the early 1950s, at a professional meeting, Rock mentioned his work with progesterone to colleague Gregory Pincus who had by then become aware of the synthesis of inexpensive progestins, artificial progesterones. Pincus's research into the effects of the progestin had in part been supported by birth control advocate Margaret Sanger. Rock agreed to Pincus's suggestion that he test the new chemicals on willing patients at Lying-In Hospital.

The drug proved very successful at preventing pregnancy in those first tests and soon after, with pills manufactured by G. D. Searle, Rock and Pincus began field studies in Brookline, Massachusetts, Puerto Rico, Haiti, and elsewhere. Because of the result of those highly successful tests, the U.S. Food and Drug Administration gave approval in 1960 for the sale of Enovid, the first hormonal contraceptive pill.

Most unusual about John Rock was his active and eager support of birth control despite the rigorous stand the Catholic Church had taken against contraception. While the Catholic Church held reproduction of children as the primary reason for sexual intercourse, Rock argued that love was the primary reason for intercourse and that people should have the means to allow that expression of love without the concern of having children, or too many children, when they could not afford to parent them well. Rock saw the use of progestin and then estrogen in contraception as an extension of a natural process rather than an interference with nature.

In 1963, Rock wrote and published *The Time has Come: A Catholic Doctor's Proposal to End the Battle for Birth Control*. He had since the 1930s been a strong advocate for the removal of anti-contraception laws in Massachusetts. By 1964, doctors were prescribing Rock and Pincus's hormonal pill to 4 million people. The Catholic Church, however, did not change its stand against birth control, to Rock's disappointment.

John Rock died 4 December 1984. By then the pill had changed greatly, from the 150 micrograms of estrogen and 10 milligrams of progestin he and Pincus had developed to the standard 50 micrograms of estrogen and 1 milligram of progestin or less, and become the most prescribed contraceptive in the world. The basic research Rock and Pincus conducted became the basis of the development of all hormonal contraceptives. *See also* COMBINED ORAL CONTRACEPTIVES; PINCUS, GREGORY GOODWIN

Further reading: Asbell, Bernard. *The Pill: A Biography of the Drug That Changed the World*. New York: Random House, 1995. McLaughlin, Loretta. *The Pill, John Rock, and the Church: The Biography of a Revolution*. Boston: Little, Brown, 1982. Rock, John. *The Time Has Come: A Doctor's Proposal to End the Battle for Birth Control*. New York: Knopf, 1963.

Roe v. Wade

On 22 January 1973, the United States Supreme Court, ruling in the case of *Roe v. Wade*, declared unconstitutional by a vote of seven to two state laws that denied women the right to abortion. This decision made abortion legal across the United States and affirmed a woman's right to privacy in choosing to end a pregnancy.

Essentially, the Court ruled that a person's right to privacy was broad enough to include a woman's decision to end a pregnancy without interference from the government. Building on rulings in *Griswold v. Connecticut* (1965), in which the Court determined that married people had a right to privacy that governed their use of contraceptives, and on *Eisenstadt v. Baird* (1972), in which the Court held unmarried people also had a right to privacy in making reproductive decisions, the Court argued that a woman's right to privacy outweighed a state's interest in that pregnancy.

The challenge to state abortion laws that would become *Roe v. Wade* began in Texas where a group of young women attorneys, including Sarah Weddington and Linda Coffee, planned the challenge before meeting a woman who would agree to be the party harmed by the Texas restrictions. When unmarried Norma McCorvey, a carnival worker, pregnant with her third child, sought help in obtaining an abortion, the attorney she contacted introduced her to Weddington and Coffee. Under the court-accepted pseudonym of Jane Roe, McCorvey agreed to sue Texas for denying her the abortion she wanted.

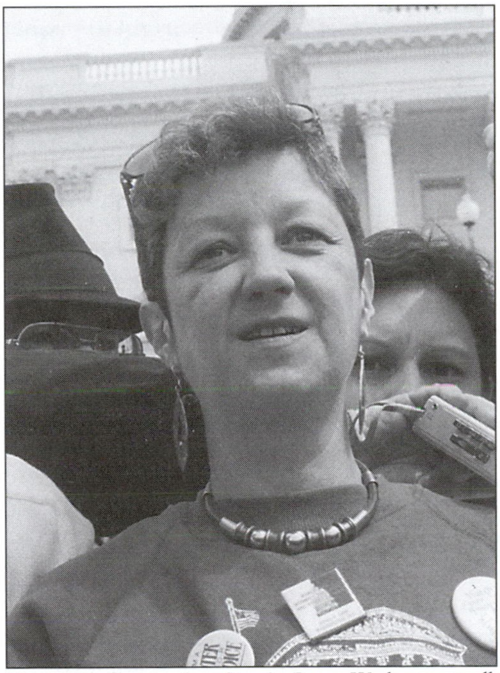

Norma McCorvey, Jane Roe in *Roe v. Wade*, eventually took a stand against abortion and in 1989 protested against the procedure. *AP/Wide World Photos*

In *Roe v. Wade*, the Court placed two limits upon that right to privacy. First it recognized a state's responsibility to regulate who was qualified to perform abortions and how abortion would be performed in order to protect the health and life of the woman. More importantly to a woman's access to abortion, the Court ruled that at some point in a pregnancy a conceptus (the biological result of a sperm fertilizing an egg) becomes a viable human being that the state has an interest in defending. The Supreme Court established that point at the end of the first trimester of pregnancy, about 24 to 28 weeks from the woman's last menstrual period. Before viability, the state could put no restrictions upon a woman's access to abortion. After that time, the state could prohibit only abortions that were not necessary to protect the woman's health and life.

Roe v. Wade began as a pair of lawsuits filed 3 March 1970, in federal court in Dallas, Texas. Attorney Linda Coffee, who filed the initial complaints, named Dallas County District Attorney Henry Wade as the plaintiff and argued that the Texas law banning abortions deprived women of the right to privacy in choosing to end a pregnancy. In *Doe v. Bolton*, Coffee argued the case for abortion on behalf of a married couple. In *Roe v. Wade*, she made the argument on behalf of all women.

The response from the Texas attorney general's office argued that the named complainants had no standing in the court since Texas law applied to people who performed abortions and not to people who would undergo them. Legal proceedings in advance of a hearing before a three-judge federal panel resulted in attorney's combining the two cases and in making *Roe v. Wade* a class action suit brought on behalf of all women who found themselves in circumstances similar to those of the two women in the initial complaint, wanting or needing an abortion but unable to obtain one in Texas. After a hearing on 22 May 1970, the panel ruled unanimously and swiftly on June 17, that the Texas law was unconstitutional and deprived women of the basic human right of privacy.

As *Roe v. Wade* proceeded through the Texas court, activists in several states had successfully worked to reform abortion laws. Abortion became legal in New York on 1 July 1970. Newly passed statutes in Colorado, North Carolina, and California in 1967 allowed therapeutic abortions to save the life and health of the woman. Nearly a dozen other legal challenges to state abortion laws were also working their way through the legal system by the time the Texas court heard the case of *Roe v. Wade*.

District Attorney Wade and the Texas attorney general announced the day after the federal panel made its decision that the state would appeal the *Roe v. Wade* ruling to the Supreme Court. There, on 13 December 1971, the Supreme Court, made up of only seven of its nine justices as the court awaited new appointments, heard for the first time the arguments against the Texas law. Earlier, the Court had decided to combine into one proceeding *Roe v. Wade* with *Doe v. Bolton,* a case that had come out of an appeal of the Georgia law requiring that abortions be performed in hospitals, that a woman secure approval from three doctors and a hospital committee, and that any woman seeking an abortion be a resident of Georgia. The supreme court ruled that both cases sought the same object, the right of a woman to decide for herself to terminate a pregnancy.

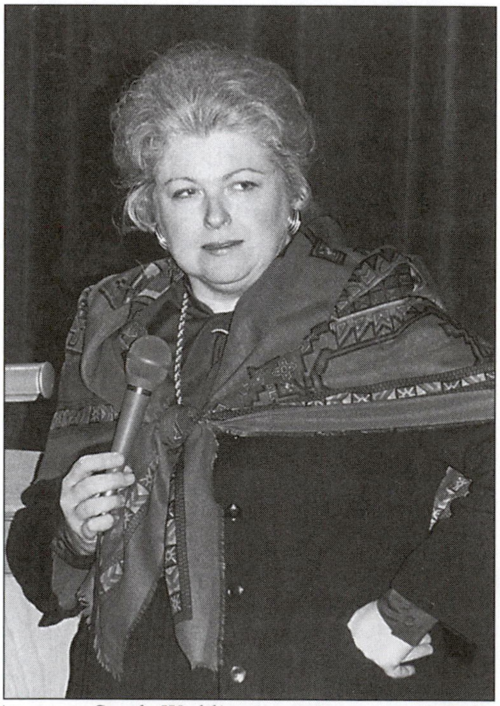

Attorney Sarah Weddington twice presented the arguments for abortion before the Supreme Court in *Roe v. Wade*. *Bettmann/CORBIS*

In November of 1971, the court had heard the case of *Eisenstadt v. Baird* where the state of Massachusetts had arrested birth control activist William Baird for giving contraceptives to unmarried college students during a lecture in Boston. The timing of that case and the timing of *Roe v. Wade* overlapped on the Supreme Court calendar, and the decision in the Massachusetts case would have a direct bearing on the Texas case.

Sarah Weddington, who with Linda Coffee had filed the original *Roe v. Wade* complaint, argued in 1971 that pregnancy had such a profound influence on a woman's life that a woman had a fundamental and basic right to decide if she wanted to continue that pregnancy. Jay Floyd, defending the Texas law, argued that because Jane Roe was no longer pregnant, the Court had no reason to be hearing a case if no harmed plaintiff could be presented. The Court, however, had already ruled that *Roe v. Wade* was a class action suit and that, given the unusual circumstances of the legal process taking far longer than the gestation period of humans, the Court would make an exception to its long-standing policy of only hearing cases in which a party could be produced who had been harmed by the law in question. Texas further argued that its responsibility to protect the human life begun at conception gave it the right to make abortion illegal.

As it considered its decision on the abortion cases, the Supreme Court issued its decision in *Eisenstadt v. Baird*, arguing that unmarried as well as married people had the right to privacy in their decision to beget and bear children. That argument signaled to the lawyers that the Court would rule in favor of allowing women the right to privacy in deciding whether to give birth once fertilization had occurred. Unwilling to make such a momentous decision without a full complement of justices, the Supreme Court announced in June 1972 to have the lawyers for *Roe v. Wade* reargue the case now that two new justices had been appointed and sworn in.

On 11 October 1972, lawyers reconvened in Washington to argue for a second time the case of *Roe v. Wade*. Drawing on *Eisenstadt* and *Griswold* and on a woman's right to privacy, Sarah Weddington repeated her arguments. Robert Flowers represented Texas and reiterated the stand of the state in protecting the right of a conceptus to be born. On 17 January 1973, in a majority opinion written by Justice Harry Blackmun, the court ruled that laws prohibiting abortion, with limits, were unconstitutional.

That law effectively overturned antiabortion laws across the United States. In the years following the ruling, attempts to propose a constitutional amendment to overturn *Roe v. Wade* were weak and ineffective. However the Supreme Court has since heard 25 cases that challenged the specifics of the *Roe v. Wade* ruling. The rulings in those cases narrowed the scope of access to abortion, particularly for adolescents and for procedures performed after the first trimester. *See also* ABORTION; *EISENSTADT V. BAIRD; GRISWOLD V. CONNECTICUT*

Further reading: Faux, Marian. Roe v. Wade: *The Untold Story of the Landmark Supreme Court Decision That Made Abortion Legal*. New York: Macmillan, 1988. Garrow, David J. *Liberty and Sexuality: The Right to Privacy and the Making of* Roe v. Wade. New York: MacMillan, 1994. United States Senate. "The 25th Anniversary of *Roe v. Wade*: Has It Stood the Test of Time?" Hearing Before the Subcommittee on the Constitution, Federalism, and Property Rights of the Committee on the Judiciary, 21 January 1998. Washington, DC: Government Printing Office, 1998.

Roman Catholic Church

The Roman Catholic Church, as a religion, as a group of people, and as a hierarchy, struggles with a significant conflict over human sexuality and modern contraception. Within the membership of this global religion, to which more than 1 billion people belong, many believe strongly that modern contraceptives violate God's natural law. Many others believe as strongly that the use of contraception is a personal choice and a social justice necessity of followers of Jesus Christ.

The structure of the Catholic Church places the pope at the top of a male hierarchy that includes cardinals, archbishops, bishops, and priests. In contrast to that official structure, a firm belief of the Catholic faith is that the people themselves, the followers of Jesus, make up the actual church. The church, in common Catholic use, refers to those billion people who have been baptized into the Roman Catholic faith.

In the use of modern, artificial forms of contraception and the place of sexual intercourse within marriage, those two aspects of the Catholic Church found themselves in conflict during the twentieth century. In 1968, Pope Paul VI wrote and distributed *Humanae Vitae*, a church encyclical or letter to his bishops, that stated emphatically that "any action which either before, at the moment of, or after sexual intercourse, is specifically intended to prevent procreation" (English translation from the Vatican) was condemned by the authority of the Catholic Church. That letter also condemned permanent or temporary sterilization, including male, female, and hormonal contraceptives, and condemned abortion under all circumstances. Paul VI confirmed for the twentieth-century Catholic Church the ban on modern contraceptive methods that had been in place for more than a century. Within the scope of the official ruling, with every act of sexual intercourse, which is only permitted between husband and wife, Catholics should be willing to accept the conception of a child as a natural outcome and do nothing to interfere with that process.

Paul VI wrote that letter five years after the development of the hormonal contraceptive pill in the United States in 1960. In those five years, many Catholics, including John Rock, a Catholic doctor who worked on the team that tested the pill, had been arguing that the pope should revise Catholic law. They hoped he would change that religion's law that denied people religiously accepted access to a growing number of modern contraceptives. After convening councils on the subject, which included lay Catholics, Paul VI took his stand on birth control. His position remained unchanged by the two popes who succeeded Paul VI after his death in 1978. Pope John Paul II reaffirmed the Catholic church's official ruling against the use of contraceptives in 1995 with the issuance of an the official proclamation "The Truth and Meaning of Human Sexuality: Guidelines for Education within the Family."

Many of the Catholic laity, particularly in Europe and the United States, however, turned quickly to modern contraceptives, including the hormonal pill. By the late 1990s estimates suggested that almost all Catholics had at some time relied on modern contraceptives to prevent pregnancy. Theologians who support the use of contraceptives argue that members of the Catholic faith have the right within the church to dissent from church doctrine after prayerful consideration. If prayer and a belief that the Holy Spirit, the third representative of God in the Catholic faith's concept of a tri-part deity, calls them to dissent from law as stated by church authorities.

Fertility rates in Europe and the United States fell rapidly in the 1960s and 1970s, an accomplishment achieved primarily through artificial contraception. By 1999, even very Catholic Italy, home to Vatican City and the seat of authority for the pope and that church, had a fertility rate of 1.2 children. In 1960 surveys in the United States, Catholic women had much higher birth rates than their Protestant counterparts. By the 1980s, Catholic and Protestant women were giving birth on average to the same number of children, and by 1996 Catholic women gave birth to 1.6 children compared to 1.9 for Protestant women. With the majority of Roman Catholics ignoring the ban on modern contraception, the pope and his administrators occasionally called on priests to be lenient with their parishioners who confessed to using contraceptives. The Vatican advised parish priests to not ask people if they did use modern birth control.

Several organizations formed within the Catholic Church as the division deepened between people who supported the papal rule and people who did not. Human Life International, founded by a Benedictine monk in 1981, takes a staunch and public stand in favor of the Vatican ban and argues that people who use contraceptives are committing serious sins that could condemn them to hell in an afterlife. Members of Catholics for a Free Choice, which formed in 1973, argue that the church is relying on old theology which papal authority itself has negated by allowing fertility awareness forms of family planning.

In some countries of the world, notably the Philippines and Ireland, the influence of the church's hierarchy and its power have restricted access to contraceptives. Insisting that people use fertility awareness, a modern version of the "rhythm" method, which calls for abstinence by married couples from sexual intercourse during and after ovulation, the Catholic Church in the Philippines has influenced the Philippine government since the late 1980s to modify family planning programs. The Catholic hierarchy also influences politics in Ireland where the use of contraceptives was banned until1980.

In other areas, including most of Central and South America, population growth rates have slowed dramatically. In Brazil, where a large portion of the population is Catholic, more than 70 percent of women of childbearing age use modern contraceptives. Overall, more than 50 percent of women in Latin America and the Caribbean used modern contraceptives as of 1999.

The authority of the pope, however, through his representative at the United Nations, and the Catholic Church has influenced international policy in drafting statements on human rights, reproductive rights, and reproductive choice. *See also* ABORTION; EUROPE; IRELAND; PHILIPPINES

Further reading: *Humanae Vitae: Encyclical of Pope Paul VI on The Regulation of Birth*. The Vatican: The Vatican, 1968. Online: http://www.vatican.va/holy_father/paul_vi/encyclicals/documents/hf_p-vi_enc_25071968_humanae-vitae_en.html, 14 November 1999. Hume, Maggie. *Contraception in Catholic Doctrine: The Evolution of an Earthly Code*. Washington, DC: Catholics for a Free Choice, 1991. Rathschmidt, Jack. "Cafeteria Catholics Don't Need to Get in Line." *U.S. Catholic* 63.1 (1998): 36–38.

RU–486. *See* MIFEPRISTONE

Russia

Turmoil in Russia's history before and after the beginning of the break up of the Soviet Union in 1989 is reflected in the country's population size and age profile. The birth rate, the abortion rate, and the rate of women's use of and access to modern contraceptives all fluctuate according to economic and social conditions in the massive country that spans eastern Europe and northern Asia.

Russia's total fertility rate, an estimate of the number of children a woman is likely to bear in her lifetime, fell dramatically through the 1990s. In 1988, Russia's total fertility rate was estimated at 2.2 children per women, a birth rate just above that needed to replace the population. By 1993 that rate had fallen to 1.4. In 1997, the Russian birth rate was 1.2 and had fallen by an average of one child per family. That rapid rate of decline occurred across Russia. Even the poorer more rural areas of Siberia and the far east showed a rapid decline in the average number of children to which women were giving birth.

Across Russia women rely heavily on abortion to control their family size. Since it became legal in 1955, abortion has been the primary method of fertility regulation in Russia. In the mid-1990s official reports showed that women underwent twice as many abortions as live births each year. The average woman in Russia is likely to undergo between two and four abortions in her lifetime.

Russia, along with former Soviet satellite countries Romania and Belarus, had the highest reported abortion rates in the world. Official statistics in 1995 showed that 68.4 of every 1,000 Russian women between the ages of 15 and 44 would undergo an abortion. In Romania in 1996 the rate was 78 for every 1,000 women and in Belarus in 1996 the rate was 67.5 women for every 1,000. Those rates have been steadily falling since 1990 when all three nations had abortion rates of more than 100 for every 1,000 women each year.

Despite having easy access to legal abortions, illegal abortions still contribute to the nation's high maternal death rate. Fifty-two women out of every 100,000 people die each year from pregnancy-related causes. That rate is between six and seven times higher than maternal mortality rates in the United States and Western Europe. Abortions account for approximately 28 percent of maternal deaths and of those deaths 90 percent were related to complications from illegal abortions. Maternal deaths are much higher in the rural areas of eastern Siberia and the far east than in the more populated northwest region of the country.

Infant mortality rates are also high in Russia and the number of deaths each year also fluctuates more than in most other nations. In 1995, 24.7 children for every 1,000 were likely to die before their first birthday. By 1997, that figure had dropped to 16.9. Those rates are two to three times greater than rates in the developed countries of Western Europe.

Russian women gained greater access to modern contraceptives in the 1990s and the use of those products was increasing. However, estimates of use vary widely. For instance, women living in more remote areas of the country have little access to modern contraceptives. Nationwide, Russia's women and men frequently use traditional and biological methods of family planning such as withdrawal and fertility awareness. Across Russia, nearly 67 percent of married women reported using family planning methods in 1994, of that proportion, 18 percent relied on traditional methods.

Most married women who used modern contraceptives relied on intrauterine devices (IUDs) to protect them from unwanted pregnancies. In 1994, 33.1 percent of married women between 20 and 49 had an IUD in place. That equals about half of Russia's married women. In part, Russian women rely on IUDs because Soviet public health officials and Soviet doctors until 1987 strongly discouraged women from using oral contraceptive pills, emphasizing a negative connection between hormonal contraceptives and cancers. Only 6 percent of Russian women used hormonal contraceptive pills as of 1994.

The economic unrest Russia began experiencing in the early 1990s as the nation began its shift from a communist to a free market economy created difficulties for women gaining access to modern contraceptives. Irregular supplies of contraceptives and unreliable quality have hindered access. Relatively high prices for contraceptives (a pack-

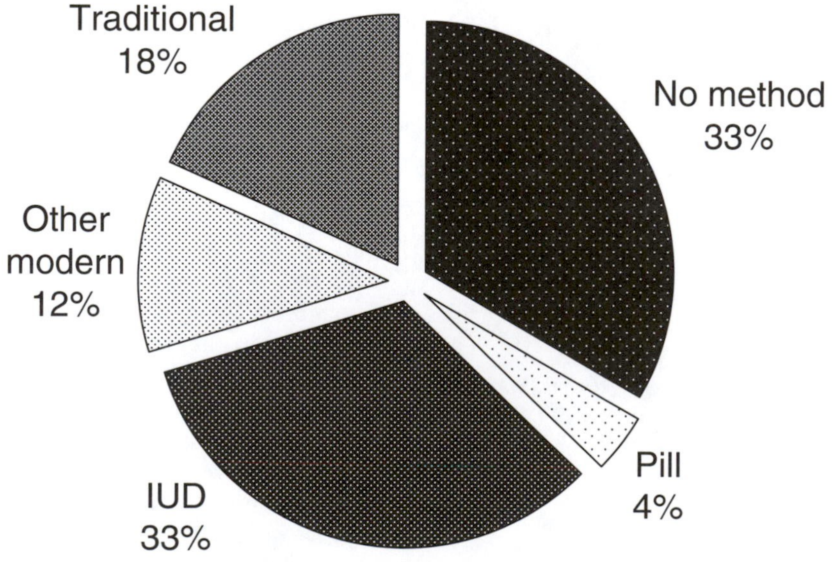

Russia: 1994 Contraceptive Use by Women Ages 15–49

Source: U.S. Census Bureau International Data Base

age of condoms may cost US$1) make modern methods unaffordable for average Russians (whose monthly income is an average of US$50). The reportedly poor quality of Russian-made products decreases contraceptive effectiveness and also helps account for Russia's high level of unmet need for methods other than abortion for preventing pregnancy.

Surveys in the mid-1990s showed that half of Russia's married women who reported not wanting to become pregnant were not using a contraceptive method, either modern or traditional, to prevent conception. However, researchers and reproductive health specialists expect women's use of modern contraceptives to rise rapidly during the first decades of the twenty-first century, because of Russia's high level of overall education. Staff at the Russian Family Planning Association, which formed in 1991 and became a member of International Planned Parenthood Federation in 1993, have seen significant decreases in the abortion rate in areas where contraceptives services and supplies have become more reliable and accessible.

Further reading: Chalmers, Beverly, et al. "Contraceptive Knowledge, Attitudes, and Use Among Women Attending Health Clinics in St. Petersburg, Russian Federation." *The Canadian Journal of Human Sexuality* 7 (1998): 129–137. Entwisle, Barbara, and Polina Kozyreva. "New Estimates of Induced Abortion in Russia." *Studies in Family Planning* 28 (1997): 14–23. Kingkade, Ward. *International Brief: Population Trends: Russia*. Washington, DC: U.S. Department of Commerce, Economics and Statistics Administration, Bureau of the Census, 1997. Mahler, K. "Rates of Modern Method Use Are High Among Urban Russian Women, Who Typically Want Small Families." *Family Planning Perspectives* 30.6 (1998): 293.

S

Safe Sex

"Safe sex" became a popular expression in the 1980s to indicate ways in which people could protect themselves from the spreading the epidemic of acquired immunodeficiency syndrome (AIDS) as well as from unplanned pregnancy. Each act of sexual intercourse between a man and a woman where neither partner uses a contraceptive brings with it the chance of a man's sperm fertilizing a woman's ovum and beginning a pregnancy. Such intercourse where the partners do not desire or seek pregnancy, then, carries with a risk of undesirable, or unsafe, consequences. Sexual activity where partners exchange bodily fluids also brings with it the risk of either partner contracting or transmitting a sexually transmitted disease (STD). While the male latex condom offers people protection from these unwanted consequences, no form of contraceptive can offer risk-free intercourse. For this reason, some critics argue that there is no such thing as safe sex, only safer sex.

No sex is safe, some people argue, except vaginal intercourse within marriage where both partners are willing to accept the pregnancy to which their union might give rise. This argument holds that only abstinence from sexual activity protects people from unwanted consequences. Proponents of abstinence-only pregnancy and disease prevention became an increasingly strong voice in the United States in the 1990s and successfully guided legislation through state and federal governments to restrict the lessons children learn in health classes regarding sex and how to remain safe from unwanted consequences. Rather than teaching the student ways to reduce risks, proponents of abstinence wanted teachers to instruct students in how to say no to intercourse.

Sex, other people argued, could and should be enjoyed simply for the emotional pleasure and not only to begin a pregnancy, but people need to be educated in ways to protect themselves from disease and unplanned pregnancy. Advocates of helping people protect themselves during intercourse stressed the need for people to learn the technique of using a condom in addition to learning the facts of its effectiveness. While pointing out that sex is part of the complex array of human emotions, advocates of safer sex stressed that if people learn skills for negotiating safety within a relationship, skills in developing lower-risk relationships, and skills in trusting and using internal value systems, they will live significantly decrease their risks for STDs and unwanted pregnancy.

The male latex condom became in the 1980s the leading defense against the spread of disease. It also offered men and women protection as a barrier contraceptive against pregnancy. While condom use has risen sharply in most nations since the late 1980s, most people use condoms inconsistently.

When they use condoms consistently and accurately, people experience a 97 percent effectiveness rate at preventing pregnancy. Success at preventing sexually transmitted diseases is less easily calculated, but laboratory and field tests have established high rates of protection for the male latex condom.

The female condom, a polyurethane sheath that lines the vagina and which received U.S. Food and Drug Administration approval in 1993, also offers people protection from pregnancy and sexually transmitted diseases. In fact, laboratory tests showed that the female condom was even better at preventing the risk of disease than the male latex condom, though it is not as effective as the male condom at preventing pregnancy.

Advocates of safer sex also began to strongly encourage that people express sexual urges through masturbation, the manipulation of a person's own sexual organs, or, by some definitions, the manipulation of another person's sexual organs. The practice of self-stimulation, however, while a natural part of human experience, remained a social and cultural taboo in many cultures where it was seen as deviant behavior. Health care providers and sexuality specialists, however, urged a reexamination by individuals of the role of masturbation in sexual expression, pregnancy prevention, and disease protection.

As of the year 2000, advocates of abstinence as the best safeguard against unwanted pregnancy and sexually transmitted diseases argued that teaching people, particularly teens, about alternatives to abstinence and sexual intercourse were increasing the risk of the those people from the very circumstances they were seeking to prevent. The best deterrent, they insist, is to wait for marriage and then to marry a person free of sexually transmitted diseases and remain the exclusive partner of that person.

Opponents of the abstinence-only approach, while conceding that there is no such thing as "safe" sex, argued that preparing people to deal with the dangers of sexual intercourse is more effective at preventing unintended consequences than is allowing people to remain ignorant. *See also* ABSTINENCE; ADOLESCENTS; SEX EDUCATION; SEXUALLY TRANSMITTED DISEASES; UNPLANNED PREGNANCY

Further reading: Larkin, Marilynn. "Easing the Way to Safer Sex." *The Lancet,* 28 March 1998, 964.
Patton, Cindy. *Fatal Advice: How Safe-Sex Education Went Wrong*. Durham, NC: Duke University Press, 1996.

Sanger, Margaret Higgins (1879–1966)

Margaret Sanger, a trained nurse and an advocate for women's rights, founded the American birth control movement and became an international advocate for women's reproductive rights. She grew up in a large, poor family and watched her mother struggle with health problems related to her many pregnancies. In her early adult years Sanger worked as a public health nurse in New York City's immigrant neighborhoods and met many poor women who also suffered from the health and financial hazards of bearing too many children too close together. These early experiences inspired Sanger to a lifelong goal of bringing contraceptive knowledge to poverty-stricken women around the world.

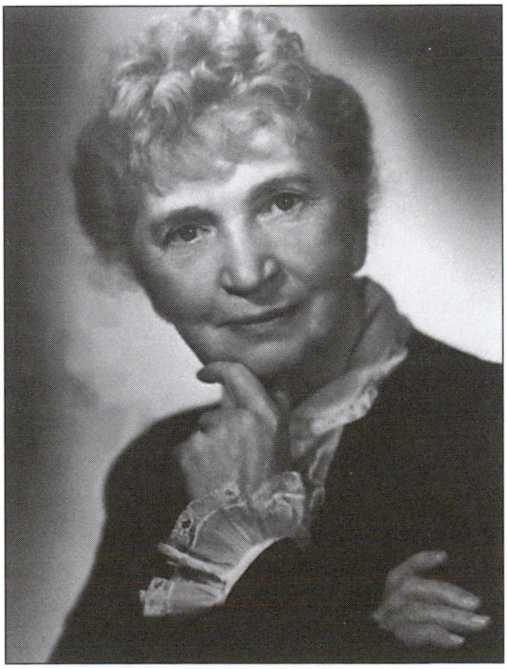

Margaret Sanger worked around the world to give all women easy access to birth control.

Born Margaret Louisa Higgins on 14 September 1879, in Corning, New York, Sanger was the child of an Irish immigrant father. After her mother's death in 1899 of tuberculosis, Margaret enrolled at the White Plains Hospital nurse's training program in Westchester County, New York. In the summer of 1902 she completed her studies at a special program at the Manhattan Eye and Ear Infirmary. That year, Margaret also met William Sanger, 28, whom she married on 18 August 1902. The birth of Margaret's and William's first son followed in 1903. Poor health—doctors diagnosed tuberculosis during her studies—required that Sanger avoid further pregnancies, and not until years after her first child was born did Margaret have another son (1908) and a daughter (1909).

In 1910 the Sangers moved to New York City. To make ends meet, Margaret took assignments as a visiting nurse in the immigrant districts of New York's Lower East Side. There she nursed women made ill by many and closely spaced pregnancies and women who suffered and died from illegal abortions.

In those early years, Sanger became involved in the growing Socialist Party in New York and developed her talents as a writer and organizer. Offering women help in preventing pregnancies became Margaret's focused objective in 1914 when she founded the radical magazine *The Woman Rebel*. At the inspiration of a friend, Margaret began using the term "birth control" to describe the field of knowledge she wanted to share with women. The term would come to mark her and the social movement she is credited with beginning. From that year on, Margaret's battle for birth control involved many struggles with the law, Congress, the Catholic Church, and with the conflict between women's desires and society's expectations.

With the first issue of *The Woman Rebel*, Sanger challenged the Comstock Laws, passed by Congress in 1873, which restricted sending obscene material through the U.S. mail, a restriction that included information on contraception. Post Office authorities confiscated her first issue and in August of 1914 she was arrested. While preparing for trial, Sanger wrote *Family Limitation*, a very popular brochure which described, with diagrams, the common forms of birth control then in use. Sanger's attorney recommended that she plead guilty to the charges and negotiate a sentence and fine, but Sanger was unwilling to compromise; she decided to leave the country. Before her trial, Margaret boarded a train for Canada under an assumed name and from there traveled to Europe. While she was abroad, her husband, William, distributed her *Family Limitation* pamphlet and in 1915 was arrested, tried, and served 30 days in jail.

For more than a year, Sanger traveled in Europe and met people involved in fledgling birth control movements. In the Netherlands, she learned of the success of an early diaphragm used with spermicidal jelly that would later become the contraceptive method provided in her clinics. She returned to the United States in 1915 to face the charges against her, but after several postponements of the trial, prosecutors dropped all charges in February 1916.

On 16 October 1916, Margaret opened the first birth control clinic in the United States in a rented storefront tenement in Brooklyn. She set the model for clinics that would become the standard around the world: independent, not-for-profit medical facilities that, in the case of this first clinic, provided contraceptive knowledge and in future clinics, the methods of contraception. In the few weeks it remained open, more than 450 women attended the clinic, but on 26 October, police arrested Margaret for distributing what they saw as obscene materials: pamphlets and diagrams and information on where to buy "pessaries," early forms of diaphragms. Found guilty of violating obscenity laws, she spent 30 days in prison.

The arrest and trial received tremendous coverage by the New York newspapers and Sanger's notoriety grew. From then on, she spent much of her career lecturing women across the United States and around the world on birth control and building networks of volunteer organizations. Supporters of the

Catholic Church, which opposed birth control, often protested and attempted to stop those lectures, but sympathetic Sanger supporters provided ways for her to share the birth control information with the women who sought it.

In 1917, Sanger began publishing the *Birth Control Review*, a small-circulation magazine. She organized the first American birth control conference, held in New York City in 1921, and in that year founded the American Birth Control League, a not-for-profit, charitable organization. By the mid-1930s this league had opened more than 300 clinics nationwide, staffed mostly by volunteers. During 1922, and again in 1930s, she traveled around the world lecturing and supporting birth control efforts. In 1923, Margaret opened her second clinic, the Birth Control Clinical Research Bureau in New York, a place to study as well as provide contraceptives.

Sanger's first marriage ended in divorce in 1921. In 1922, she married millionaire James Henry Noah Slee, who would provide significant financial and business assistance to Margaret's cause until the Depression depleted his fortune.

Through the 1930s and 1940s, Sanger remained an active lobbyist for birth control reform and struggled in the face of Catholic opposition to convince Congress to support, then pass, a bill that would give public support to birth control efforts. She founded the *Journal of Contraception* in 1935, and wrote *My Fight for Birth Control* in 1931 and *Margaret Sanger: An Autobiography* in 1938. Though constrained by the Depression and then World War II, Sanger continued to spread knowledge around the world. She opened a clinic in London and supported a network of clinics worldwide. In 1953, Margaret became the first president of the International Planned Parenthood Federation.

In 1951, when she met Gregory Pincus, a biologist researching the hormonal control of reproduction, Sanger began her support for what would be her last significant contribution to the birth control movement. Sanger persuaded Pincus to devote the energy and talent of his staff at the Worcester Foundation for Experimental Biology to developing a hormonal contraceptive, and through her significant fund-raising talent helped pay for that research. Over the next six years, Pincus and gynecologist John Rock developed the first hormonal contraceptive pill, which relied on artificial forms of progesterone and estrogen to simulate pregnancy and prevent ovulation. The U.S. Food and Drug Administration gave the contraceptive its approval and it reached the U.S. market in 1960. With this event, Sanger saw fulfilled her goal to provide women with an easy, convenient contraceptive that did not need to be used during intercourse.

Sanger also saw fulfilled her efforts to build a network of clinics as a community of women working together to improve their personal lives. Throughout her career, Sanger struggled to keep birth control efforts under women's influences and from becoming a medically controlled aspect of women's lives. She failed in that goal, however, when changing attitudes of medical professionals and court rulings shaped birth control as a medical issue.

Margaret Sanger died 6 September 1966, in Tucson, Arizona, after seeing the revolution in birth control brought about by the combined oral contraceptive pill and after having seen birth control and population concerns become public issues of significant importance around the world. *See also* COMBINED ORAL CONTRACEPTIVES; PINCUS, GREGORY GOODWIN; ROCK, JOHN CHARLES

Further reading: Chesler, Ellen. *Woman of Valor: Margaret Sanger and the Birth Control Movement in America*. New York: Anchor-Doubleday, 1992. Sanger, Margaret Higgins. *Margaret Sanger: An Autobiography*. 1938. Elmsford, NY: Maxwell Reprints, 1970. Steinem, Gloria. "Margaret Sanger: Her Crusade to Legalize Birth Control Spurred the Movement for Women's Liberation." Time 100: Leaders and Revolutionaries of the 20th Century. *Time,* 13 April 1988, 93–94.

Semen

The milky white fluid of the semen carries mature sperm out of a male's body and into a female's body. This fluid provides nourishment for the sperm cells, chemicals that improve the sperm's ability to swim, and chemicals that neutralize acidic secretions in the woman's vagina and thus increase the chances of the sperm surviving in a woman's body.

Semen is made by the seminal vesicles, the prostate gland, the testes and the bulbourethral gland, parts of a man's internal reproductive system. During sexual arousal, sperm, which is created in the testicles and store in the epididymides, travels through the two vas deferens and mixes with the semen in the urethra, which the vas deferens join near the top of the prostate gland.

Sperm in men who have their vas deferens severed in a vasectomy never reaches the glands that make semen. However, a man who has had a vasectomy still produces semen and that semen still erupts from his body upon ejaculation. *See also* REPRODUCTIVE SYSTEM—MALE; SPERM; VAS DEFERENS

Sex

Depending on the subject people are discussing, the term "sex" can have a variety of specific meanings. In all contexts, however, "sex" refers to some aspect of being a man or a woman.

In nonscientific discussions, "sex" refers first to the biological characteristics of being male or female. Second, "sex" refers to the physical and emotional acts that satisfy the person's biological urge to produce children. "Sex" also refers to the gametes, the egg cells produced in the woman's ovaries and the sperm cells produced in the man's testes, each of which contains half of the genetic material needed to produce a new human life.

"Sex" often refers to the whole range of sexual expression, from hugging and kissing to an inventive variety of forms of genital stimulation. "Sex" is also commonly used to refer specifically to vaginal-penile intercourse, often referred to as sexual intercourse, when a man inserts his erect penis into a woman's vagina.

The broad term "sex" is not adequate for determining the contraceptive needs of a male and female couple, because not all sexual acts lead to reproduction. Scientists and scholars often use the precise term "coitus." This Latin word means the entry and penetration of the male's penis into the woman's vagina. It is this act of sexual expression that gives rise to the need for birth control, for it is during coitus that a man ejaculates his sperm into the woman's vagina, thus allowing the sperm to travel through her reproductive system and perhaps reach and fertilize a mature egg that has been ejected from one of her ovaries. Should people choose to experience the intimacy and pleasure of coitus, but not wish to conceive children, they must use some form of birth control to decrease the chance of the sperm reaching the egg.

Sex and sexuality involve the identities, relationships, perceptions, and expectations of people as they deal with their biological drives to produce offspring. The entire physical, emotional, and social process of being sexually active and responding to sexual desires is a complex, confusing, exciting, and often frightening reality of adult life. For the purpose of discussing birth control and contraception, however, only the one central act that can mingle sperm and eggs requires clear and emphatic discussion. *See also* BIRTH CONTROL; CONCEPTION; REPRODUCTIVE SYSTEM—FEMALE; REPRODUCTIVE SYSTEM—MALE

Further reading: Michaels, Stuart, and Alain Giami. "Sexual Acts and Sexual Relationships: Asking About Sex in Surveys." *Public Opinion Quarterly*. 63 (1999): 401–420.

Sex Education

How people learn about sexuality and reproduction influences their ability to choose when to have children. Worldwide, the low levels of sex education adults and children receive concern reproductive health professionals and public health advocates. They point out that scholars have not studied the impact of sex education, or its lack, on people's reproductive behavior. While studies measure individual knowledge of the basic factors of sex—when ovulation occurs, the relationship between sexual intercourse and pregnancy, contraceptive knowledge, awareness of sexually transmitted disease—research has not established the link between education and reproduction.

Providing sex education to children in schools has been a concern for societies since the 1960s and 1970s when governments in the United States and Europe began requiring that teachers present students with information on human sexuality. The definitions of human sexuality, the role of the government in assigning that task to schools and taking it out of the hands of parents, and the exact nature of the education children are to receive has all led to confusion, controversy, and curriculum experimentation and no definitive understanding of effective teaching.

In the United States, each state has the responsibility to determine the curriculum that will be taught in public schools, including the curriculum in sex education classes. The actions the governments of the 50 states have taken have varied from simply stating the requirement that classes be taught to specifying training requirements for teachers and curriculum standards for students. As of 1998, 19 states and Washington, DC, required that public school coursework contain classes in sexuality education and sexually transmitted diseases and acquired immunodeficiency syndrome (AIDS). Fifteen states required only education on sexually transmitted diseases and AIDS, while 16 states required no teaching of any aspect of human sexuality in their schools.

Sex education from the 1970s through the middle of the 1990s was typically based upon a model that encouraged a wide range of topics including human biology, reproductive health, and the emotional aspects of human sexuality. These topics included discussions of contraceptives, their uses, their success and failure rates, and their limitations in helping students prevent pregnancy. While this was the model, the specifics varied widely. Some schools offered very little classroom time; some had full courses equivalent to a mathematics or social studies course. Many teachers were underprepared for their assignments, never having been required to take courses in how to teach sex education during their teacher training.

While this variety in focus and quality of teaching persisted into the 1990s, that decade brought with it a new issue in sex education in the United States, the rise of the "abstinence-only" curriculum in sex education. This course material stresses for students that the only way to protect themselves from unwanted pregnancies is by abstaining from sexual intercourse. Proponents of abstinence-only education successfully advocated at federal, state, and local levels that schools be required to teach only sexual abstinence to their students. Discussions of contraception and health and hygiene, as well as the full range of sexual expression, were banned from school districts in North Carolina and Mississippi. Virginia also attempted to impose a ban. Even at the federal level, proponents helped pass a law requiring that states receiving education funds for teaching sex education had to teach an abstinence-only curriculum if they spent that money on classroom teaching.

Proponents of a thorough curriculum in sex education from the elementary grades through high school argue that only through an in-depth understanding of human sexuality can children grow up understanding fully their responsibilities to their own reproductive health. Opponents of sex education in the schools argue that parents need to teach their children that material, as well as a moral and ethical value of sexuality that includes sex within marriage. Proponents of school sex education argue that abstinence-only education leads to teenagers having unprotected sex, to a greater incidence of sexually transmitted diseases, and a greater number of unwanted teen pregnancies and abortions. Opponents of sex education that contains more than abstinence-only course materials argue that the only effective prevention from any of those consequences is to teach children to say no to sex. The debate continues as both sides take credit for a 17 percent decrease in the number of teen pregnancies from 1990 to 1996 and the continuing decline in the teen pregnancy rate.

Sex education efforts in Europe also vary greatly from country to country and even school to school. While conferences in the 1970s and 1980s advocated comprehensive sex education that included biology, family life education, and information on sex roles, family planning, and reproductive health, reports in the 1990s suggested that the advice from that early planning hadn't been applied across the continent. In Ireland in 1999, only half of the schools were teaching a planned curriculum in relationships and sexuality education. In Italy, surveys showed that most teens still learned of sex from their friends.

Innovations in Europe include the Netherlands where educators teach teens how to protect themselves from unwanted pregnancy and sexually transmitted disease. In Hungary, specially trained students teach younger students about sex education, allowing the younger students to open up with volunteers close to their age in ways they would not discuss sex with adults.

Still, researchers point out that most sex education in Europe, as in the United States, focuses too heavily on biology and not enough on the expression of human emotion and the communication of sexual behavior. Adolescents still learn more about sex from friends, who often have incorrect information, than they learn from their schools. This lack of knowledge prevents them from effectively choosing contraceptives, and, as in developing countries, individuals around the world need adequate knowledge to make decisions concerning reproductive health. *See also* ABSTINENCE; SAFE SEX; SEXUALLY TRANSMITTED DISEASES

Further reading: Donovan, Patricia. "School-Based Sexuality Education: The Issues and Challenges." *Family Planning Perspectives* 30 (1998): 188–193. Nadler, Richard. "Birds, Bees, and ABCs." *National Review,* 13 September 1999, 8. Sears, James T. *Sexuality and the Curriculum: The Politics and Practices of Sexuality Education*. New York: Teachers College Press, 1992.

Sexually Transmitted Diseases

More than 20 infections fall into the medical category of sexually transmitted diseases (STDs), which pass between people through the exchange of body fluids such as semen and blood or with physical contact through the touching of infected areas on another person's body. Once commonly known as venereal diseases, that term is rarely used to refer to these diseases in modern medical discussions and has been replaced by STDs, which health care workers suggest more accurately describes the nature of the spread of these infections. Some medical researchers further argue that the phrase "sexually transmitted infections" offers still greater precision in describing the health problems increasingly faced by people around the world.

Included in the list of the common STDs are human immunodeficiency virus (HIV), the cause of acquired immunodeficiency syndrome (AIDS); chlamydial diseases, a rapidly growing group of diseases caused by a parasite; genital herpes, an incurable viral infection and very common STD; syphilis, a life-threatening disease; gonorrhea, one of the most commonly reported communicable diseases in the United States; human papilomavirus, also known as genital warts; and pelvic inflammatory disease (PID), a group of infections that can be caused by a combination of circumstances.

Only one modern contraceptive, the male condom, offers couples protection from sexually transmitted diseases in addition to protecting them from unwanted pregnancies, which is a contraceptive's primary purpose. Health care professionals and researchers, however, see a strong link between these two consequences of sexual intercourse and work is underway to develop products that are designed to simultaneously protect against unwanted pregnancy and STDs.

The modern latex condom provides couples with the best present protection, other than sexual abstinence, from STDs, including human immunodeficiency virus (HIV), but that protection is not perfect and success depends significantly on people consistently and accurately using a condom during intercourse. If used properly, condoms could reduce the rates of STD infections by nearly

50 percent. Condoms prevent contact with the sores common with STDs and keep to a minimum the sharing of body fluids that carry bacteria, viruses, and other infectious particles.

People, however, are inconsistent in how and when they use condoms. They often improperly apply the sheath to the man's penis, or apply it after enough genital contact has occurred between the couple to pass diseases between bodies. Condoms must be used with each and every act of sexual intercourse to protect against sexually transmitted diseases. Only 16 percent of women who used condoms in 1994 reported using them every time they had sex. Another 56 percent of sexually active men and women reported occasionally using condoms. The remainder did not use condoms at all. All couples who occasionally use condoms or who don't use them with every act of intercourse are exposed to the same risk of STDs as people who never use condoms.

In addition, not all condoms offer protection against STDs. Those made of animal membranes offer little if any protection, because the material is too porous. Tiny holes in the surface can allow diseases to pass through the condom while still blocking the path of semen from the penis during ejaculation. Animal membrane condoms are often used by those with allergies to latex condoms.

Condoms made of new materials, though, may provide even more protection against sexually transmitted diseases than do latex condoms and offer people more choice. Polyurethane, a type of plastic, and a natural rubber under study would work like latex in preventing disease organisms from passing through them during sexual intercourse. A polyurethane condom reached the U.S. market in the mid-1990s.

The female condom, also known as the vaginal pouch, offers similar protection to that of the male condom. Made of polyurethane and inserted into the woman's vagina before intercourse, the condom's walls prevent the spread of disease while helping prevent pregnancy. The single-use product was approved in the United Kingdom in 1992 and the United States in 1993 and is slowly being marketed in countries in Africa and South America.

Modern spermicides seem to offer some help in preventing the spread of some sexually transmitted disease. Studies suggest that nonoxynol-9, the most commonly used spermicide in the United States, may help protect people from chlamydia and gonorrhea. Spermicides are often used with diaphragms and vaginal sponges. Some condoms also contain small amounts of spermicides. However, nonoxynol-9 used in too large a dose irritates the lining of the vagina and may destroy microorganisms necessary for the woman's health. Health care workers worry that doses high enough to protect people from sexually transmitted diseases would create pain, irritation, and damage to the woman's vagina.

Hormonal contraceptives offer women no protection against most sexually transmitted diseases; however, medical research has established that combined oral contraceptives do decrease a woman's risk of contracting pelvic inflammatory disease, particularly the more severe forms.

Microbicides seem to offer the most promise for giving women a product to protect them from sexually transmitted diseases, rather than requiring the women to expect the man to use a condom. Research on about 40 microbicidal products is underway and 15 were being tested on humans in 1999. Researchers did not expect products to reach the market before 2001. Essentially, microbicides target specific diseases and leave the natural and healthful organisms of the vagina in tact. Some of the products under development would combine protection from unwanted pregnancy with protection from sexually transmitted diseases. Others would offer only STD protection.

Public opinion polls taken in the United States suggest that women of all ages would welcome the arrival on the market of a protection from STDs that could be applied hours before intercourse, that could be purchased over the counter at a drugstore, like condoms, and that could be used privately.

Some STDs, such as herpes and genital warts, can be transmitted through parts of the body other than the genitals, and condoms, spermicides, and microbicides cannot protect people from diseases passed from person to person through contact in these areas.

Abstinence, in the late twentieth century, was still the safest way for people to protect themselves both from sexually transmitted diseases and unwanted pregnancy. However, people's willingness to take risks with their health and their lives through unprotected sexual intercourse has led to what health care professionals have called an epidemic of most STDs, and recommend regular examinations of men and women for symptoms of these diseases.

In fact, many pharmaceutical companies and organizations have shifted from studying contraception to studying and developing microbicides as responses to the public health concern of fighting rising rates of sexually transmitted diseases. *See also* ACQUIRED IMMUNODEFICIENCY SYNDROME (AIDS); CONDOM—FEMALE; CONDOM—MALE; SAFE SEX

Further reading: Larkin, Marilynn. "Easing the Way to Safer Sex." *The Lancet,* 28 March 1998, 964. Nevid, Jeffrey S., and Fern Gotfried. *Choices: Sex in the Age of STDs.* Boston: Allyn and Bacon, 1995. Stephenson, Joan. "Report Offers Vision for Microbicide Development." *Journal of the American Medical Association* 281 (1999): 405.

Side Effects

All forms of birth control and contraception have the potential to cause unintended reactions in the people who use them. These side effects, when they occur, tend to be personally uncomfortable, unacceptable, and the primary reasons people stop using specific methods of contraception. In contrast, medical professionals and experts use the term "risk" to refer to the potentially life-threatening or physically damaging consequences of using birth control methods; generally, "side effects" are viewed as not life threatening and occasionally advantageous to the person using the method.

Some people see the side effects of contraception as nuisances they are willing to tolerate for the protection the device provides against unwanted pregnancy. Other people find those same side effects to be intolerable and reasons to seek other protection. By the end of the twentieth century, however, the major modern artificial means of preventing pregnancy provided people with enough variety that they could find similar products that did not have the same side effects. Combined oral contraceptives (COCs) are currently available in a wide range of dosages of both estrogen and progestin. If a progestin level causes breakthrough bleeding for a woman, she can consult her doctor for a pill that contains progestin levels that prevents the problem. One formulation might cause a headache where another will not. Condoms also come in loser-fitting models than were previously available to increase the sensations men feel during intercourse. Researchers are working to develop new spermicides that do not cause irritation to the vagina or penis with repeated use.

While a nuisance side effect may not prevent a person from trying a specific contraceptive method, those side effects may lead her or him to stop using the method. Compliance with the directions provided by product manufacturers and health care providers forms an important criteria for the effectiveness of a contraceptive. With perfect use, hormonal contraceptives are more than 99 percent effective at preventing pregnancy, but a woman's experience with headaches or nausea can cause her to decide to take a break from the pill. During this break she may neglect to use an alternative birth control method and risk pregnancy. In order to increase the success of a method and help the woman achieve her contraceptive goals, experts who advise clients will discuss the side effects and the woman's likelihood of experiencing them. This education, in turn, helps women recognize and report side effects and their reactions to them so that the experts can use their knowledge and resources to modify the woman's contraceptive method.

Package directions deal with physical side effects of birth control methods; however, emotional or cultural side effects may also influence the success of a product. Women who feel uncomfortable touching their vaginas may experience emotional discomfort while using a female barrier contraceptive. The possible embarrassment of being found carrying contraceptive pills may cause some women to miss taking their pills. Even cultural issues, such as the importance of menstruation as a sign of good health, can make a specific method that interferes with her monthly period unacceptable to a woman. Even fertility awareness methods of contraception, which relies on periods of abstinence from intercourse, may strain the emotional relationship between a woman and a man.

Most contraceptive users, however, do not experience side effects. Hormonal contraceptives have the greatest chance to cause side effects since they alter a woman's normal hormonal balance. Even so, women who experience nausea, fluid retention, and breast tenderness as they begin using the pill commonly find that these side effects subside and disappear with continued use and within a few months. Following package directions and following advice for conditions that can lead to side effects can also prevent many discomforts caused by contraceptives.

Some side effects of hormonal contraceptives have led to uses of them for conditions other than prevention of pregnancy. The progestins in COCs are known to have a positive effect on acne and oily skin and often reduce the impacts of these conditions in women once they begin taking the contraceptive. In addition, women using COCs tend to have less intense menstrual cramps, more regular periods, and shortened periods. The incidence of ovarian cysts also decreases, by 80 to 90 percent, for women using COCs.

Learning about and discussing side effects with trained professionals before choosing a contraceptive method helps men and women effectively use their chosen method, and helps them realize when a side effect is preventing them from being successful at preventing pregnancy. *See also* RISK

Further reading: "Compliance with Oral Contraceptives." *The Contraception Report* 5, special report (1995): 3–23. Goldzieher, Joseph W., and Nesaam M. Zamah. "Oral Contraceptive Side Effects: Where's the Beef?" *Contraception* 52 (1995): 327–335.

Smoking

For women, smoking poses extra risk to their reproductive health, especially if they use combined hormonal contraceptives containing synthetic estrogen.

Smoking has been shown to increase a woman's risk from cervical cancer and ectopic pregnancy. It can cause the early onset of menopause, delay conception, and decrease a woman's fertility.

A woman's smoking significantly influences her choice of contraceptives. Combined oral contraceptives (COCs) contain doses of synthetic estrogen. Intense scientific research since the first COCs became publicly available in 1960 have demonstrated a clear connection between the estrogen in COCs and smoking and cardiovascular problems. Women who smoke have been shown to be at higher risk from heart attack and circulatory problems than COC users who do not smoke (for whom the risk of heart attack is the same as or even less than for nonsmoking women who do not use COCs).

Among smoking women who use COCs, those who smoke fewer than 15 cigarettes a day are at three times the risk from heart attack than those who do not smoke. Women who smoke more than 15 cigarettes a day are at 21 times the risk from heart attack as those who do not smoke. Age increases that risk further to the point that women over 35 who smoke at all are at significantly higher risk of heart disease than nonsmoking COC users of the same age.

Decreasing the estrogen component in COCs directly decreases a smoking woman's risk from heart attack. Modern very low dose pills contain 20 micrograms of estrogen. The most commonly prescribed pills contain 50 micrograms. The less estrogen, the less the risk to smokers. This formula, however, does not hold for women over 35.

Prescribing information and information provided to and by the physicians who prescribe COCs advise women under the ages of 35 who smoke to use very low estrogen dose pills. Women 35 and older who are light smokers and who use COCs to prevent pregnancy are safest using very low dose estrogen pills. However, experts strongly recommend that women over 35 should quit smoking or not use the estrogen containing combined oral contraceptives of any dose.

Smoking also puts women at greater risk of suffering from thromboembolisms, or deep vein blood clots, which can cause death. Again, choosing a COC with a low estrogen dose reduces a woman's risk from this illness.

While the very low dose combined oral contraceptives have significantly reduced the risk from heart attack and circulatory diseases for younger women who smoke, they have not decreased the risk for women over 35 whether they are light or heavy smokers. Required drug information, client counseling, and physician education efforts in the 1990s all aimed at encouraging women who smoke and want to use combined oral contraceptives to stop smoking by the time they reached that risk age. In contrast, progestin-only contraceptives, such as Norplant, depot medroxyprogestrone acetate, and mini-pills, offer women long-term contraceptive options to combined oral contracrptives. *See also* COMBINED ORAL CONTRACEPTIVES; RISK

Further reading: Castelli, William P. "Reducing Risk in OC Users Who Smoke." *Contemporary Obstetrics/Gynecology* 41 (1996): 118–126.

South Africa

A greater percentage of women in South Africa, which is located at the southern tip of the African continent, use modern contraceptives than in any other African country. As of 1999, 55 percent of married South African women used modern contraceptives and 49 percent of all women did so. With a total fertility rate, the average number of children a woman could expect to give birth to, hovering at 3.0, the nation's growth rate stood at 1 percent each year, also low for sub-Saharan Africa. Researchers predict that the total fertility rate will fall to 2.0 by 2010 and annual growth through births will slow until it stops. In its success at limiting growth to encourage economic development, South Africa is held by many reproductive health and social advocates as well as population policy analysts as a model for its African neighbors to follow.

In 1994, the first democratically elected government began governing South Africa. With that government came a new constitution that guaranteed to people the "right to

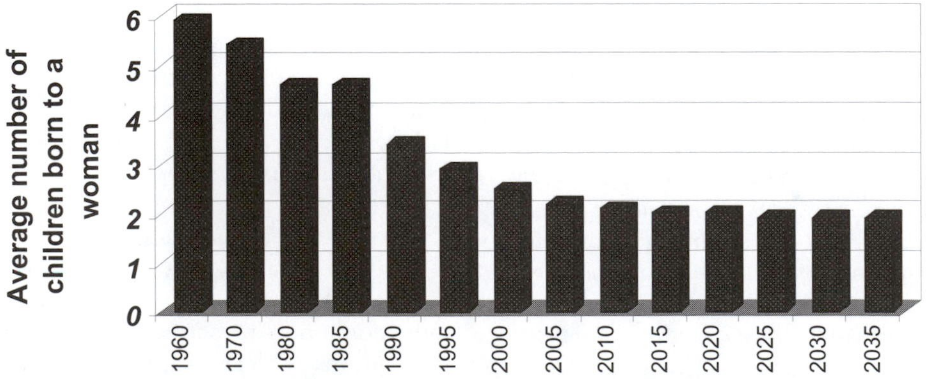

South Africa: Total Fertility Rate: Actual and Projected

Source: U.S. Census Bureau International Data Base

make decisions about reproduction and the right to reproductive health care." With that goal in mind, the government provided free health care to pregnant women and children under the age of six.

The relationship between the women of South Africa and modern birth control methods grew out of and is still influenced by the practices of the white-ruled apartheid government in place when modern methods first became available in the late 1960s and 1970s. In 1974, the apartheid government began a family planning program aimed primarily at the black population. By 1989, when apartheid was ending, 44 percent of the nation's black women used modern contraceptives, including the pill and Depo-Provera. The fertility rate had dropped from 6 children per women of reproductive age to 4.6. Despite the government's racist motivations for making contraceptives available, many black women turned voluntarily to these methods to prevent pregnancy. As men left their homes to work on farms, women were left to care for families. Resources also became scarce for black women and they found that modern contraceptives helped them prevent unwanted pregnancies, which could lead to them losing their jobs and to having too many children to feed and care for.

Women in South Africa still face a high incidence of death due to the complications of pregnancy and childbearing. At 44 maternal deaths for every 100,000 women, South African health professionals became concerned that deficiencies in the supply of contraceptives led to unsafe abortion practices. In an effort to decrease that number, and also to grant women the right to a legal termination of a pregnancy, South Africa's legislature passed into law in 1997 the Choice on Termination of Pregnancy Act. The law faced a constitutional challenge in 1998, but the high court in Pretoria ruled that the act was consistent with the constitution. South Africa is now the only African nation to have made abortion legal without restrictions during the first 12 weeks of pregnancy.

The new South African government has found that women still expect and use the contraceptive services provided in that country. While many women seem to be suspicious of the government's support of abortion, the government is working to bring a wide range of contraceptive and family planning options to its people. In general, however, South Africans have more convenient access to condoms, oral contraceptives, intrauterine devices, and female sterilization than any other African nation. Vasectomies are also increasing in availability. *See also* AFRICA

Further reading: Bennett, Trude. "Reproductive Health in South Africa." *Public Health Reports* 114 (1999): 88–90. *Center for International Health Information Health Statistics Report: South Africa*. Center for International Health Information, 29 October 1999. Online: http://www.cihi.com/PHANstat/SOUTH_AFRICA, 12 November 1999.

Sperm

A sperm, the male sex cell, carries half the chromosomes necessary to begin a new human life.

At puberty, a male's testicles begin making sperm in the seminiferous tubules and his body continuously makes the cells throughout his life. The sperm move to the epididymis, a long coiled tube resting on top of the testicles, where they mature and wait until sexual arousal causes them to travel through two more tubes in the male reproductive system, the ductus deferens, and into the urethra. As the urethra passes through the prostate gland, the sperm mix with semen, which has been produced by the seminal vesicles, prostate gland, testes, and the bulbourethral gland. With each ejaculation at the end of sexual intercourse, a man sends between 200 million and 400 million sperm from his body; they travel in 2 to 6 millimeters of semen. Only one of those sperm cells is needed to fertilize a female ovum.

Each sperm cell is made up of a large head and a long whiplike tail. The action of that tail propels the sperm through the female reproductive system. If the sperm meets with a mature ovum, the head penetrates the outer layer of the egg and transfers the 23 sex chromosomes to the egg where they combine with the female's chromosomes. Fertilization has occurred.

Commonly used contraceptives stop sperm along their path to the ovum. In a vasectomy, a surgeon cuts or ties the vas deferens. A condom covers the penis and captures the semen as it leaves the man's body. Other barriers inserted into the woman's vagina either prevent sperm from entering the uterus or kill the sperm in the vagina.

Several chemical methods of male contraception, such as enzymes that alter the sperm's structure and testosterone injections to suppress the manufacture of sperm, are now being studied and tested. *See also* MALE CONTRACEPTIVES; PROSTATE GLAND; REPRODUCTIVE SYSTEM—MALE; SEMEN; VAS DEFERENS

Spermicides

Spermicides use strong chemical reactions to block the path of sperm in the vagina and kill sperm on contact. Most often spermicides are used with barrier contraceptives, such as the diaphragm, cervical cap, and vaginal sponge, to increase their effectiveness. Many varieties of condoms also include spermicides to increase their effectiveness.

As foams, creams, gels, suppositories, and tablets, spermicides are available without prescription in drug stores and many convenience stores. All spermicides must be inserted into the vagina to be effective. Rules for use vary but all packaging is required to include clear instructions, that users need to follow carefully for full effect. Two spermicides—nonoxynol-9 and octoxynol—are in common use in the United States.

When used alone, spermicides have a reported effectiveness rate ranging from 6 percent with perfect use to 21 percent with typical use, though there is disagreement on these figures, due primarily to the wide variety of forms in which spermicides are manufactured. Films can slip out of place and tablets and suppositories need time to dissolve in the vagina before the man inserts his penis. Verifying the effectiveness of spermicides alone is also complicated by its common use with diaphragms, cervical caps, and condoms. Most commonly, clinicians recommend spermicides be used with other barriers and only be used alone in an emergency, such as if a condom breaks.

Many people who use spermicides often report irritation of the woman's vagina or the man's penis from the chemicals, though not all brands have the same reported level of irritation. Frequent use of spermicides, two or three times a week, has been linked to increased risk of urinary track infections in women.

Research efforts are underway to develop less caustic spermicides that immobilize sperm but that do not work like detergents to wash off the outer layer of the sperm. The ingredients of common spermicides that kill sperm also can cause the irritation that many users report.

Some spermicides have been shown to protect women against sexually transmitted diseases. However, current formulations of spermicides are known to kill natural occurring organisms in the woman's vaginal, as well as sperm, and diminish the spermicide's effectiveness against disease. Scientists hope that ongoing research will lead to effective chemicals that inhibit sperm while not destroying the natural state of the vagina.

Scientists are also trying to develop spermicides that would require far smaller concentrations to effectively kill sperm. Study is still underway and yielding mixed results of the effectiveness of spermicides to protect people from sexually transmitted diseases, though some of the spermicides under development contain antimicrobial agents that would kill diseases as they stop sperm. *See also* BARRIER CONTRACEPTIVES; SEXUALLY TRANSMITTED DISEASES

Further reading: Harrison, Polly F., and Allan Rosenfield, eds. *Contraceptive Research and Development: Looking to the Future.* Washington, DC: National Academy Press, 1996. Hatcher, Robert, James Trussel, Felicia Stewart, and others. *Contraceptive Technology.* 16th rev. ed. New York: Irvington, 1994. Vergano, D. "The Trouble with Condoms." *Science News,* 14 September 1996, 165.

Sterilization

Sterilization acts as a contraceptive by permanently blocking or interrupting the reproductive tracts and permanently preventing pregnancy. Current methods of surgical sterilization are highly effective, and research is underway around the world to develop nonsurgical methods of blocking the reproductive tract. In developing as well as developed countries, sterilization has become one of the most frequently chosen forms of contraception.

Contraceptive methods of sterilization involve, in women and men, blocking the tubes that carry sex cells through the reproductive tract. In women, the two fallopian tubes that lead from the ovaries to the uterus are cut, tied, or blocked in a tubal sterilization. In men, the two vas deferens, which lead from the testicles to the penis, are also cut or blocked in a vasectomy. Surgical procedures performed for reasons other than contraception also may leave a person sterile. The removal of a woman's uterus in a hysterectomy or removal of the prostate in men result in the inability of those people to conceive children.

Tubal sterilization has a reported success rate, for typical and perfect use, of 99.6 percent; four women out of every 1,000 are likely to become pregnant within one year of the operation. Vasectomy has a higher success rate at 99.85 percent with typical use and 99.9 percent with perfect use. Failures seem to result most when women are pregnant before undergoing the procedure and when men fail to wait the minimum of three months after a vasectomy to have unprotected sexual intercourse for all of the sperm to finally be cleared from their reproductive tracts. Recent studies, however, have called into question the high success rate of female sterilization, noting that different methods of blocking the fallopian tubes lead to different rates of preventing pregnancy and that the woman's age when she was sterilized also influences its effectiveness.

In developed countries both tubal sterilization and vasectomy are typically performed in outpatient settings, with vasectomies performed in medical offices and tubal sterilization performed in surgical centers. Access to both procedures is spreading slowly and steadily in developing countries but is most often performed in hospitals.

A man's vasectomy involves far less surgical risk during the procedure than does a woman's tubal sterilization. A vasectomy requires that a surgically trained medical practitioner puncture or slit the thin skin of the testicles to reach the vas deferens. A tubal sterilization, in contrast, requires that a surgically trained practitioner cut through the abdominal wall, including skin and muscle tissue, to reach the fallopian tubes. Despite the safety and greater ease of performing vasectomy, more than twice as many women undergo tubal sterilization than men undergo vasectomies.

In the United States, married women were twice as likely to have undergone a sterilization procedure than were their husbands. According to the 1995 National Survey of Family Growth, 26 percent of married women had undergone tubal sterilization, whereas 12 percent of the husbands of married women had undergone vasectomy. In all subgroups of women, including groups determined by age, race, education, and household income, tubal sterilization was significantly more common than vasectomy.

That trend in the frequency of female sterilization over male sterilization occurred around the world according to similar national surveys and United Nations statistics. In many countries, the use of tubal sterilization far outnumbered the use of male vasectomy. In Latin America, 21percent of sexually active adults had undergone female sterilization and 1 percent had undergone male sterilization. In Asia, 23 percent of the sexually active adults had undergone female sterilization compared to 6 percent having undergone vasectomy. For all developed countries, 8 percent had undergone female sterilization and 4 percent had undergone male sterilization.

In the United States and other developed countries, increasing numbers of younger women seemed to be choosing this form of permanent sterilization over temporary methods. Research showed that the younger a woman was when she first had a child, the more likely she was to have a sterilizing operation. Some family planning specialists and medical professionals see this trend as a clear indication that much research needs to be done to provide young women with highly effective, convenient, and safe, but easily reversible, forms of contraception.

To make permanent sterilization available to people who do not have easy access to hospitals and the sterile settings needed for surgical procedures, scientists are working to develop methods of nonsurgical sterilization. All concentrate on inserting substances into the tubes to scar or otherwise block these passages. While tests are under way for studying balloons, chemicals, such as quinacrine, and plastic plugs for men and women, none was expected to result in a publicly available procedure until well into the twenty-first century. *See also* HYSTERECTOMY; QUINACRINE; TUBAL STERILIZATION; VASECTOMY

Further reading: Barnet, Barbara. "Search for Nonsurgical Sterilization Continues." *Network* 18.1 (1997). Online: http://resevoir.fhi.org/en/fp/fppubs/network/v18-1/nt1815.html, 25 June 1999. Moore, M. "Most U.S. Couples Who Seek Surgical Sterilization Do So for Contraception: Fewer Than 25 Percent Desire Reversal." *Family Planning Perspectives* 31 (1999): 102.

Stopes, Marie C. (1880–1958)

In 1921, scientist, writer, and social reformer Marie C. Stopes founded the first free birth control clinic in Great Britain. At a time when people believed that human sexuality and birth control were unfit topics for public and private discussion, Stopes became a powerful leader in the fight for women's rights and a woman's right to control when and if she conceived children.

Born 15 October 1880, in Edinburgh, Scotland, to Henry Stopes, an architect and amateur paleontologist, and Charlotte Carmichael, a Shakespeare scholar and advocate for women's rights. Through her father's interests, Marie developed a passion for science and in 1904 became the first woman to receive a PhD in botany from Munich University. In 1905, she became the youngest person to earn a doctor of science degree in Great Britain. Marie was the first woman to serve on the science faculty at Manchester University. Her continuing research and articles and lectures on botany earned Marie international acclaim for her scholarship.

In an attempt to understand her own feelings and to explain the failure of her first marriage, which was annulled in 1916 for non-consumation, Marie applied her scientific skills to a study of human sexuality. She made charts and notes of her sexual reactions and desires and carefully studied other women's feelings and impulses. She also studied the collection of scientific materials on human sexuality that were kept in a nonpublic area of the British Museum.

This personal and scientific study led Marie to write *Married Love* (1918), an in-depth discussion of sexuality that contained a detailed description of intercourse. The tremendous popularity of that book and the poor and middle class women it brought her in contact with increased Stopes's concern for women and the hardships they faced when burdened with unwanted pregnancies. Her influence in the women's suffrage movement and the growing birth control movement increased dramatically and on 17 March 1921, with the help of her second husband, Stopes took the daring step of opening the Mother's Clinic for Constructive Birth Control in north London. Her purposes, and those of her supporters, were to help the poor, to test the attitudes of the working class towards birth control, to gather data about contraception, and to collect data on the sex lives of women.

Stopes staffed the clinic with women: a midwife to examine the clients, a female doctor to consult with patients with abnormal cases, and nurses to fit the pessaries—vaginal plugs—or early diaphragms. While the first year saw only a few women each day at the clinic, it remained open, and over the years public demand for the services grew. By 1930, approximately 14 free birth control clinics were open in Great Britain, birth control clinics affiliated with Stopes's were open in much of the British Empire, and a horse-drawn mobile birth control facility served England's rural areas. Stopes drew criticism from the medical community, both male and female, for not being a physician, and experienced conflict with members of the Roman Catholic Church, but also experienced strong popular demand for her clinics' services.

Stopes believed passionately in the rights of poor women to have access to birth control. She saw firsthand and often received letters from women burdened by too many children and women who suffered physically from too many pregnancies. Stopes abhorred abortion and considered it an "evil" and "murderous" practice. She saw birth control and education on human sexuality as a solution to the miseries of poverty, a humane alternative to abortion, and a recourse for women who wanted to have greater control over their lives.

Her two books of advice to married couples, *Married Love* and *Wise Parenthood* (1918), and her work to establish birth control as a topic of public discussion established Stopes as the leading advocate in the social movement that brought issues of human sexuality and the scientific study of birth control into the public realm. She died 2 October 1958, of breast cancer.

Today, Marie Stopes International, a worldwide charity, continues the work Stopes started and offers services in reproductive health care. *See also*: DENNETT, MARY WARE; SANGER, MARGARET HIGGINS

Further reading: Hall, Ruth. *Passionate Crusader: The Life of Marie Stopes.* New York: Harcourt Brace Jovanovich, 1977. Rose, June. *Marie Stopes and the Sexual Revolution*. London: Faber and Faber, 1992.

Sweden

Sweden's society and government has since the middle of the 1900s strongly supported contraception for family planning, school-based sex education for children, and social programs that encourage the education, equality, and advancement of women.

Women in Sweden can expect to give birth to an average of 1.6 children in their lifetimes. Well below the replacement level of 2.08 children, that birth rate is one of the highest in western Europe, a rapidly aging and slowly

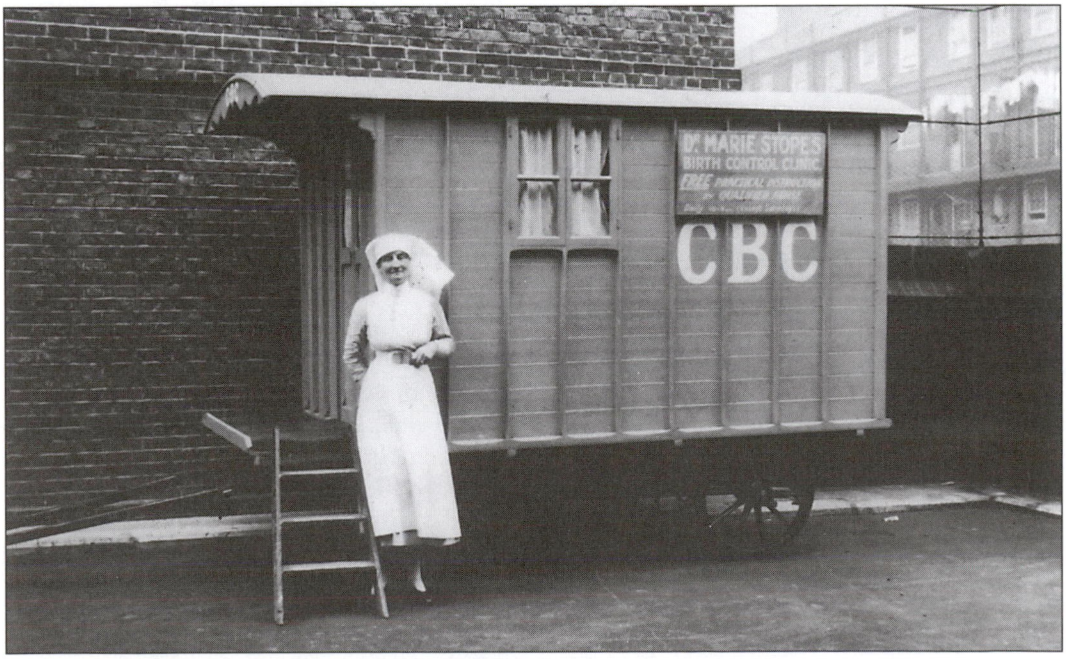

By 1930, horse-drawn mobile birth control facilities established by Marie Stopes and her clinic staff served England's rural areas. *Courtesy Marie Stopes International*

reproducing area of the world. Sweden's population at the end of the twentieth century was neither growing nor decreasing at a flat zero percent annual growth rate.

The Swedish government passed laws in 1938 removing restrictions on providing full information on contraceptives and on distributing and selling birth control devices. Since the 1970s, newspapers have run ads in that country for condoms. Ads and billboards promote awareness of birth control and emphasize a person's responsibility to their sexual partners to take precautions against unwanted pregnancy and sexually transmitted diseases.

Contraceptive use in Sweden is virtually universal. All sexually active people, including teens, have easy and often free access to the full variety of modern contraceptives. Use of condoms by men is extremely high. People can easily buy condoms in gas stations, grocery stores, and pharmacies. Teens do not need their parents' permission to buy contraceptives or to receive prescriptions for contraceptives. Their doctors may encourage teens to discuss contraception with their parents, but doctors cannot inform parents that their daughter or son has received advice and a prescription.

Abortion has been officially legal in Sweden since 1975, when a new law made abortion legal within the first 12 weeks of pregnancy and available upon the request of the woman. That law specified that from the thirteenth through the eighteenth week the woman must apply for an abortion and between the eighteenth and twenty-third week the National Board of Health must approve the abortion. This law applies equally to teens and adults. Without her specific permission, a physician or social worker may inform no one of a teen or adult's decision to undergo the abortion.

The teen birth rate in Sweden is very low, about 13 for every 1,000 women between the ages of 15 and 19. That low rate, far lower than the U.S. rate at 64 births for every 1,000 teens of the same age, is believed to result from policies regarding education and access to birth control and abortion. Sweden provides comprehensive sex education in the schools that emphasizes explicit contraceptive education. Most schools also have within them gynecological clinics where teens, mostly girls, receive reproductive health care, including contraceptives, without requiring parental permission. Finally, teens have the same rights to abortion services as do adults and abortions within the first 12 weeks are paid for by the government. Experts believe these three approaches have resulted in fewer teen pregnancies, fewer teen abortions, and fewer teen births.

Women make up a large percentage of the members of Sweden's parliament, 41 percent after the 1994 elections. Half of the nation's cabinet members were women in 1994. Women also make up nearly half of the labor force in Sweden. As women moved into Sweden's government, they exercised their power to lead the government to provide social services that support a woman's, man's, or couple's decision on when and if to have children. Women and men now share almost equally in the decision to have children.

Sweden's social innovations have decreased fertility, though not to the lows seen in Italy where women and children receive little government support but where the total fertility rate was 1.2 in the late 1990s. In Sweden, social policies support child-bearing decisions, women and men then feel they are better able to financially and socially afford to raise the number of children they choose to bear. Through social policy and support of the family, Sweden has encouraged a balanced population growth rate that will not lead to overpopulation or to too few children being born to meet the needs in society. In Italy, by contrast, a lack of social support for family needs leads people to choose not to have children. With its fertility rate, Sweden has maintained such low growth that demographers expect its population to grow by only 400,000 by 2025.

The education and social empowering of women account for both the low fertility rate and the very high prevalence of use of modern contraceptives in Sweden. *See also* EUROPE

Further reading: Chenais, Jean-Claude. "Fertility, Family, and Social Policy in Contemporary Western Europe." *Population and Development Review* 22 (1996): 729–739. Santow, Gigi, and Michael Bracher. "Explaining Trends in Teenage Childbearing in Sweden." *Studies in Family Planning* 33 (1999): 169–182. Trost, Jan E. "The Family Planning Rights of Minors in Sweden." In *The Adolescent Dilemma: International Perspectives on the Family Planning Rights of Minors,* edited by Hyman Rodman and Jan Trost. New York: Praeger, 1986.

T

Testicles

The two testicles are the primary male sex organs. They contain the basic cells that evolve into sperm, the male sex cells. They also produce testosterone, the primary male sex hormone.

The oval-shaped organs are 5 centimeters (2 inches) long and 3 centimeters (1.25 inches) in diameter, about the size of a large olive. They hang in the scrotum, a small sac of skin that hangs behind the penis outside of the lower end of a man's abdomen.

As a male fetus grows, the testicles form inside of the abdomen and shortly before birth travel down through a narrow canal and out of the boy's body to take up their permanent position suspended in the scrotum. The temperature inside the human body would prevent the sperm cells from maturing, but the cooler temperatures outside of the abdominal cavity allows the full development of the sperm.

Beginning in puberty, a man's testicles continuously create sperm. From the testicles, the sperm moves to the attached epididymis, a long, coiled tube that rests on top of the testicles inside the scrotum. Each epididymis is connected to a testicle at one end and a vas deferens, a tube that leads to the urethra in the penis, at the other. *See also* REPRODUCTIVE SYSTEM—MALE; SPERM; VAS DEFERENS

Testosterone

Testosterone, the primary and most potent male sex hormone, governs the development of the male reproductive tract and the creation of sperm. It is manufactured in a man's testicles, the same organ that produces sperm cells.

A steroid hormone, testosterone performs its functions by connecting to receptor molecules in target cells. Those functions include inducing puberty in boys, stimulating sperm growth throughout a man's adult life, and maintaining his secondary sex characteristics, such as facial hair, enlarged muscles, and enlarged sex organs.

During fetal growth, testosterone helps develop male characteristics in a fetus, but production of this hormone stops several weeks after birth. It resumes when a male body grows to the point of entering adulthood when the endocrine system triggers the renewed production of testosterone. From puberty on, the man's testicles produce high levels of this hormone. However, by age 40, testosterone levels begin to decrease, and by age 80 most men produce about one-fifth of their peak levels.

Several artificial forms of testosterone are manufactured by pharmaceutical companies. They are used primarily to treat a variety of diseases in both men and women. In the 1990s, researchers began experimenting with male contraceptives that alter testosterone levels and thus decrease sperm production. However, low levels of testosterone change a man's secondary sex characteristics and cause a decrease in a man's sex drive.

Other glands secrete small amounts of testosterone, but the functions of these glands are not yet fully understood by scientists. Cells of the adrenal cortex, at the top of the adrenal glands which sit on top of each kidney, produce testosterone both in men and women. It is believed that both sexes convert these testosterone hormones into estrogens, the primary female hormone. *See also* HORMONES—SEX; HORMONES—SYNTHETIC; MALE CONTRACEPTIVES; REPRODUCTIVE SYSTEM—MALE

Further reading: Jones, Richard, E. *Human Reproductive Biology.* San Diego, CA: Academic Press–Harcourt Brace Jovanovich, 1991.

Total Fertility Rate

The statistical calculation of a nation, region, or people's total fertility rate represents one way to attempt to understand population growth. An estimate, the total fertility rate is the average number of children born alive to a woman, or a group of women, during her, or their, lifetime. It is a statistic that adds the age-specific rates easily calculated for women, where the number of children born to women in a specific age or range of ages, is divided by the number of women in that age group.

By using contraceptive methods, people control the number of children to which they give birth and influence the total fertility rate of the populations to which they belong. Generally the greater the number of people who use contraceptives, the lower a nation's total fertility rate.

Demographers, who study the statistics of population, use total fertility rate as an indication of the current levels and trends in fertility. A total fertility rate of 2.0 indicates a population that is neither growing or shrinking. Women would be giving birth to two children, a number considered replacement, for themselves and the fathers of their children. Numbers higher than 2.0 indicate a growing population and with rates below 2.0 the population is shrinking.

In India, for example, the total fertility rate in 1999 was 3.5 for the entire nation. That figure varied greatly from state to state; in Kerala, a southwestern state, the total fertility rate stood at 1.7 and in Uttar Pradesh, a northern state, it stood at 5.2. Italy, with a total fertility rate of 1.2 in 1999, had the lowest fertility rate in the world, matched only by Spain.

Demographers have detected a flaw in using the total fertility rate to estimate the rate of population growth and decline. By the late 1990s many women were using birth control methods to delay childbirth. That delay was causing "tempo effects" in fertility rate calculations, which, in varying ways, were distorting a true picture of the rate at which women were having children. *See also* POPULATION GROWTH

Further reading: Bongaarts, John. "The Fertility Impact of Changes in the Timing of Childbearing in the Developing World." Policy Research Division Working Paper No. 120. New York: Population Council, 1999.

Toxic Shock Syndrome

Toxic shock syndrome is a rare but serious illness seen most frequently in women who use tampons during menstruation. A woman who uses barrier birth control devices that are inserted into her vagina is also at slight risk from this illness. Most commonly a bacterial infection causes toxic shock.

The labeling and packaging on diaphragms, vaginal sponges, and cervical caps, warn women of the risk of toxic shock, though that risk is very low. Two or three cases of toxic shock develop each year for every 100,000 women using barrier contraceptives. The chance of death from the disease is much rarer for those not using barrier contraceptives at only 0.18 deaths for every 100,000 women. Teens and young women, between 15 and 24 years old, have been shown to be at greater risk of toxic shock than older women.

Doctors and clinicians, who must prescribe the diaphragm and cervical cap, also council patients on the risks of toxic shock. A careful and detailed discussion between the woman and health care provider concerning symptoms and actions to take if symptoms occur decreases the risk of toxic shock even further.

The disease causes a fever over 102 degrees Fahrenheit, headaches, sore throat, vomiting or diarrhea, dizziness and lightheadedness, cramping, confusion, and a sunburn-like rash on the bottom of the feet or the palms. Women who experience these symptoms are instructed to remove the diaphragm, sponge, or cap and contact their health care provider immediately. Treatment for the bacterial infection includes antibiotics and medication to reduce the fever.

Use of oral contraceptives have been shown to reduce a woman's risk from toxic shock. *See also* RISK

Further reading: Hatcher, Robert, James Trussel, Felicia Stewart, and others. *Contraceptive Technology*. 17th rev. ed. New York: Ardent Media, 1998. Schwarts, Benjamin, et al. "Nonmenstrual Toxic Shock Syndrome Associated with Barrier Contraceptives: Report of a Case-Control Study." *Reviews of Infectious Diseases* 11, Supplement 1 (1989): S43–S49.

Traditional Methods of Contraception

In many studies of contraception, writers interchange the terms "natural" and "traditional," using them to set apart these older methods of trying to prevent pregnancy from modern manufactured and surgical forms of pregnancy prevention. Around the world and throughout history, women have turned to herbs, plants, and natural substances to limit the number of children born. These traditional methods of contraception often pass from generation to generation through word of mouth. Many are still used by populations around the world, from the Appalachian Mountains of the United States to rural South America and Africa.

In the United States, women have reported using the crushed seeds of Queen Anne's lace, a commonly grown herb, to prevent conception after intercourse. Historical records also show that European women used this herb as recently as the seventeenth century. In developing countries, even where modern contraceptives are easily available and often used, such as Jamaica and Egypt, women continue using herbal contraceptives to influence their fertility. Often, as modern contraceptives become more available in developing countries, women will use both the scientifically developed and studied contraceptive in conjunction with that passed down through their culture. Sociological research suggests that older, less educated, and poorer women may rely on such traditional methods to prevent pregnancy, while younger, more educated women in such traditional societies turn to modern contraceptives.

Concern among some researchers that policy makers and family planning programs were ignoring the possibility that traditional methods of fertility control had value and effectiveness in women's lives led in the 1990s to reconsideration of traditional methods. Anthropological and sociological researchers in the 1990s began calling for careful scientific study of the chemicals at work in traditional contraceptives and for study of their effectiveness and safe, appropriate methods for their use. The World Health Organization also advocated the study and acceptance of traditional herbal methods of contraception as ways to help women achieve their goals in family planning.

Part of this increased interest among scientists stemmed from the rise in popularity of natural family planning methods, such as the Billings Method and the lactation amenorrhea method (LAM) of contraception. Both received careful study in the 1980s and 1990s and scientists found fertility awareness methods and LAM to be highly effective when used perfectly. Both, however, had high failure rates when couples did not carefully follow them. However, the study of the Billings Method, which uses secretions of a woman's cervical mucus to determine when ovulation occurs, and LAM, which relies on the suppression of ovulation through a child breastfeeding, proved that a precise method greatly improved their success. Researchers began arguing that the same careful study of traditional contraceptives could lead to clear, precise knowledge that women who choose these traditional methods could rely on when making this family planning choice.

Douching, too, has long been seen as traditional contraceptive, but scientific study of this process of rinsing the vagina immediately after sexual intercourse has been found to be ineffective for preventing pregnancy. Sperm travel quickly into the uterus following ejaculation, needing only seconds to reach the safety of the uterus; a woman cannot douche soon enough after ejaculation to destroy them. Scientific study of the human reproductive system also taught people that amulets and charms worn outside of the body would not prevent pregnancy. However, some devices, such as herbal compounds and animal skins, used as vaginal plugs or condoms, could have effects similar to modern contraceptive barriers in blocking the path of sperm.

Anthropological studies have suggested ways to combine women's acceptance of traditional contraceptive methods with modern products and with research into highly effective contraceptive methods. Researchers seek ways of joining cultural and social expectations concerning reproduction and fertility with social goals of reducing population and encouraging development and suggest that close study of traditional contraceptive methods might help people accept more readily highly effective contraceptive methods. *See also* BIOLOGICAL METHODS OF CONTRACEPTION; MODERN CONTRACEPTIVE METHODS

Further reading: Agadjanian, Victor. "Women's Choice between Indigenous and Western Contraception in Urban Mozambique." *Women and Health* 28.2 (1998): 1–17. Bull, Sheana S., and L. Mercedes Melian. "Contraception and Culture: The Use of Yuyos in Paraguay." *Health Care for Women International* 19 (1998): 49–60. Newman, Lucile F., ed. *Women's Medicine: A Cross-Cultural Study of Indigenous Fertility Regulation.* New Brunswick, NJ: Rutgers University Press, 1985. Riddle, John M. *Eve's Herbs: A History of Contraception and Abortion in the West.* Cambridge, MA: Harvard University Press, 1997.

Tubal Sterilization

A form of permanent birth control, tubal sterilization involves surgery to cut or block a woman's two fallopian tubes through which a mature egg must travel and where it is fertilized by the male sperm cells. Cutting or blocking the tubes prevents eggs and sperm from joining.

While tubal sterilization costs more and has more risks associated with it, this form of sterilization was far more common around the world in the late 1990s than was vasectomy, the surgical procedure that cuts or blocks a man's vas deferens, the tubes through which sperm travel. Results of a study by Population Action International showed that, in the developed world, twice as many women were sterilized as men. In 1995, in the United States, 24 percent of married women using a form of contraception reported having had a tubal ligation compared with 15 percent who said their husbands had had a vasectomy.

Because a woman's fallopian tubes are located in her abdomen below her abdominal muscles, tubal sterilization is more complicated than the man's vasectomy, where the vas deferens is cut just below the skin of the scrotum. Modern techniques, however, have reduced the invasiveness of female sterilization and made it a more convenient operation than it had been before the early 1980s.

Tubal sterilization most frequently takes place in a surgical center on an outpatient basis and no longer requires an overnight hospital stay. The surgery is performed by surgically trained medical professionals. Surgeons commonly use one of two methods of reaching the fallopian tubes. A third, commonly used before the development of less invasive techniques, requires major surgery and hospitalization.

Most women undergo a laparoscopy. This procedure can be performed at almost any time, though it is not recommend soon after a pregnancy. Women commonly need only a two- to three-day recovery time and have few reported side effects other than cramping soon after surgery and minor bleeding. The surgeon makes a tiny incision below the naval and inserts a laparoscope, a thin, hollow flexible tube with a tiny camera on the front end. This device sends pictures to a television screen the doctor watches during the 20–

30 minute procedure. Often the medical team will insert an additional tube through the incision to pump harmless gas into the patient's abdomen. This expands the space and gives the surgeon more room in which to work. A doctor may choose to insert the tiny tools needed to isolate, cut, or block the tubes through the first incision or make another small incision just above the pubic hairline through which to insert the surgical instruments.

Guided by the images transmitted by the tiny camera, the surgeon cuts the tubes and fastens the ends shut with rings or clamps. Damage done to the ends of the tubes with these devices helps prevent the cut tubes from reconnecting. When finished, the surgeon removes the instruments and stitches the incision shut.

Doctors can perform a procedure known as a mini-laparotomy within a few weeks following childbirth. This technique takes advantage of the higher position in the abdomen of the uterus and fallopian tubes. Here the surgeon makes a small incision and lifts the tubes out of the body for cutting and most commonly tying with a suture. Once tied, the doctor tucks the tubes back into the abdomen and stitches the incision closed.

Generally, the patient receives a local anesthetic during either the mini-laparotomy and the laparoscopy. Recovery time to normal activities, including sexual intercourse, is a few days.

The now sterilized woman should experience no changes in her reproductive biology. except that she will be very unlikely to get pregnant. Menstruation and ovulation proceed normally, and there is no change in libido. Even menopause proceeds normally. While some women have reported some changes to their menstrual cycles, recent studies have suggested that most changes are due to stopping the use of an alternative contraceptive method, such as the birth control pill, rather than to the surgery.

Several other procedures for reaching the fallopian tubes are being performed and are undergoing study. An incision through the vagina allows doctors to clearly see the fallopian tubes. Researchers are also experimenting with methods for injecting chemicals, such as quinacrine, into the tubes through the cervix.

Success rates for tubal sterilization are very high. Only 0.4 percent of the women who undergo surgical sterilization become pregnant. Most of these rare cases are the result of a pregnancy that had started before the operation. Approximately 30-50 percent of the failures relate to surgical error, though care in choosing the method of blocking or tying off the tubes greatly reduces this chance of failure. In the case of error, the tubes may become reattached, a very rare occurrence. To decrease the chance of performing an operation on a woman who may be pregnant, many doctors are now requiring a pregnancy test less than 48 hours before surgery.

Tubal sterilization presents few risks to the woman. Complications occur in less than 1 percent of the procedures. Deaths from tubal sterilization result in fewer than 4 for each 100,000 operations.

At this point, tubal sterilization is permanent. A woman will be unable to conceive a child once her tubes are severed. While research is underway to develop methods of temporarily blocking the tubes, science has not yet found a method or procedure for reversible sterilization. Researchers have developed very expensive surgical techniques for trying to reconnect the tubes but this requires expensive major surgery and involves complications and risks from that procedure.

The cost for the tubal sterilization varies. Many insurance companies will cover all or part of the cost and in many states a woman may qualify for federal assistance in paying for the procedure.

Some women experience strong regret after the procedure. Counseling by the medical staff before the operation, including discussions with the woman's partner, can help make the decision to have or not to have a tubal sterilization operation easier for the woman to make and live with. Such counseling also helps determine if surgery is necessary, and often includes tests for fertility to assure the patient and doctor that the woman or her partner are fertile and at risk of pregnancy. If the couple is infertile for other reasons, doctors would not recommend the risk of a sterilization operation. *See also* HYSTERECTOMY; REPRODUCTIVE SYSTEM—FEMALE; STERILIZATION; VASECTOMY

Further reading: Chandra, A. "Surgical Sterilization in the United States: Prevalence and Characteristics, 1965–1995." Vital and Health Statistics: Series 23, 20. National Center for Health Statistics, 1998. Department of Health and Human Services—Public Health Service. *Information for Women: Your Sterilization Operation.* U.S. Department of Health and Human Services, 1991. Grimes, David A., et al., eds. *Modern Contraception: Updates from The Contraception Report.* Totowa, NJ: Emron, 1997. Hatcher, Robert, James Trussel, Felicia Stewart, and others. *Contraceptive Technology*. 16th rev. ed. New York: Irvington, 1994.

U

United Kingdom

The United Kingdom, an island nation lying to the northwest of continental Europe, offers its citizens free reproductive health care through its national health system and works to increase contraceptive options throughout the region. Formed from the union of England, Scotland, Wales, Northern Ireland, and several outlying islands, the United Kingdom struggles with conflicting beliefs concerning abortion and difficulty with teen pregnancies.

As an industrialized western nation, the national birth rate began declining in the United Kingdom in the early 1800s. By 1998, women could expect to give birth to an average of 1.7 children in their lifetimes, well below the replacement level of 2.0. Nearly 65 percent of the women of reproductive age used modern contraceptives. Another 7 percent relied on natural methods to attempt to prevent pregnancy.

Modern contraceptives are widely available and prescriptive forms are free through the U.K.'s National Health Service. Efforts by some government members in the mid-1990s to change that policy and begin charging for birth control failed. Making contraceptives more difficult to obtain, opponents successfully argued, would increase already high rates of teen pregnancy and result in dramatic increases in abortion.

In 1997, women turned most frequently to contraceptive pills to help them prevent pregnancy; 26 percent of women under 50 used the contraceptive pill. While that proportion of women who use hormonal pills has remained steady since the early 1990s, the number of women between the ages of 35 and 39 who use hormonal pills doubled from 1986 to 1993 and increased to 20 percent by 1997. New information on the safety of hormonal contraceptives is believed to have influenced that number.

Condom use in the United Kingdom rose steadily in the early 1990s from 13 percent to 21 percent. People reported that awareness of acquired immunodeficiency syndrome (AIDS) had increased their concern with sexually transmitted diseases and their willingness to use condoms.

Women and men also relied on the male condom and male and female sterilization to prevent pregnancy. Both methods combine to account for 21 percent of the contraceptive choice of women under 50. Overall, 11 percent of women and 10 percent of men had undergone sterilization procedures as of 1997. More than 43 percent of contracepting women ages 40 to 45 reported that they or their partner had been sterilized. That percentage had risen from 35 percent in 1989.

Contraceptive access in the United Kingdom, though supported by government programs, is not evenly provided throughout the island nation. Poorer women, including teens, have poorer access to contraceptives than do people with higher incomes. These poorer women experience a greater number of pregnancies and a greater number of abortions than do their wealthier counterparts. Nearly one-fifth of the United Kingdom's single mothers live at or near the poverty level, and these are the women who have trouble obtaining contraceptives.

Teens in the United Kingdom experience more pregnancies and more abortions than any country in western Europe. Thirty-three women for every 1,000 between the ages of 15 and 19 give birth each year in Britain. Approximately twice as many teens undergo abortions. While sex education is required in Britain's schools for children ages seven to16, government action in late 1999 suggested that education was inadequate. The Prime Minister proposed then that the nation begin work to revise its national sex education curriculum and urged schools to emphasize the importance of marriage and family values.

Access to abortion services, however, is inconsistent. Generally, government programs pay for abortions, but approximately 70 percent are performed in public clinics while the other 30 percent are performed in private clinics, at the patient's expense. Some health districts meet 90 percent of the demand for abortions while others meet only 40 percent of local demand. Funding also varies from one district to the next when local officials give lower priority to providing abortion services than do officials in other districts.

In 1968, abortion became widely available in the United Kingdom, except Northern Ireland, which was allowed to remain exempt from the law due to religious and social concerns. That law provided for abortion through the first 24 weeks of pregnancy for health or social and economic reasons. British women do not have unrestricted access to abortion, however. Doctors may decide if a woman's request for an abortion meets those criteria and can reject a request for an abortion. Twenty percent of conceptions in the United Kingdom end in abortion. More than two-thirds are for women under the age of 30.

Efforts are underway to update the abortion law. Public opinion polls conducted in the late 1990s suggest that 60 percent of the United Kingdom's adult population believe that abortion should be available at the request of the woman, as it is in most of western Europe. The United Kingdom's abortion law was considered in 1968 to be a progressive reform toward providing services for women, though it still limited a woman's right to abortion. Now all but six European na-

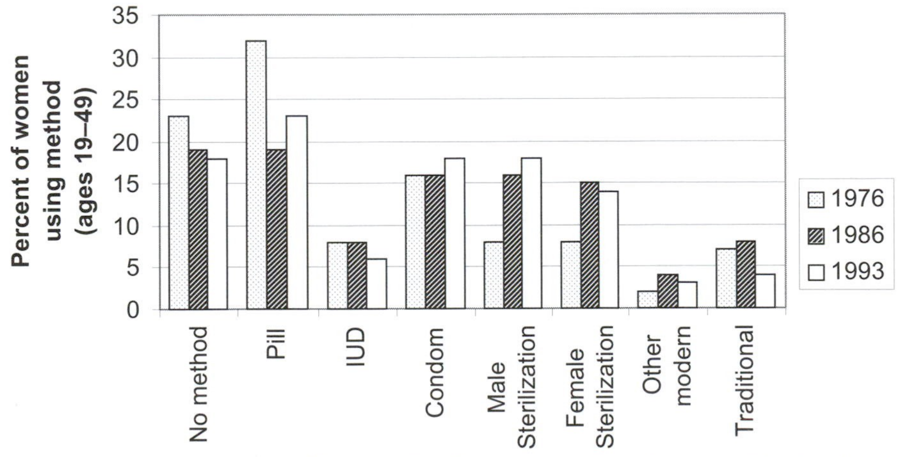

United Kingdom: Change in Contraceptive Use by Method

Source: U.S. Census Bureau International Data Base

tions, two of them the governments of Ireland, provide for legal unrestricted abortions early in a pregnancy. Advocates in the United Kingdom want their nation to join with their European Union partners in providing this service. *See also* EUROPE; IRELAND

Further reading: Barker, Paul. "Statistics to Gladden the Heart." *New Statesman,* 5 February 1999, 23. Department of Health (U.K.) Web site: http://www.doh.gov.uk.

United Nations Fund for Population Activities

The United Nations Fund for Population Activities (UNFPA), commonly referred to as the United Nations Population Fund, works to improve reproductive health and access to family planning around the world.

The fund, a special unit of the United Nations General Assembly, began its work in 1969. With directions from the United Nations Economic and Social Council given in 1973 and then in 1993, UNFPA works first to build knowledge among people concerning population and family planning and then to help people meet their family planning needs. UNFPA also promotes awareness in developed and in developing countries of the problems caused by population growth and helps them devise plans for dealing with population concerns. Within the UN, the Population Fund coordinates projects in support of population issues, including organizing the 1994 International Conference on Population and Development, a special session of the United Nations Assembly, held in Cairo, Egypt.

In 1997, the UNFPA was working with 168 countries and oversaw one-fourth of the donated funds used worldwide for population assistance. Since it was started, the fund has provided more than $4.3 billion to population programs, reaching nearly all developing countries.

UNFPA receives funding from voluntary contributions and no funds from the United Nations budget. In 1997, 95 countries, most of them developing countries, were contributing to UNFPA's budget. Japan, Denmark, and the Netherlands were the fund's largest contributors. The UNFPA's total income for that year was $309 million.

The Population Fund spends most of its assistance on reproductive health care, family planning, and sexual health programs. Sixty-three percent of its 1997 budget supported reproductive health. None of its funds, however, support abortions or abortion-related activities, which the staff at UNFPA does not consider a form of family planning. To help solve the world's problems caused by unsafe abortion, the fund directs its efforts at increasing people's access to birth control and family planning methods.

To achieve its goals, UNFPA often works directly with nongovernmental organizations (NGOs) in the countries it supports. In the early 1980s, the fund began working with organizations within societies, rather than only with governmental offices. By the end of the 1990s, more than 15 percent of UNFPA's funding efforts to help people achieve their family planning goals provided financial support, resources, and expertise to nongovernmental organizations. The UNFPA worked with NGOs in more than 130 countries by 1997. In Nepal, 600 NGOs ran country-level family planning projects. In Senegal, a woman's organization runs an informational project, providing people with information concerning family planning, health, hygiene, and environmental projects. *See also* WORLD HEALTH ORGANIZATION

Further reading: Nafis, Sadik. "Itself Far from Public Eye, UNFPA Looks towards the Future." *UN Chronicle* 35.4 (1998): 36–37. Population Action International. *Fact Sheet No. 3: Why The United States Should Restore Funding for UNFPA.* Washington, DC: Population Action International, 1999. United Nations Funds for Population Activities Web site: http://www.unfpa.org

United States

By 1999, many of the birth control related problems in the United States that leaders of the birth control movement in the 1920s had fought against had been resolved. For the most part, contraceptives were easily available in pharmacies, even gas stations. Family planning clinics had spread across the country and its citizens had easy access to information on birth control and family planning. Women on average gave birth to two children in their lifetimes and the nation's population was growing at only 0.6 percent a year, much of that due to immigration.

Still, this wealthy developed nation, which contributed billions of dollars to nations and organizations around to world to support family planning, reproductive health, and efforts to decrease population, faced subtle and intricate social problems that continued into the twenty-first century to challenge people's access to contraception, abortion, and reproductive health care.

The United States in the middle of the twentieth century was home to much of the innovation that lead to the wide variety of contraceptives available around the world. In the 1950s, U.S. scientists developed the world's first combined oral contraceptive pill. After U.S. Food and Drug Administration (FDA) approval in 1960 pharmacists quickly began manufacturing, doctors began prescribing, and women began requesting the pill. By the mid-1990s, more than 70 million women around the world used this method to prevent pregnancy. Research by leading universities in that country continued to develop highly effective barrier contraceptives and intrauterine devices.

The American birth control movement of the 1920s, led in its early days by Margaret Sanger, spread its influence around the world from the 1930s to the 1950s and spawned the creation of the International Planned Parenthood Federation, which by 1999 provided reproductive services to more than 190 countries and in many countries led efforts to increase access by men and women to modern contraception.

By 1999, more than 90 percent of sexually active women who did not want to become pregnant used modern contraceptives. Contraceptive use among U.S. teens had increased by 23 percent in the 1990s. By 1995, 78 percent of teens used a contraceptive the first time they had sexual intercourse; two-thirds of those people used condoms. At the same time, the number of sexually active teens fell below 50 percent in the late 1990s, and teens were engaging in first intercourse later in their adolescent years. Almost 20 percent did not experience their first intercourse until they were older than 19.

U.S. women most frequently turned to hormonal contraceptive pills, female sterilization, and condoms to prevent pregnancy. Women in their 20s and teens most often used hormonal contraceptive pills. Nearly 27 percent of American women used hormonal pills in 1995; 49 percent of women ages 15 to 19 relied on the pill and only 6 percent of women 40 to 44 did so. Half of all women ages 40 to

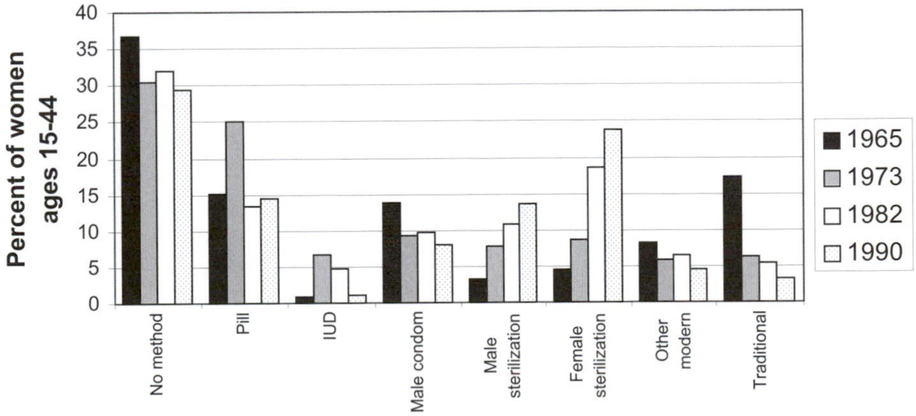

United States: Change in Contraceptive Use by Method

Source: U.S. Census Bureau

44 had undergone female sterilization as of 1995 and 20 percent of the women in that age group lived with men who had undergone vasectomies. Condom use rose from 13 to 38 percent among teens from 1982 to 1995, and from 6 percent to 33 percent among women ages 20 to 24. Condom use by older women fell from 18 percent of women 25 to 29 years old to 9 percent of women 40 to 44.

Intrauterine devices accounted for less than 1 percent of all U.S. contraceptives being used in 1995. In 1982, 8.2 percent of contracepting women had an IUD in place. That decline is believed to be based primarily upon the concerns aroused by the serious health problems caused by the Dalkon Shield in the 1970s. Research on IUDs in the late 1990s suggested that modern IUDs were very safe, and gynecological medical associations hoped to improve the reputation of the IUD in the United States to give women another long-term contraceptive option.

Use of hormonal implants and injectable contraceptives, which were approved for use in early 1990s, accounted for 4.3 percent of the contraceptive users.

In the United States, women and families have relatively easy access to medical services that provide reproductive health care, and with a wide variety of manufacturers making condoms, birth control pills, and spermicides, both women and men have fairly easy access to contraceptives. Gynecologists increasingly have access to better barrier methods, IUDs, and long-term hormonal contraceptives. In general, access to contraception and the overall desire among women and men to have few children work together in the United States, in addition to its wealth, to keep nationwide fertility rates low.

However, the United States, as one of the world's developed nations, where industrialization in the 1800s led to fertility declines that preceded modern birth control methods, faces challenges in providing reproductive health care that distinguish it from the developed countries of western Europe. Insurance coverage of birth control is inconsistent, with some plans fully covering contraception and others covering none. Debates over how to educate children limit their access to birth control information, and inconsistency in medical service, especially to poor and minority populations, hinders their access to birth control options.

As a result, women in the United States experience a greater rate of unplanned pregnancy than most developed nations, including the rate of unintended pregnancies among teens. In 1997, 57 percent, or 3 million of all pregnancies were unplanned. That compares to 39 percent in Canada and 6 percent in the Netherlands, the lowest unplanned rate among western nations. Teens contribute to that high rate. Of the 1 million adolescent U.S. women who become pregnant each year, 80 percent do not plan that pregnancy. Considering the high rate of contraceptive use among women, the high unplanned pregnancy rate has challenged and even confused reproductive health care professionals. The 10 percent of sexually active women who do not want to become pregnant but who do not use contraceptives account for 53 percent of the unplanned births. The remainder are caused by contraceptive failure, often the result of misuse. Recent studies suggest that both education on contraceptive use and the cost of contraceptives contribute significantly to the U.S. unplanned pregnancy rate.

Of those unplanned pregnancies, 1.4 million, or 43 percent, end in abortion. The United States has a very high abortion rate compared to other western developed countries. Made legal by the 1973 ruling of the Supreme Court in the case of *Roe v. Wade*, abortion ends almost one-fifth of all pregnancies in the United States. Women in their early 20s turn most frequently to abortion, but greater proportions of pregnant women younger than 19 and older than 40 choose abortion than choose birth. Significant social conflict in the United States since the legalization of abortion has limited its availability to teens, and 15 percent of the nation's counties offer no abortion services. Reproductive health advocates foresee a significant decline in that abortion rate when the chemical abortion drug, mifepristone, becomes available in the United States; approval from the U.S. Food and Drug Administration was expected in 2000. Reducing the rate of unplanned pregnancy to 30 percent, which is more in line with other industrialized nations, could result in 200,000 fewer unwanted pregnancies and 800,000 fewer abortions each year.

The United States also had the highest incidence of sexually transmitted diseases (STDs) and reproductive tract diseases of any industrialized country. More than 15.3 million new cases of STDs were reported in 1996. Chlamydia reached epidemic proportions in the late 1990s. Deaths from acquired immunodeficiency syndrome (AIDS) fell by 47 percent in the late 1990s, but the rate at which people contracted human immunodeficiency virus (HIV), the virus that leads to AIDS, continued to rise.

Changing family patterns in the United States also influence contraceptive use. Opinions also conflict on how to educate the young, and adults, about reproduction and pregnancy prevention. Some U.S. schools have banned all sex education, others have limited that education to abstinence-only courses, and still others provide thorough instruction in all aspects of a person's sex life. That decline in access to education concerns many health care professionals, who worry that teen pregnancies will stop their decline and once again start to increase.

As women and men wait until their mid-20s to marry and until their 30s to have children, more people are turning to contraceptives to help them time the birth of children. More people are also choosing to never marry, but many of them are choosing to have children outside of marriage. Many health care providers worry that adult lack of understanding of fertility, the result of poor education in school, contributes to the high rate of unplanned pregnancies.

While the United States provides expertise, policy support, contraceptives, and money to support the family planning and reproductive health programs in other countries around the world, it also struggles with its own problems of equity, especially among its many racial groups and between rich and poor, in providing adequate and demanded reproductive health care to its citizens. *See also* AFRICAN AMERICANS; HISPANICS; NATIVE AMERICANS

Further reading: Casterline, John B., Ronald D. Lee, and Karen A. Foote, eds. *Fertility in the United States: New Patterns, New Theories*. Supplement to Population and Development Review, 22. New York: Population Council, 1996. Mosher, William D., and Christine A. Bachrach. "Understanding U.S. Fertility: Continuity and Change in the National Survey of Family Growth, 1988–1995." *Family Planning Perspectives* 28 (1996): 4–12. Piccinino, Linda J., and William D. Mosher. "Trends in Contraceptive Use in the United States: 1982–1995." *Family Planning Perspectives* 30 (1998): 4–12.

Unmet Need (for Contraception)

Women and men have an "unmet need" for family planning and contraception when they want to choose the timing of the births of their children or have no more children but have sexual intercourse without using a method for preventing a sperm from fertilizing an egg. The conflict between their expressed goals and their actions to achieve those goals present women and men with a reproductive health problem that they may not know how to solve or feel is unsolvable. Knowledge of the biology of reproduction or of methods of preventing pregnancy, access to contraceptives, and the availability of methods that suit people's preferences all influence people's ability to set or achieve family planning goals. Reproductive health and policy researchers and program developers seek to help women and men achieve their family planning goals and see meeting these needs as a primary goal of current efforts to improve reproductive health worldwide.

Before the invention of modern birth control methods, people relied upon the relatively ineffective methods of abstinence and withdrawal as well as herbal contraceptives to try to avoid unwanted pregnancies. With the development of more effective barrier methods in the 1800s, and nearly 100 percent effective hormonal contraceptives and intrauterine devices in the 1950s and 1960s, and refined procedures for surgical sterilization throughout the twentieth century, more and more people have gained access to highly effective ways to prevent or delay pregnancy. Research in the 1960s first identified the gap between a woman's desire to control pregnancies and a lack of action by her or her partner to achieve that goal. Despite technical advances of the twentieth century, many people around the world, but mostly in developing countries, still do not use available means of contraception though they want to prevent pregnancy. Understanding why these people still do not use contraceptives provides a challenge to policy makers and researchers.

Lack of knowledge of modern contraceptives represents the primary reason women give for their unmet need. While women and men may be aware of a modern method of preventing pregnancy, that knowledge is often sketchy and inaccurate for people who say the do not want to become pregnant but who do not take preventive measures. Health concerns and a husband's disapproval of family planning rank second and third as the reasons women who do not want to become pregnant do not use contraceptives. Further research, however, suggests that women who say they need contraceptives but do not use them have more difficulty in discussing family planning with their husbands than do women who use family planning methods. Concern with the health aspects of contraceptives appears to be closely linked to the accuracy of the knowledge a woman has concerning modern contraceptives.

Measuring unmet need is a difficult task. Most research into contraceptive use and knowledge is based upon surveys of women who are or who have ever been married. Estimates as of 1999 show that 120 million married women worldwide want to limit pregnancies but do not use contraceptives. Sub-Saharan Africa as a region has the greatest unmet need among married women. India, with more than 39.6 million women reporting an unmet need for contraceptives, ranks highest among nations for the level of unmet need.

These commonly accepted and often quoted statistics, however, do not represent unmarried women. In many nations, including developed nations, unmarried women have a greater desire to prevent pregnancy than do married women. Discovering the sta-

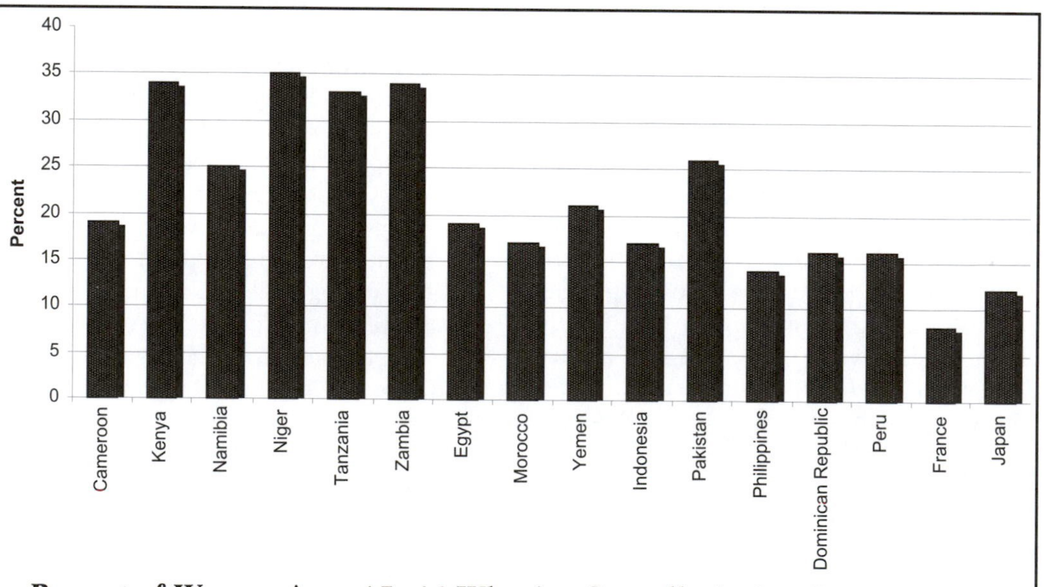

Percent of Women Ages 15–44 Who Are Sexually Active, Do Not Want Pregnancy, But Use No Birth Control: 1995

Source: Alan Guttmacher Institute

tistics for that group of women is an area of research underway.

Around the world, people face varying barriers to gaining contraceptives. In some nations the barriers are the cost and delivery of medical services, in some they are cultural restrictions on influencing pregnancy, and in others they are government support for family concerns. These barriers can conflict with personal goals and even mask personal unmet needs, since ignorance prevents people from knowing about the services to which others have access.

Increasingly, men have been found to have an unmet need for family planning methods and services. Men, too, have a choice in risking pregnancy during intercourse, and understanding why they have sexual intercourse without using a method that will prevent pregnancy challenges societies as well as researchers.

For women and men, single or as couples, the need for family planning varies throughout their lives as they move into and out of wanting and not wanting to give birth. This movement causes problems for statisticians who attempt to identify the problem of unmet contraceptive need and researchers have had to accept that the calculation of unmet need is at best an approximation. *See also* ACCESS (TO CONTRACEPTIVES)

Further reading: Bongaarts, John, and Judith Bruce. "The Causes of Unmet Need for Contraception and the Social Content of Services." *Studies in Family Planning* 26.2 (1995): 57–75. Dixon-Mueller, Ruth, and Adrienne Germain. "Stalking the Elusive 'Unmet Need.'" *Studies in Family Planning* 23 (1992): 330–335. Ngom, Pierre. "Men's Unmet Need for Family Planning." *Studies in Family Planning* 28 (1997): 192–202.

Unplanned Pregnancy

Women and men risk experiencing an unplanned pregnancy during intercourse when neither partner uses a contraceptive. As modern family planning methods became increasingly more available during the twentieth century, women, families, nations, and international organizations became increasingly more concerned with the rate at which women were becoming pregnant when they did not wish to. As reproductive rights and reproductive health received in the 1980s and 1990s support from nations worldwide, the beliefs that every child should be a wanted child and that unplanned pregnancies should be rare occurrences became policy goals of more and more nations, organizations, and families.

An estimated 210 million women become pregnant each year. Of those pregnancies, about 38 percent are unplanned and 22 percent end in abortions. The statistics for less developed and more developed countries are similar. In developed countries, 49 percent of the 28 million pregnancies are unplanned and 36 percent end in abortion. In developing countries, 36 percent of the 182 million pregnancies are unplanned and 20 percent end in abortion. Worldwide, about 26 million women have legal abortions and 20 million have illegal abortions each year.

Most of those unplanned pregnancies and a large proportion of abortions are the result of a couple who uses no contraceptive during intercourse. In the United States the 10 percent of all women who use no birth control methods experience most of the unintended pregnancies. Failure of a contraceptive, such as a broken condom or a forgotten pill, also leads to unplanned pregnancies. Poor access to contraceptives, whether that poor access is the result of living in a hard-to-reach rural setting or the result of a person's inability to afford to buy contraceptives, also causes unplanned pregnancies.

Unplanned, unintended, mistimed, or unwanted pregnancies bring with them several conditions that reproductive health professionals and policy makers see as problems. Women who do not want to be pregnant tend not to receive the prenatal attention that can best lead to successful birth of a healthy child. Even in the United States and other affluent countries, most children who are born from unwanted pregnancies are born into poverty, a condition that puts the children and their mothers at greater risk from illness and death than they would be if the birth had been planned.

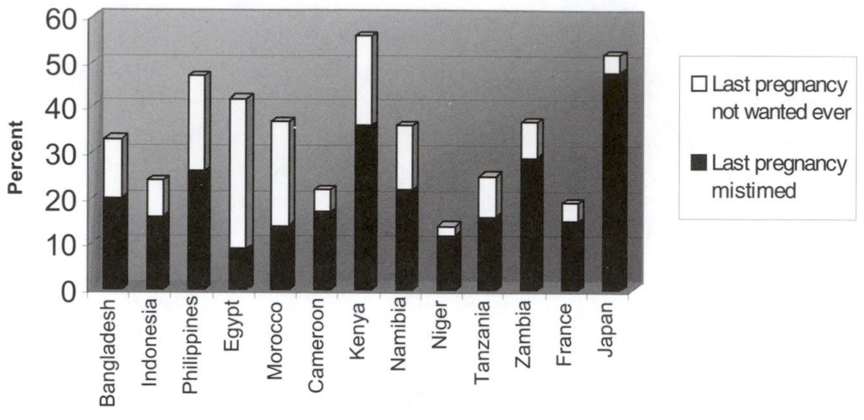

Unplanned Pregnancy Percentages for Developed and Developing Nations: 1995

Source: Alan Guttmacher Institute

In nations where abortion is illegal or restricted, women often turn to illegal means of abortions to end an unplanned pregnancy, and this action puts them at serious risk of infertility, disability, and death. Abortion is also a highly controversial social issue for many nations and, whether legal or illegal, creates conflict that could be eased by decreasing the number of unplanned pregnancies women experience.

Doctors and analysts also cite the limited number of contraceptive methods available to couples as a cause of unplanned pregnancies. Despite the availability of barrier, hormonal, and chemical contraceptives, many individuals often have trouble finding a contraceptive that suits their needs and their lives. Rather than experience side effects of hormonal pills or tolerate inserting vaginal barriers, people will risk having intercourse while not using a birth control method.

United Nations population estimates suggest that if the number of unplanned pregnancies worldwide could be reduced, if women and men had greater access to contraceptives, the world population could stabilize at 7 billion by about the year 2020. Not reducing the levels of unplanned pregnancy could lead to a population of more than 8 billion by 2020 and that level could steadily increase past 10 billion by 2050.

Economically developed nations face the challenge of identifying why women with relative easy access to contraception still put themselves at risk from unplanned pregnancy. In developing countries, part of the challenge is providing easier access to contraceptives to women who want to control when they become pregnant. In both settings, education, access to information, and the availability of a wide range of contraceptives also influence a woman's ability to prevent unplanned pregnancies.

In the United States, where 49 percent of pregnancies were unplanned according to statistics in 1994, inadequate insurance coverage of contraceptives approved by the U.S. Food and Drug Administration keeps many women from being able to afford effective methods of contraception. In that country, federal health care programs that fund family planning methods cover only some of the women who qualify for overall assistance. That leaves a large segment of the nation's poorer women unable to afford the contraceptives they want to use. Ineffective sex education, for people when they are teens and adults, also prevents women and men from fully understanding the risk of pregnancy they face during intercourse; in one year a couple not using contraception during sexual intercourse has an 85 percent chance of beginning a pregnancy.

Critics of abortion as a resolution to an unplanned pregnancy often site adoption as a more moral and ethical choice for the woman, family, and society. Adoption, however, presents social obstacles as well, argue critics of adoption as a workable solution to unplanned pregnancy. In some nations, adoption laws limit who can become an adoptive parent, in others adoption is unacceptable for kinship and cultural reasons. Though it is often raised by advocates of antiabortion policies as a means of helping women deal with unplanned pregnancies, adoption is rarely raised by antiabortion advocates or by public health and reproductive rights advocates as a means of preventing unwanted pregnancies.

Of the more than 120 million married women in developing countries who are not using contraceptives, many want to choose when and if they have children. Many more millions of unmarried women also want this choice. Health care programs, governmental initiatives, assistance from volunteer and nongovernmental organizations, and research by pharmaceutical companies and nonprofit groups that target the causes of unplanned pregnancies are seeking to provide them with that choice. *See also* ADOPTION; CHILD MORTALITY; INSURANCE; MATERNAL MORTALITY; UNMET NEED (FOR CONTRACEPTION)

Further reading: Henshaw, Stanley K. "Unintended Pregnancy in the United States." *Family Planning Perspectives* 30 (1998): 24–29. Hogue, Carol J. Rowland. "Missing the Boat on Pregnancy Prevention: Teenage Pregnancy Grabs the Headlines, but Most Unintended and Unwanted Pregnancies Occur among Adults." *Issues in Science and Technology* 13.4 (1997): 41–45. McDevitt, Thomas M. *World Population Profile: 1998*. Washington, DC: U.S. Department of Commerce, Bureau of the Census, 1999.

Urology

Medical specialists who choose to specialize in urology study and treat the urinary tracts of men and women and the reproductive systems of men, which share some of the same duct work as men's urinary systems.

Most frequently, urologists perform vasectomies. This surgical procedure sterilizes a man and is often performed for contraceptive purposes. It is most frequently performed on an outpatient basis and is done in the doctor's office.

Urologists also assist men who have fertility problems and study sperm production and transportation as well as the hormonal system that governs the reproductive process in men.

Researchers who emphasize urology are exploring forms of temporary male contraceptives and methods of reversible sterilization. *See also* ANDROLOGY; VASECTOMY

U.S. Agency for International Development

Since its creation by executive order of U.S. President John F. Kennedy in 1961, the United States Agency for International Development (USAID) has carried out humanitarian and economic assistance programs to other countries.

Through its Program for Population, Health, and Nutrition, USAID works to stabilize the world's population and protect human health. By its spending levels alone in the 1980s and 1990s, USAID was the largest international donor helping countries with family planning and population concerns. Working in sub-Saharan Africa, Asia, Latin America, the Caribbean, and Europe, this branch of USAID spent $10.5 billion in assistance from 1985 to 1997. Its budget for 1998 was $935 million dollars.

The Office of Population provides help to countries in obtaining contraceptives and in designing programs to give access to those contraceptives to the people who need them. This office also works on providing family planning and reproductive health services to countries receiving help from USAID. The research division of the Office of Population works to develop new fertility control methods and to increase understanding of the workings and effectiveness of current contraceptives.

The USAID office of Women in Development provides countries with assistance to improve the economic status of women, expand education to women, and improve women's rights, all of which have a direct impact on a nation's population and on a woman's ability to choose when and if to have children.

According to its own reports, by the end of the twentieth century more than 50 million couples worldwide were using family planning methods provided through the financial and expert help of USAID. The average number of children in each family in the 28 countries with the largest USAID programs had fallen from 6.1 in the mid-1960s to 4.2 in the late 1990s. The overall health of people in countries receiving assistance from USAID also improved. The number of years people could expect to live rose and the child and infant mortality rates fell in the last half of the twentieth century by 50 percent. Literacy rates and school attendance also grew significantly.

USAID has come under criticism for its efforts and the local organizations and government it chooses to work with. For example, the ethics of the agency came under scrutiny in 1998 when reports from Peru indicated that USAID money had helped support that country's government's efforts to coerce or trick women into being surgically sterilized. Attacks from the conservative members of the U.S. Congress have also called into question the role of USAID in family planning efforts. *See also* CONTRACEPTIVE RESEARCH AND DEVELOPMENT PROGRAM (CONRAD)

Further reading: Russell, Keith. "Does the U.S. Back Sterilization? Alleged Involvement in Involuntary Sterilization Program in Peru." *Insight on the News,* 23 March 1998, 18–19. "USAID Office of Women in Development." *Women's International Network News* 24 (1998): 19–20.

U.S. Food and Drug Administration

The United States Food and Drug Administration (FDA) is charged with approving the development and marketing of new drugs and medical devices, including contraceptives and abortion methods. In addition to its oversight of the safety of the food supply and cosmetics in the United States, this governmental agency, a part of the U.S. Department of Health and Human Services, also monitors products already on the market to ensure their continuing safety.

Birth control methods, such as medical devices and drugs, have undergone varying degrees of regulation depending on when they were developed and the U.S. laws in effect then and the definitions of "drug" and "device" in effect at that time. The combined oral contraceptive (COC) pill, for example, as a new use for an existing product—Enovid, the first COC approved for sale in 1960 had received FDA approval in the mid-1950s as treatment for menstrual disorders—quickly received FDA approval based upon tests conducted in the United States, Puerto Rico, Haiti, and other places and its history of previous use, a faster approval, scholars suggest, than it would have received 20 years later. All medical devices, such as intrauterine devices, needed no FDA approval until 1976. By the 1990s, all new drugs and medical devices, including contraceptives, received such close FDA scrutiny that critics and product developers complained loudly of FDA interference.

While federal control of the nation's drug supply began in the mid-1800s and the FDA as a named agency began enforcing laws in 1931, it was not until the passage in 1938 of the Federal Food, Drug, and Cosmetic Act that the agency received the power, among other responsibilities, to require proof of a new drug's safety before it could be sold. With that law, the FDA also received authority to conduct inspections of drug manufacturing factories, and the ability to obtain court injunctions to stop manufacturers it found in violation of the law. Amendments to that 1938 law passed in October of 1962 increased the FDA's authority. With their passage, manufacturers were required to prove not only the safety but the effectiveness of new drugs before marketing them. The 1976 Medical Device Amendments to the 1938 act finally gave the FDA the same authority and responsibility over medical devices, which had proliferated after World War II, that it had over drugs. In 1990, the Safe Medical Devices Act increased further the FDA's ability to control the effectiveness and safety of new products and to monitor those already sold.

The size, scope, and slowness of the FDA and its cautious approach to regulation brought it under close scrutiny and intense criticism in the 1980s and 1990s. New drug applications required three carefully researched phases of approval and could take more than a decade to pass through FDA bureaucracy and testing. Definitions of "new product" included manufacturers switching the factories in which they made their products, which meant new and long applications for FDA approval. The research steps required by FDA officials have been credited by contraceptive and public health experts with slowing the pace at which organizations research and develop new contraceptive methods and new drugs.

Spurred on in part by the medical needs of people suffering from acquired immunodeficiency syndrome (AIDS), a worldwide epidemic, and by research aimed at curing cancer, the U.S. Congress passed and President Bill Clinton signed in November 1997 the Food and Drug Modernization Act, a detailed revision of the 1938 laws. Many of the new amendments were aimed at streamlining the organization and its drug approval and monitoring processes. In the first year after its passage, the requirements of the Modernization Act reportedly cut the approval time of new drugs in half and expanded its review of existing low-risk medical devices by allowing outside experts, rather than FDA staff inspectors, to conduct the reviews.

The FDA's staff of more than 9,000 employees maintains 157 regional offices around the United States. That staff monitors the safety of $1 trillion of products each year and inspects 95,000 regulated businesses. Through the Obstetrics and Gynecology Devices Branch of the Center for Devices and Radiological Health, the FDA oversees devices used in reproductive medicine. Its Office of Women's Health provides coordination between the divisions and offices that deal in products for women, including contraceptives.

In many ways the United States Food and Drug Administration is seen as the world's leading overseer of the safety of drugs and medical devices and an advocate for research and development, yet it is also seen as a hindrance to the timely and efficient development of new drugs and devices. In February 1997, FDA staff took the step of encouraging manufacturers of combined oral contraceptive pills to package them specifically for emergency contraception and established that it already had ample evidence to support such an application . Despite the availability of such products in Europe, American manufacturers had resisted developing the product in attempts to avoid public controversy. In September 1998, the FDA approved the sale of PREVEN, that nation's first emergency contraceptive pill.

Critics blamed the FDA for overzealous– ness and for maintaining overly restrictive regulations when, after FDA inspections Whitehall-Robins removed its "Today" contraceptive sponge from the market in 1995 after FDA inspectors found bacteria in the water of the only plant to manufacture the sponge. To fix the problem according to FDA rules, Whitehall-Robins would have needed to reapply for approval for the Today sponge, a long and costly testing process. Citing financial constraints in light of those rates Whitehall-Robins stopped manufacturing the sponge. In the early 1970s, the FDA came under fire for not calling for the removal of the Dalkon Shield intrauterine device against which evidence of harm to patients and ineffectiveness were mounting rapidly. Then, the FDA, without the provisions of the Medical Device Amendment of 1976 to support it, had argued that it could not legally prevent the manufacturers from making the device.

Despite its shortcomings, critics maintain that the job the FDA has been given is monumental and while it is understandable that a government agency is conservative in its estimations of safety and effectiveness, the contraceptive and medical needs of the twenty-first century will demand a flexible, efficient, and cooperative oversight agency in order to bring new products to the market in a timely manner. *See also* DALKON SHEILD; RESEARCH (CONTRACEPTIVE)

Further reading: Burkholz, Herbert. *The FDA Follies*. New York: BasicBooks/HarperCollins, 1994. "Law to Reform Food, Medical Product Regulation: President Clinton Signs FDA Modernization Act into Law." *FDA Consumer* 32.2 (1998): 3. Merrill, Richard A. "Regulation of Drugs and Devices: An Evolution." *Health Affairs* 13.3 (1994): 47–69.

Uterus

The central organ in the female reproductive system, the uterus provides the cushioned place for a fertilized egg to grow. The uterus is small, almost pear-shaped organ located inside a woman's pelvis above and behind the bladder and in front of the rectum. The two fallopian tubes, which receive the mature eggs once they are ejected from the ovaries, attach to the top and either side of the uterus.

This organ is made of the larger, upper, bulbous portion known as the corpus or fundus and the longer, narrow "neck" or cervix located at the bottom of the uterus. The cervix rests in the vagina, a canal that connects the inner organs with the outside. The inner wall of the corpus, the endometrium, fills with blood each month in preparation to receive a fertilized egg. Should no egg implant in that wall, the blood drains from the lining and out of the body through the cervix and vagina.

The uterus, when a woman is not pregnant, is 7 centimeters long (2.75 inches), 5 centimeters wide (2 inches), and, at its roundest point, about 2.5 centimeters (1 inch) in diameter. Its size changes as the woman's body goes through its monthly reproductive cycle. The uterus is a round, bulky organ when the endometrium is filled with blood and awaiting the arrival of fertilized egg. It is flat and empty after the blood has been shed in menstruation and before the cycle begins again. The uterine muscles stretch greatly while a woman is pregnant.

Disrupting the function of the uterus provides an opportunity for people to prevent pregnancy. The intrauterine device (IUD) prevents eggs from implanting in the uterine wall by twisting and scraping the wall. Recently, a surgical procedure designed to prevent unusually and unhealthy menstrual bleeding, known as endometrial ablation, has been discussed as a means of birth control. *See also* ENDOMETRIAL ABLATION; INTRAUTERINE DEVICE; REPRODUCTIVE SYSTEM—FEMALE

V

Vaccine

Since the mid-1970s, researchers have experimented with methods of birth control that work like a vaccine to prevent pregnancy. By the late 1990s, however, no research avenue had produced a product that was convenient, safe, and as effective as hormonal contraception.

Such a birth control vaccine would cause the immune system to respond to a hormone or chemical vital to the reproductive process as if that hormone or chemical were a foreign substance in the body. The vaccine would prevent the hormone from functioning normally and thus prevent pregnancy.

In the early 1970s, scientists in India and the United States began developing a vaccine process that focused on human chorionic gonadotropin (hCG), a hormone produced by the placenta. By attaching a version of the tetanus virus to a portion of the hCG chain, they hoped to stimulate the immune system to attack hCG and prevent it from maintaining the corpus luteum (the portion of the structure that supports a maturing egg that remains on the ovary after the egg ruptures from the sack and begins its journey down the fallopian tube). While early tests proved successful at interfering with hCG, scientists encountered difficulty with providing effective pregnancy prevention for more than a few months.

Research on vaccines aimed at hCG continues, but because this hormone is produced by the placenta, which forms after a fertilized egg implants in the uterus, hCG-based vaccines are considered by many people to be abortifacients and thus morally unacceptable as a way of regulating fertility. This aversion to interrupting the reproductive process after fertilization of an egg by a sperm rather than before fertilization has deterred some organizations from spending time and money to develop an hCG-based vaccine and has led others to stop funding vaccine research.

Alternate approaches to contraception based on immunological responses that target process preceding fertilization are also underway. Researchers look for ways to alter through the immune system both male and female fertility.

Several processes under investigation would alter the outer cell membrane of an egg, the zona pellucida, to prevent sperm from interacting with the egg and sharing its chromosomes during fertilization. Other research studies the possibility of causing women's bodies to treat sperm as invading organisms and destroy them before they reach the fallopian tubes and a mature egg.

Vaccines aimed at the male reproductive system would interact with the two pituitary hormones, luteinizing hormone-releasing hormone (LHRH) and follicle-stimulating hormone (FSH), and prevent those hormones from acting on the testicles where they encourage sperm production.

Research to discover an immunological approach to contraception and fertility control has lead to significant detailed scientific understanding of the reproductive process, though none has yet led to an effective method of pregnancy prevention that would be convenient and easy to use. Products based upon this research may one day be developed but experts expect none to be developed until well into the twenty-first century.

Further reading: Aitken, R. John. "The Complexities of Conception." *Science,* 7 July 1995, 39–40. Mukerjee, Madhusree. "Gursaran Prasad Talwar: Pushing the Envelope for Vaccines." *Scientific American,* July 1996, 38–39. Online: http://www.sciam.com/0796issue/0796profile.html, 7 March 2000. Richter, Judith. "'Vaccination' Against Pregnancy: The Politics of Contraceptive Research." *The Ecologist* 26.2 (1996): 53–60.

Vagina

The canal that is the vagina leads from outside the woman's body to the base of the uterus in the female reproductive system. It is about 9 centimeters (3.5 inches) long and receives the male's erect penis during sexual intercourse. The vagina also conveys uterine discharge out of the body during menstruation and transports a baby into the world during childbirth.

Usually, the front and back wall of this canal touch, effectively closing the vagina. The walls of the vagina contain blood vessels that fill and enlarge during sexual intercourse. The glands of the vagina secrete a mucous that lubricates the vagina during intercourse and child birth.

The secretions of the vagina and the male's semen, the fluid in which the sperm travel through the male's penis and into the woman's body, resemble those of the mucous discharged by the cervix when a mature egg is traveling through a woman's reproductive system. The visual similarity of these fluids can make the recognition of cervical mucous difficult and cause difficulty for people who use observation of cervical mucous as a means of predicting the onset of a woman's fertile days.

The vagina also provides access to the internal female reproductive organs for inserting forms of birth control devices that present barriers to the sperm, such as the cervical cap. This canal provides a place for women to insert before intercourse spermicidal jellies and vaginal sponges that contain chemicals that kill sperm. *See also* BARRIER CONTRACEPTIVES; FERTILITY AWARENESS; REPRODUCTIVE SYSTEM—FEMALE; VAGINAL SPONGE

Vaginal Ring

Thin plastic vaginal rings now being developed and tested in the United States, Great Britain, and several other countries combine the control over contraception many women desire with the high effectiveness of hormonal contraceptives.

Now under study and development by the Population Council, the small plastic flexible vaginal rings resemble the outer rim of a diaphragm, although unlike the diaphragm, they are open in the middle. The rings fit snugly in place high into the vagina and work by slowly releasing synthetic sex hormones into the woman's body.

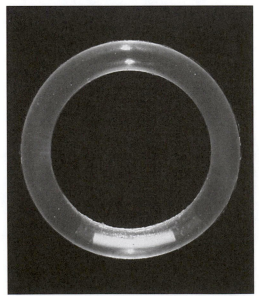

Vaginal rings made of silicone rubber fit snugly into the vagina and release synthetic hormones. *Population Council*

Several different rings are now being tested. One contains levonorgestrel, an older form of manufactured progesterone. Another contains only Nestorone, a newer artificial progesterone. A third contains Nestorone and a synthetic estrogen.

The rings now being tested vary in how long a woman may leave them in place in the vagina. The Nestorone-only ring may be used continuously for six months before it needs to be replaced. The levonorgestrel ring may be used for three months. The Nestorone and estrogen ring was designed to be worn for three weeks, then removed during menstruation.

As with oral contraceptive pills, the rings work by altering the hormonal signals that control the reproductive cycle in women. Tests underway include studying the lowest dose needed to prevent ovulation and studying the side effects of wearing the ring, including changes the rings may cause to the vagina.

The Population Council and investigators in the United States and Great Britain expect to have fully approved, factory manufactured vaginal rings available to the public early in the twenty-first century. *See also* FUTURE METHODS OF CONTRACEPTION; HORMONAL CONTRACEPTIVES; HORMONES—SYNTHETIC

Further reading: "Future Contraceptive Methods." *The Contraception Report* 5 (1994): 4–11.

Vaginal Sponge

The modern vaginal sponge, a descendent of linen devices used in ancient Egypt, is an easy-to-insert contraceptive that fits snugly over the cervix. The vaginal sponge is currently available from pharmacies in Canada and through mail order in the United States without prescription.

Made of polyurethane, the small pillow-shaped barrier contraceptive blocks the path of sperm and contains a spermicide to kill sperm. A woman can insert the small round device well before having intercourse or moments before. It must be left in place at least six hours after intercourse for it to provide maximum protection and may be left in place for up to 30 hours.

If used properly and consistently, sponges can have an effective pregnancy prevention rate as high as 90 percent. Studies show they are more effective for women who have never been pregnant than for women who have given birth. Overall, sponges are less effective than diaphragms and female condoms at preventing pregnancy.

Vaginal sponges are popular with women who need and want an occasional rather than a constant method of birth control, or who want more control over their protection than they receive from a condom alone and from the willingness of their partners to use condoms.

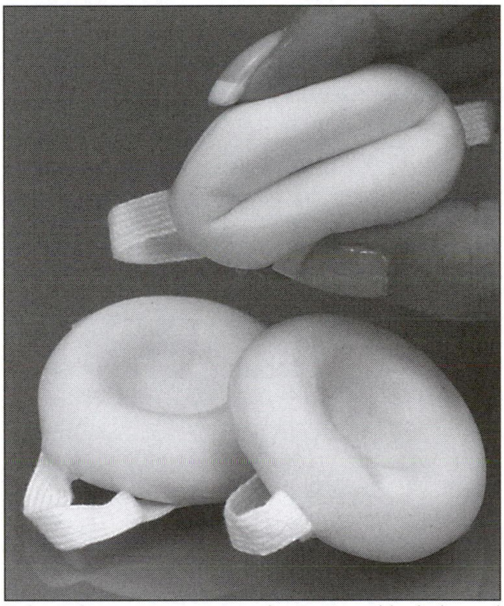

Polyurethane sponges cover the cervix to block the path of sperm. *Allendale Pharmaceuticals*

Toxic shock is a possible side effect of vaginal sponges. While very rare, this disease is associated with devices inserted into the vagina, such as tampons and barrier contraceptives.

In February 1996, Protectaid, a new vaginal sponge, became available in drugstores to women in Canada. It is also available through the mail in the United States and is offered for sale on the Internet. Protectaid replaced the "Today" sponge, which had been manufactured in the United States from 1983 until January 1995 when its manufacturer stopped making the device for economic reasons and while involved with the U.S. Food and Drug Administration inspection requirements. According to the manufacturers, the lower doses of spermicide in Protectaid make it less irritating to users than had been the Today sponge. Protectaid is reported to be 90 percent effective. Allendale Pharmaceuticals purchased the rights to the Today sponge in 1998 and as of mid-2000 was working to obtain FDA approval to reintroduce it in the United States.

Another sponge containing an alternative spermicide is available to women in Europe. *See also* BARRIER CONTRACEPTIVES; SPERMICIDES; TOXIC SHOCK SYNDROME

Further reading: Hatcher, Robert, James Trussel, Felicia Stewart, and others. *Contraceptive Technology*. 16th rev. ed. New York: Irvington, 1994.

Vas Deferens

The vas deferens form the major portion of the sperm transportation system. One of the two tubes connects each testicle to the remainder of the male reproductive system.

The two vas deferens are internal tubes that connect the sperm-storing epididymides, which rest on the upper portion of the testicles on the outside of a man's body, to the urethra that travels through the man's penis.

After they are made in the testicles, sperm are stored in the epididymis, a coil-like structure that rests on top of each testicle. The vas deferens, 45-centimeter-long (18 inch) tubes, travel up and into the pelvic cavity, behind the ureters, over the front of the bladder, to the top of the prostate gland. Here the two tubes widen and join with the ducts from the seminal vesicles and the prostate, which produce the semen, the fluid that carries the sperm into and through the urethra and out of the body.

During ejaculation, muscle contractions rapidly push the sperm from the epididymis into the vas deferens. Contractions along this cordlike structure move the sperm and the semen through the reproductive system.

Because of their role as the sperm transportation system, the vas deferens provide a place where sperm can be stopped in the journey toward a mature egg. In a vasectomy, both tubes are surgically severed through a small incision in the scrotum, the sack that holds the two testicles. This procedure results in permanent sterilization of the man. *See also* REPRODUCTIVE SYSTEM—MALE; VASECTOMY

Vasectomy

A vasectomy, the permanent severing or blocking of a man's vas deferens, the tubes that carry the mature sperm from the epididymides to the penis, provides a safe, nonreversible form of sterilization that is growing steadily, but slowly, in popularity around the world.

During a vasectomy, a medical professional with surgical training makes an opening in the man's scrotum through an incision or puncture, then lifts each of the two vas deferens, one at a time, through the opening. Several methods are now in use for blocking or severing these thin tubes. Commonly, the doctor cuts the vas deferens and fastens off the ends with a non-biodegradable thread.

A method known as a "no-scalpel vasectomy" gained prominence around the world during the 1990s. Developed in China in 1974, the method involves puncturing the man's scrotum rather than cutting it with a scalpel. The doctor first locates the vas deferens from outside the scrotum, then encircles them with a special forceps. The doctor uses another special forceps to puncture the skin of the scrotum and stretch it slightly. Once the doctor pulls the vas through this puncture hole, he or she lifts it out for severing. This method is known to be less painful, result in fewer complications, and heal faster than a vasectomy done through an incision

The no-scalpel vasectomy is now the standard practice in China and is growing in popularity in India, Thailand, and Indonesia. In the United States in 1997, 29 percent of all vasectomies used the no-scalpel method.

As more doctors are trained in this technique around the world, it is likely to become the method of choice for a vasectomy.

Vasectomies are usually performed at a clinic or doctor's office, require no hospital stay, and use only a local anesthetic. A man likely experiences a day or two of discomfort from the surgery, then returns to his normal physical routine.

Because a man is not sterile immediately following surgery, doctors recommend that he use alternative forms of birth control, such as a condom or a female barrier, for three months after the vasectomy. Mature sperm travel from the testicles through the male reproductive system to the penis and on the day the man has surgery, he will have sperm in his entire system. After the surgery, it may take up to 15 ejaculations to clear sperm out of the man's reproductive tract.

A vasectomy is more than 99 percent effective at preventing pregnancy. Only 0.15 percent of women whose partner has had a vasectomy become pregnant within the first year after the operation. Most of these failures are due to the couple not using another form of contraceptive before all sperm has been eliminated from the semen. Researchers have not established the failure rate of the actual severing of the vas deferens.

Medical workers council patients that vasectomy is permanent and needs to be seen as permanent. Though doctors have developed procedures for refastening cut vas deferens, known as vasovasostomy, this surgery is very expensive and requires highly technical skill from the physician. Success rates vary but average about 50 percent for men who go through the reversal surgery. The longer the time between the vasectomy and the attempt to reconnect the tubes, the less likely this operation is to be successful.

Vasectomies, in general, cost less than half as much as female sterilization methods and can cost as little as three-quarters less. Vasectomies also involve less risk to the patient and are more effective than female sterilization. Despite ease, effectiveness, and cost differences, however, more women world wide were surgically sterilized than men.

In Africa in 1997, of the 12 percent of the population that used contraception, 1 percent were women who had been sterilized and 0.1 percent were men who had had vasectomies. In Asia in 1997, 23 percent of the people using contraception were sterilized women and 6 percent were men who had been sterilized. The trend toward more female sterilization continued in the developed world where 8 percent of the contracepting population had undergone female sterilization surgery and 4 percent had undergone male sterilization surgery. Cultural issues and access to medical professionals capable of performing sterilization as well as education of those desiring contraception seems to influence this pattern of more female sterilization than male sterilization. *See also* REPRODUCTIVE SYSTEM—MALE; STERILIZATION; TUBAL STERILIZATION

Further reading: Department of Health and Human Services, Public Health Service. *Information for Men: Your Sterilization Operation.* U.S. Department of Health and Human Services, 1991. Hearts, Jack. "How to Get Fixed." *Men's Health,* July–August 1993, 58–60. Knowles, Jon, and Marcia Ringel. *All About Birth Control: A Personal Guide.* New York: Three Rivers–Crown, 1998. Rakel, Robert E., ed. *Saunders Manual of Medical Practice.* Philadelphia, PA: W.B. Saunders, 1996.

Very Low Dose Pills

Very low dose pills reached the prescriptive contraceptive market in the United States in the late 1990s and offer women combined oral contraceptive (COC) pills with doses of estrogen and progestin much lower than most COCs. The very low dose pills represent the culmination of efforts by biochemists and pharmacologists to prevent pregnancy using the least amount possible of synthetic sex hormones.

In 1997, Wyeth-Ayerst Laboratories received U.S. Food and Drug Administration approval to market "Alesse," the first very low dose COC. The pill contains 100 micrograms of levonorgestrel, a progestin, and 20 micrograms of ethinyl estradiol, an estrogen. The conventional COCs prescribed in the 1990s contained between 5 and 15 times more progestin and 15 more micrograms of estrogen. Tests leading up to FDA approval established that the very low dose pills have a pregnancy prevention success rate better than 99 percent when used according to directions, the same as the higher dose pills.

Side effects of the very low dose pills were much milder and less frequent than with the stronger conventional COCs, though more women did experience irregular bleeding. Because they use the same artificial hormones, very low dose pills present risks to women who smoke as well as women at risk of deep vein blood clots.

The very low dose pills should be very effective for women in perimenopause—the few years that precede menopause when a woman's periods stop and she is no longer produces mature eggs. While perimenopausal women still risk pregnancy, they require lower amounts of progestins and estrogens to protect them from unwanted pregnancy than women younger than 35. *See also* COMBINED ORAL CONTRACEPTIVES

Further reading: "Combination Birth Control Pill Formulation Available in One-Third Lower Dose." *Cancer Weekly Plus,* 11 August 1997, 13.

Vietnam

Government action in Vietnam since 1976 led to dramatic increases in the number of people who use contraceptives, decreases in the nation's total fertility rate, and a total population of 5 million fewer people than the southeast Asian country would have had without strong governmental support.

Vietnam, a long thin country on the western shore of the South China Sea, is one of the most populated countries in the world (77 million in 1999). Though fertility rates had begun to decline during the war between North and South Vietnam in the 1960s, policies established by the communist government after the country was reunified in 1975 increased citizens' knowledge, awareness, and use of contraceptives.

Due in part to the decision by the government to increase spending by eight times what it was in 1979 and in part due to the establishment of a "one-or-two-child" policy in 1988, Vietnam's total fertility rate fell from 4.8 to 2.8 births per woman from the late 1970s to the late 1990s. Contraceptive use in that time rose from 35 percent to 66 percent. The nation's annual growth rate fell from 4.7 percent in 1980 to 1.2 percent in 1999. Much of its present growth rate is the

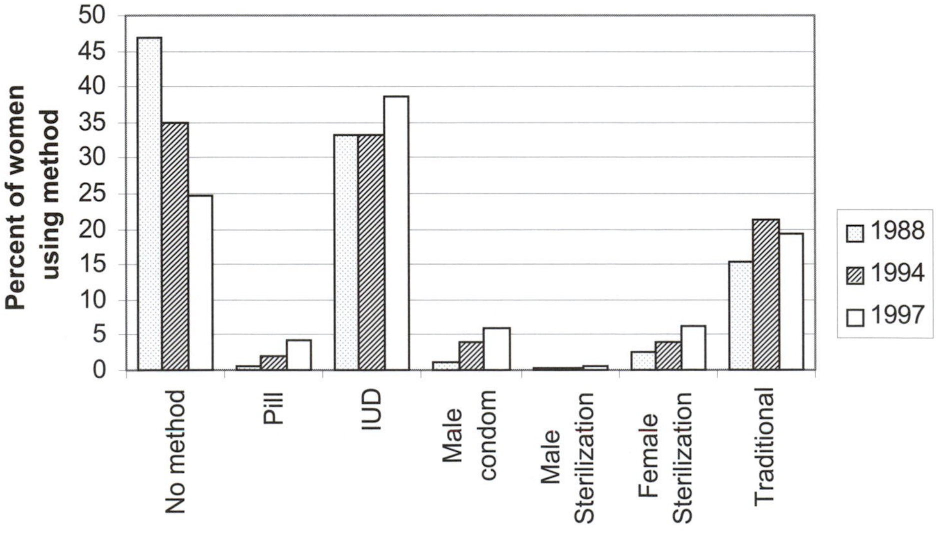

Vietnam: Change in Contraceptive Use

Source: U.S. Census Bureau International Data Base

result of the momentum created by the larger family sizes of the mid-twentieth century and experts expect Vietnam's growth rate to continue to fall.

Enforcement of the nation's one-or-two-child policy, less strict than neighboring China's "one-child" population policy, and billboard campaigns to persuade parents, as well as efforts to improve the educational levels of women, aim to change social attitudes. While Vietnamese women, especially those with more than an elementary education, say they prefer families of one or two children, very few report that they want to have no children.

Vietnam stands out in the developing world for the number of women who use or have used intrauterine devices to prevent pregnancy. By 1994, almost half of the women in Vietnam who had ever been married had used an IUD. As of 1996, 33 percent of married women of reproductive age were using IUDs. That rate is not exceeded by any of the 119 countries for which the United Nations tracks this data and is matched only by China and Cuba. Vietnam's government support of family planning programs had since the 1970s advocated the use of IUDs and provided them to women.

As other modern contraceptives have become available in Vietnam, the predominance of IUDs has begun to fade. The use of modern contraceptive methods increased by 6 percent from 1988 to 1994, all of it the result of increase in methods other than IUDs, and most of it in the use of contraceptive pills and male condoms.

Vietnam's government reported high abortion rate indicated that 100 of every 1,000 women each year have an abortion, which is legal in Vietnam. That figure, however, includes a procedure for removing the contents of the uterus, known as menstrual regulation, that is performed within six weeks of the woman's last period and is meant to bring on menstruation. It is often performed on women before pregnancy is confirmed by tests and may be performed when no egg has been fertilized.

Most people in Vietnam live in rural villages and communes. They make their livings as farmers, producing the world's third largest crop of rice. This emphasis on farming, however, results in a low gross national product of $290 for each residence. Despite this poverty, the government has worked to increase access to family planning knowledge and resources. The Vietnam government makes contraceptives and abortion widely available as part of the public health care program and funds access to family planning and abortion services. Vietnam's population policy resulted in significant financial savings by the end of the twentieth century. Accounting reports suggest that in 1995 the country began saving more money as a result of family planning efforts than it spent on those efforts. *See also* ASIA; CHINA

Further reading: Goodkind, Daniel M. "Vietnam's One-or-Two-Child Policy in Action." *Population and Development Review* 21 (1995): 85–111. Johansson, Annika, et al. "Population Policies and Reproductive Patterns in Vietnam." *The Lancet,* 1 June 1996, 1529–1532. Van Phai, Nguyen, John Knodel, Mai Van Cam, and Hoang Xuyen. "Fertility and Family Planning in Vietnam: Evidence from the 1994 Inter-censal Demographic Survey." *Studies in Family Planning* 27 (1996): 1–17.

W

Withdrawal

A very old method of attempting to prevent pregnancy during sexual intercourse, withdrawal requires that a man quickly remove his penis from a woman's vagina immediately before he ejaculates. Technically, withdrawal is known as *coitus interruptus*, a Latin term that means interrupting vaginal-penile intercourse.

Withdrawal, or "Onanism," most likely dates to times when human understanding of reproduction led to the awareness that ejaculation of semen into the vagina caused pregnancy. According to the biblical story of Onan, son of Judah, Onan did not want to impregnate the widow of his dead brother, as custom dictated, and poured "his seed upon the ground" during sexual intercourse (Gen. 38:6–10). This early recording of an act of withdrawal gave this man's name to the method.

Withdrawal is seen by many people as a "better than nothing" method of birth control. While some people describe it as a natural method of contraception, others argue that there is nothing natural about a man pulling his penis out of the woman's body just at the moment his body is prepared to eject sperm. In fact, biologists point out that at the moment of ejaculation, the man naturally thrusts his penis deeper into the woman's body in an attempt to ensure that the semen ejects as close as possible to the woman's cervix, the opening to her uterus. Scientists also point out that during the height of sexual stimulation and orgasm, which precedes ejaculation, men and women experience a euphoric clouding of consciousness, making withdrawing very difficult for the man.

The success rate for withdrawal is uncertain and difficult to determine, since it is difficult to study if all semen has been ejaculated outside of the vagina. Estimates put the range of success between 96 percent success rate with perfect use and 65 percent success with imperfect use. However, when used in conjunction with fertility awareness by couples committed to the method, withdrawal can be useful in preventing pregnancy. Withdrawal has several distinct advantages as a contraceptive. It costs nothing, has no known medical side effects, and is always available as a back-up contraceptive.

According to the 1995 National Survey of Family Growth, in the United States 40.7 percent of women between ages 15 and 44 reported ever using withdrawal as a contraceptive method and 6.8 percent said they used withdrawal during their first experience with intercourse. Only 2 percent of the women who were trying to avoid pregnancy at the time of the survey used withdrawal as their current method of contraception.

Worldwide, withdrawal is used as a traditional form of contraception and is still widely practiced where modern contraceptives are less available. Use of withdrawal is dwindling as people gain access to modern methods of contraception increases. *See also* FERTILITY AWARENESS; INTERCOURSE; REPRODUCTIVE SYSTEM—MALE; TRADITIONAL METHODS OF CONTRACEPTION

Further reading: Santow, Gigi. "Coitus Interruptus in the Twentieth Century." *Population and Development Review* 19 (1993): 767–792. Winikoff, Beverly, and Suzanne Wymelenberg. *The Whole Truth about Contraception*. Washington, DC: Joseph Henry Press, 1997.

World Health Organization

As part of its mandate, the World Health Organization (WHO), through its Department of Reproductive Health Research, conducts research into reproductive health issues, provides technical assistance to nations as they work to improve their population's health, and publishes numerous books, pamphlets, and research papers to share knowledge around the world in an effort to solve reproductive health problems and assist individuals to reach the highest possible level of good health.

As part of the health systems and community health activities of the World Health Organization, the Department of Reproductive Health Research works in two directions: technical support and research initiatives. Technical support for nations focuses on maternal and newborn health, family planning and population issues, and reproductive tract infections. WHO funding and staff efforts have supported the development and study of all aspects of contraception, from the natural methods using lactational ammenorhea and fertility awareness, to the experiments in male contraceptives and techniques to influence conception at the molecular level. The WHO provides support around the world for better health facilities, affordable methods of family planning to the people who want or need it, efforts to improve maternal health and childbearing safety, and an increasing variety of research projects. Given its focus on overall reproductive health, the WHO also works to allow men and women faced with infertility to conceive children.

The World Health Organization was founded in 1948 when its constitution was ratified by the members of the United Nations. That year the WHO held its first World Health Assembly in Geneva, where it now maintains its headquarters. The seeds for this worldwide cooperative to improve the health of people were planted in 1851 when nations gathered for the First International Sanitary Conference in Paris in an attempt to deal with the cholera epidemic that had been devastating Europe since early in that century. Today, WHO is governed by the World Health Assembly, which itself is made up of the health ministers from 191 nations. In 1999, the new director general of the WHO, Dr. Gro Harlem Brundtland, began an effort to reform the organization of the WHO to make it more able to meet the modern health needs of the world.

In its history, WHO researchers developed, studied, and saw approved around the world a wide variety of contraceptive methods including intrauterine devices, combined oral contraceptive pills, injectable contraceptives, condoms, and vaginal barriers. WHO scientists also work on developing future contraceptives including those based upon immunization-like approaches to influencing male, as well as female, reproductive biology. WHO publications include scientific studies published in leading scholarly journals, handbooks for workers in family planning clinics around the world, and pamphlets and books aimed at educating non-scientists concerning reproductive health.

WHO policy experts help countries develop the family planning services that will aid their countries and assist nations in developing laws and institutions that will support the reproductive health goals of their citizens. *See also* RESEARCH (CONTRACEPTIVE)

Further reading: "The Brundtland Era Begins." *The Lancet* 351.9100 (1998): 381. Robbins, Anthony. "Brundtland's World Health Organization: A Test Case for United Nations Reform." *Public Health Reports* 114 (1999): 30–39. World Health Organization. *The World Health Report 1998: Life in the 21st Century: A Vision for All*. Geneva: World Health Organization, 1998. World Health Organization Web site. http://www.who.org

Y

Yuzpe Regimen

The Yuzpe regimen is a combination of oral contraceptives taken according to a precise timing scheme shortly after a woman has unprotected sex. Together, the pills and timing can greatly reduce the chances of a woman becoming pregnant.

In the mid-1970s, Canadian physician A. Albert Yuzpe discovered that two extra-strong doses of oral contraceptives taken within 72 hours of unprotected sex and 12 hours apart protected women against unwanted pregnancies. The treatment is 75 percent effective.

The Yuzpe regimen, as it came to be known, was the first described use of contraceptive pills to provide emergency contraception. Several other combinations have been developed since the early 1970s that use different combinations and strengths of the hormones found in birth control pills. The Yuzpe regimen has proven to be a fairly effective method for preventing pregnancy, and, with other forms of emergency contraception, has been prescribed extensively in the United States in hospital emergency rooms, reproductive health clinics, and university health centers, though no products have been individually marketed in the United States as they have been in Europe. *See also* COMBINED ORAL CONTRACEPTIVES; EMERGENCY CONTRACEPTION

Further reading: Food and Drug Administration. "Report on Certain Combined Oral Contraceptives for Use As Postcoital Emergency Contraception." Online: http://www.fda.gov/opacom/fedregister/cd96107.htm, 1 June 1999. Yuzpe, A. A., H. J. Thurlow, I. Ramzy, and J. L. Leyshon. "Postcoital Contraception—A Pilot Study." *Journal of Reproductive Medicine* 13 (1974): 53–58.

BIBLIOGRAPHY

Abma J., Chandra A., Mosher W., Peterson L., and Piccinino L. *Fertility, Family Planning, and Women's Health: New Data from the 1995 National Survey of Family Growth*. Vital and Health Statistics 23, 9. National Center for Health Statistics: 1997.

"Achievements in Public Health, 1900–1999, Healthier Mothers and Babies." *Morbidity and Mortality Weekly Report,* 1 October 1999, 849–858.

Adlakha, Arjun. *Population Trends: India*. Washington, DC: U.S. Department of Commerce, Economics, and Statistics Administration, Bureau of the Census, 1997.

Adshead, Gwen. "A Trancient Frenzy?" *British Medical Journal* 317 (1998): 356.

Agadjanian, Victor. "Women's Choice between Indigenous and Western Contraception in Urban Mozambique." *Women and Health* 28.2 (1998): 1–17.

Aitken, R. John. "The Complexities of Conception." *Science,* 7 July 1995, 39–40.

Alan Guttmacher Institute. *Hopes and Realities: Closing the Gap between Women's Aspirations and Their Reproductive Experiences*. New York: Alan Guttmacher Institute, 1995.

———. *Into a New World: Young Women's Sexual and Reproductive Lives*. New York: Alan Guttmacher Institute, 1998.

———. *Sharing Responsibility: Women, Society and Abortion Worldwide*. New York: Alan Guttmacher Institute, 1999.

Alexander, Nancy J. "Beyond the Condom: The Future of Male Contraception." *Scientific American Presents: Men,* Summer 1999, 80–84.

———. "Future Contraceptives: Vaccines for Men and Women Will Eventually Join New Implants, Better Spermicides, and Stronger, Thinner Condoms." *Scientific American* 273.3 (1995): 136–141.

"Aletta Henriette Jacobs." In *Notable Women in the Life Sciences,* edited by Benjamin F. Shearer and Barbara S. Shearer. Westport, CT: Greenwood Press, 1996.

Alexander, Ivym. "Contraceptive Options for Perimenopausal Women." *Contraceptive Technology Update* 20 (1999): 122.

"Another Option: Contraceptive Patches Are Now Under Research." *Contraceptive Technology Update* 20 (1999): 113.

Asbell, Bernard. *The Pill: A Biography of the Drug That Changed the World*. New York: Random House, 1995.

Asso, Doreen. *The Real Menstrual Cycle.* London: John Wiley, 1983.

Austin, C. R., and R. V. Short, eds. *Hormonal Control of Reproduction*. 2nd ed. Reproduction in Mammals 3. Cambridge, England: Cambridge University Press, 1984.

Back, Kurt W. *Family Planning and Population Control: The Challenges of a Successful Movement.* Boston: Twayne, 1989.

Baird, Bill. "The People Versus Bill Baird: Struggling for Your Right to Privacy." *The Humanist,* March–April 1997, 39–40.

Barker, Paul. "Statistics to Gladden the Heart." *New Statesman,* 5 February 1999, 23.

Barnett, Barbara. "Family Planning Use Often a Family Decision: Better Ways Are Needed to Involve Relatives, Who May Influence Contraceptive Choices." *Network* 18.4 (1998). Online: http://www.resevoir.fhi.org/en/fp/fppubs/network/v18-4/nt1843.html, 8 October 1999.

———. "Search for Nonsurgical Sterilization Continues." *Network* 18.1 (1997). Online: http://resevoir.fhi.org/en/fp/fppubs/network/v18-1/nt1815.html, 25 June 1999.

Bartholet, Elizabeth. "Adoption Rights and Reproductive Wrongs." In *Power and Decision: The Social Control of Reproduction,* edited by Gita Sen and Rachel C. Snow, 177–203. Boston: Harvard University Press, 1994.

"Battle of the Bulge: Population." *The Economist,* 3 September 1994, 23–25.

Baulieu, Etienne-Emile. *The "Abortion Pill:" RU-486, A Woman's Choice.* New York: Simon and Schuster, 1991.

"Baulieu, Etienne-Emile." *Current Biography–1995.* New York: H. W. Wilson, 1995.

Bennett, John P. *Chemical Contraception.* Columbia Series in Molecular Biology. New York: Columbia University Press, 1974.

Bennett, Trude. "Reproductive Health in South Africa." *Public Health Reports* 114 (1999): 88–90.

Berke, Matthew. "Jews Choosing Life." *First Things: A Monthly Journal of Religion and Public Life,* April 1999, 34.

Best, Kim. "Contraceptive Update: Experimental Male Methods Inhibit Sperm." *Network* 18 (1998). Online: http://resevoir.fhi.org/en/fp/fppubs/network/v18-3/nt1835.html, 24 September 1999.

———. "Disabled Have Many Needs for Contraception." *Network* 19 (1999). Online: http://resevoir.fhi.org/en/fp/fppubs/network/v19-2/nt1924.html, 25 June 1999

———. "Mental Disabilities Affect Method Options: Many Factors Involving a Psychiatric Condition or Mental Retardation Influence Contraceptive Decisions." *Network* 19 (1999). Online: http://resevoir.fhi.org/en/fp/fppubs/network/v19-2/nt1925.html, 25 June 1999.

Bhatia, Rajani, and Anne Hendrixson. "The Quinacrine Controversy." *The Network News,* May 1999, 3.

Biddlecom, Ann E., and Bolaji M. Fapohunda. "Covert Contraceptive Use: Prevalence, Motivations, and Consequences." Studies in Family Planning 29 (1998): 360–732.

Biddlecom, Ann E., John B. Casterline, and Aurora E. Perez. "Spouses' Views of Contraception in the Philippines." *International Family Planning Perspectives* 23 (1997): 108–115.

Billings, Evelyn, and Ann Westmore. *The Billings Method: Controlling Fertility without Drugs or Devices.* New York: Random House, 1980.

Birth Control Options. Philadelphia: Wyeth-Ayerst Laboratories, 1995.

"Bitter Pill: Japan." *The Economist* 8 (November 1997): 42–43.

Blaney, Carol Lynn. "Contraceptive Update: Contraceptive Needs after Age 40." *Network* 18 (1997). Online: http://resevoir.fhi.org/en/fp/fppubs/network/v18-1/nt1811.html, 25 June 1999.

Bledsoe, Caroline, Fatoumatta Banja, and Allan G. Hill. "Reproductive Mishaps and Western Contraception: An African Challenge to Fertility Theory." *Population and Development Review* 24 (1998): 15–57.

Blumberg, Joan Jacobs. *The Body Project: An Intimate History of American Girls.* New York: Random House, 1997.

Bongaarts, John. "The Fertility Impact of Changes in the Timing of Childbearing in the Developing World." Policy Research Division Working Paper No. 120. New York: Population Council, 1999.

Bongaarts, John, and Judith Bruce. "The Causes of Unmet Need for Contraception and the Social Content of Services." *Studies in Family Planning* 26.2 (1995): 57–75.

Bonn, Dorothy. "Male Contraceptive Research Steps Back into Spotlight." *The Lancet* 353.99149 (1999): 302.

———. "What Prospects for Hormonal Contraceptives for Men?" *The Lancet* 347.8997 (1996): 316.

Brady, Margaret. "Female Genital Mutilation." *Nursing* 28.9 (1998): 50–51.

"Brazil 1996: Results from the Demographic and Health Survey." *Studies in Family Planning* 29 (1998): 88–92.

Brooks, Marlies. "Men's Views on Male Hormonal Contraception: A Survey of the Views of Attenders at a Fitness Centre in Bristol, UK." *British Journal of Family Planning* 24 (1998): 7–17.

Brown, Cecelia. "In Memory of Mary Steichen Calderone." *The Journal of Sex Research* 36 (1999) 218–219.

"The Brundtland Era Begins." *The Lancet* 351.9100 (1998): 381.

Bull, Sheana S., and L. Mercedes Melian. "Contraception and Culture: The Use of Yuyos in Paraguay." *Health Care for Women International* 19 (1998): 49–60.

Bureau of the Census. *Population Trends: Brazil*. Washington, DC: U.S. Department of Commerce, Economics and Statistics Administration, Bureau of the Census, 1993.

———. *Population Trends: Egypt*. Washington, DC: U.S. Department of Commerce, Economics and Statistics Administration, Bureau of the Census, 1994.

———. *Population Trends: Indonesia*. Washington, DC: U.S. Department of Commerce, Economics and Statistics Administration, Bureau of the Census, 1992.

———. Report WP/98. *World Population at a Glance: 1996 and Beyond*. Washington, DC: U.S. Government Printing Office, 1996.

———. Report WP/98. *World Population at a Glance: 1998 and Beyond*. Washington, DC: U.S. Government Printing Office, 1999.

———. Report WP/98. *World Population Profile: 1998*. Washington, DC: U.S. Government Printing Office, 1999.

Burkholz, Herbert. *The FDA Follies*. New York: BasicBooks/HarperCollins, 1994.

Carlson, Margaret. "A Girl's Best Friends: Alma Powell and Elayne Bennett, One Pro-choice, the Other Pro-life, Find Common Ground on Teens and Sex." *Time,* 22 January 1996, 32.

Carr, Bruce R., and James E. Griffin. "Fertility Control and Its Complications." *Williams Textbook of Endocrinology,* 9th ed., edited by Jean D. Wilson and others, 901–925. Philadelphia: W. B. Saunders, 1998.

Cassen, Robert, ed. *Population and Development: Old Debates, New Conclusions*. New Brunswick, NJ: Transaction, 1994.

Castelli, William P. "Reducing Risk in OC Users Who Smoke." *Contemporary Obstetrics/Gynecology* 41 (1996): 118–126.

Casterline, John B., Ronald D. Lee, and Karen A. Foote, eds. *Fertility in the United States: New Patterns, New Theories*. Supplement to Population and Development Review 22. New York: Population Council, 1996.

"Centchroman." *Contraceptive Advances*. Baltimore: Johns Hopkins University, Reproductive Health Online,1999. Online: http://www.reproline.jhu.edu/english/1fp/1advances/1centch/ceorvw.htm, 22 June 2000.

Center for International Health Information Health Statistics Report: Philippines. Center for International Health Information, 29 October 1999. Online: http://www.cihi.com/PHANstat/PHILIPPINES.html, 12 November 1999.

Center for International Health Information Health Statistics Report: South Africa. Center for International Health Information. 29 October 1999. Online: http://www.cihi.com/PHANstat/SOUTH_AFRICA, 12 November 1999.

Chalmers, Beverly, et al. "Contraceptive Knowledge, Attitudes, and Use Among Women Attending Health Clinics in St. Petersburg, Russian Federation." *The Canadian Journal of Human Sexuality* 7 (1998): 129–137.

Chandra, A. "Surgical Sterilization in the United States: Prevalence and Characteristics, 1965–1995." Vital and Health Statistics 23, 20. National Center for Health Statistics: 1998.

Chandra, Anjani, and Elizabeth Hervey Stephen. "Impaired Fecundity in the United States: 1982–1995." *Family Planning Perspectives* 30 (1998): 34–42.

Chandrasekhar, Sripati. *India's Abortion Experience*. Rev. ed. Philosophy and the Environment 4. Denton, TX: University of North Texas Press, 1994.

Chen, Constance M. *"The Sex Side of Life": Mary Ware Dennett's Pioneering Battle for Birth Control and Sex Education*. New York: New Press, 1996.

Chenais, Jean-Claude. "Fertility, Family, and Social Policy in Contemporary Western Europe." *Population and Development Review* 22 (1996): 729–739.

Chesler, Ellen. *Woman of Valor: Margaret Sanger and the Birth Control Movement in America*. New York: Anchor-Doubleday, 1992.

Chez, Ronald A., and Daniel R. Mishell, Jr. "Control of Human Reproduction: Contraception, Sterilization, and Pregnancy Termination." Chap. 34 in *Danforth's Obstetrics and Gynecology*. 7th ed. Philadelphia: J. B. Lippincott, 1994.

Cohen, Joel E. *How Many People Can the Earth Support?* New York: W.W. Norton, 1995.

Cohen, Susan A. "The Role of Contraception in Reducing Abortion." *Issues in Brief (Alan Guttmacher Institute)* 19 (1998). Online: http://www.agi-usa.org/pubs/ib19.html, 11 September 1999.

Colker, Ruth. *Abortion and Dialogue: Pro-choice, Pro-life, and American Law.* Bloomington, IN: Indiana University Press, 1992.

The Columbia University College of Physicians and Surgeons Complete Home Medical Guide. 3rd. ed. Crown, 1995.

"Combination Birth Control Pill Formulation Available in One-Third Lower Dose." *Cancer Weekly Plus,* 11 August 1997, 13.

Committee on Contraceptive Research and Development, Division of Health Sciences Policy, Institute of Medicine. *Contraceptive Research and Development: Looking to the Future.* Eds. Polly Harrison and Allan Rosenfield. Washington, DC: National Academy Press, 1996.

"Compliance with Oral Contraceptives." *The Contraception Report* 5, special report (1995): 3–23.

"Contraception for Men." *A Research Agenda for the Reproductive Sciences Branch of the NICHD.* National Institute of Child Health and Human Development, 1995. Online: http://www.nichd.nih.gov/publications/online_only/agenda/contents.htm, 8 September 1999.

Contraceptive Advances. Online: http://www.reproline.jhu.edu/english/1fp/1advances/1advance.htm, 22 June 2000.

Correa, Sonia. "Norplant in the Nineties: Realities, Dilemmas, Missing Pieces." In *Power and Decision: The Social Control of Reproduction,* edited by Gita Sen and Rachel C. Snow, 287–309. Boston: Harvard University Press, 1994.

Craig, John M. "'The Sex Side of Life': The Obscenity Case of Mary Ware Dennett." *Frontiers* 15 (1995): 145–166.

Cupp, Malanie Johns. "Melatonin." *American Family Physician* 56 (1997): 1421–1426.

Curran, Charles. "Fertility Control: Ethical Issues." In *Encyclopedia of Bioethics,* rev ed., edited by Warren Thomas Reich. New York: Macmillan, 1995

Cushman, Linda F., et al. "Condom Use Among Women Choosing Long-Term Hormonal Contraception." *Family Planning Perspectives* 30 (1998): 240–243.

Dailard, Cynthia. "U.S. Policy Can Reduce Cost Barriers to Contraception." *Issues in Brief*. New York: Alan Guttmacher Institute, 1999. Online: http://www.agi-usa.org/pubs/ib_0799.html, 6 October 1999.

"The Dalkon Shield Story: A Company Rewarded for Its Faulty Product." *Health Facts,* May 1996, 1.

Darroch, Jacqueline E. *Cost to Employer Health Plans of Covering Contraceptives.* New York: Alan Guttmacher Institute, 1998. Online: http://www.agi-usa.org/pubs/kaiser_0698.html, 8 October 1999.

Darroch, Jacqueline E., and Jennifer J. Frost. "Women's Interest in Vaginal Microbicides." *Family Planning Perspectives* 31.1 (1999): 16–23.

David, Henry P. "Abortion in Europe, 1920–1991: A Public Health Perspective." *Studies in Family Planning* 23 (1992): 1–222.

Davis, W. Marvin. "Andrology: Pharmacotherapies for Men Only." *Drug Topics* 141 (1997): 86–95.

Delbanco, Suzanne, et al. "Public Knowledge and Perceptions about Unplanned Pregnancy and Contraception in Three Countries." *Family Planning Perspectives* 29 (1997) 70–75.

Dennett, Mary Ware. *Birth Control Laws: Shall We Keep Them, Change Them, or Abolish Them?* 1926. New York: Da Capo Press, 1970.

Department of Health and Human Services, Public Health Service. *Information for Men: Your Sterilization Operation.* U.S. Department of Health and Human Services, 1991.

———. *Information for Women: Your Sterilization Operation.* U.S. Department of Health and Human Services, 1991.

Department of Health (U.K.), http://www.doh.gov.uk

Dickey, Richard P. *Managing Contraceptive Pill Patients.* 8th ed. Durant, OK: Essential Medical Information Systems, Inc. 1994.

Dixon-Mueller, Ruth. *Population Policy & Women's Rights: Transforming Reproductive Choice*. Westport, CT: Praeger, 1993.

Dixon-Mueller, Ruth, and Adrienne Germain. "Stalking the Elusive 'Unmet Need.'" *Studies in Family Planning* 23 (1992): 330–335.

Djerassi, Carl. *From the Lab into the World: A Pill for People, Pets, and Bugs*. Washington, DC: American Chemical Society, 1994.

"DMPA at a Glance." *The Population Reports* 23 (1995): S1–S2.

Donovan, Patricia. "School-Based Sexuality Education: The Issues and Challenges. *Family Planning Perspectives* 30 (1998): 188–193.

Drennan, Megan. "New Perspectives on Men's Participation." *Population Reports* 26.2 (1998).

Eberstadt, Nicholas. "Asian Population Change: What It Means for Policy." *Current* 409 (1999): 33–39.

Elias, Marilyn. "The Mysteries of Melatonin." *Harvard Health Letter* 18 (1993): 6–8.

Ellertson, Charlotte, Beverly Winikoff, Elizabeth Armstrong, Sharon Camp, and Pramilla Senanayake. "Expanding Access to Emergency Contraception in Developing Countries." *Studies in Family Planning* 26 (1995): 251–263.

"Emergency Contraception Kit Approved." *Journal of the American Medical Association* 280 (1998): 1472.

Entwisle, Barbara, and Polina Kozyreva. "New Estimates of Induced Abortion in Russia." *Studies in Family Planning* 28 (1997): 14–23.

Faden, Ruth R., and Tom L. Beauchamp. *A History and Theory of Informed Consent*. New York: Oxford University Press, 1986.

Fargues, Philippe. "State Policies and the Birth Rate in Egypt: From Socialism to Liberalism." *Population and Development Review* 23 (1997): 115–138.

Faundes, Anibal. "Opinion: Women Deserve Accurate Information." *Network* 16, 2 (1996).

Faux, Marian. Roe v. Wade: *The Untold Story of the Landmark Supreme Court Decision That Made Abortion Legal*. New York: Macmillan, 1988.

Feldman, David M. *Birth Control in Jewish Law: Marital Relations, Contraception, and Abortion As Set Forth in the Classic Texts of Jewish Law*. 2nd ed. Northvale, NJ: Jason Aronson, 1998.

"The Female Condom." *The Contraception Report.* Patient Update 6, vol. 5, no. 6.

"Female Condom Becomes Available Nationwide." *The Contraception Report* 5 (1995): 11–13.

"Female Genital Mutilation." *Fact Sheets*. April 1997. World Health Organization, Online: http://www.who.int/inf-fs/en/fact153.html, 26 March 2000.

"Fertility Control." In *Encyclopedia of Bioethics,* rev. ed., edited by Warren Thomas Reich. New York: Simon and Schuster/Macmillan, 1995.

"FHI Receives USAID Contract for Research in Africa." *Africa News Service,* 15 December 1999.

Fishel, Joy. "Contraceptive Technologies: How Much Choice Do We Really Have?" *The Zero Population Growth Reporter,* March/April, 1997. Online: http://www.zpg.org/Reports_Publications/Reports/report40.html, 6 March 2000

Fleeger, Carolyn A., ed. *United States Pharmacopeial Dictionary of United States Adopted Names and International Drug Names: 1996.* Rockville, MD: United States Pharmacopeial Convention, 1995.

Food and Drug Administration. *Estrogens*. Rockville, MD: Department of Health and Human Services, 1993.

———. "FDA Approves Application for PREVEN Emergency Contraceptive Kit." FDA Talk Paper, 2 September 1998. Online: http://www.fda.gov/bbs/topics/ANSWERS/ANS00892.html, 9 June 1999.

———. "Report on Certain Combined Oral Contraceptives for Use As Postcoital Emergency Contraception." Online: http://www.fda.gov/opacom/fedregister/cd96107.htm, 1 June 1999.

Foster, Daniel. "Miraculous Melatonin." *Cosmopolitan,* July 1999, 102–103.

Fowler, Dorothy G. *Unmailable: Congress and the Post Office*. Athens, GA: University of Georgia Press, 1977.

Francome, Colin. "Attitudes of General Practitioners in Northern Ireland Toward Abortion and Family Planning." *Family Planning Perspectives* 29 (1997): 234–236.

Fraser, Laura. "The Abortion Pill's Grim Progress." *Mother Jones,* January 1999, 41.

Freidenreich, Harriet Pass. "Aletta Jacobs in Historical Perspective." Afterward to *Memories: My Life as an International Leader in Health, Suffrage, and Peace,* by Aletta Jacobs. Trans. Annie Wright. New York: The Feminist Press at the City University of New York, 1996.

"Future Contraceptive Methods." *The Contraception Report* 5 (1994): 4–11.

Gammon, Marilie D., Joan E. Bertin, and Mary Beth Terry. "Abortion and the Risk of Breast Cancer: Is There a Believable Association?" *Journal of the American Medical Association* 275 (1996): 321–322.

Garcia, Sandra Guzman, Rachel Snow, and Iain Aitken. "Preferences for Contraceptive Attributes: Voices of Women in Ciudad Juarez, Mexico." *International Family Planning Perspectives* 23 (1997): 52–58.

Garrow, David J. *Liberty and Sexuality: The Right to Privacy and the Making of* Roe v. Wade. New York: Macmillan, 1994.

Ginsburg, Faye D., and Rayna Rapp, eds. *Conceiving the New World Order: The Global Politics of Reproduction*. Berkeley: University of California Press, 1995.

Glaser, Anna. "Levonorgestrel for Emergency Contraception." *International Planned Parenthood Federation Medical Bulletin* 32.6 (1998): 6–7.

Glass, Nigel. "Infanticide in Hungary Faces Stiffer Penalties." *The Lancet,* 13 February 1999, 570.

Goldsmith, Marsha F. "Researchers Amass Abortion Data." *Journal of the American Medical Association* 262 (1989): 1431–1432.

Goldstein, Leslie Friedman. *Contemporary Cases in Women's Rights*. Madison, WI: University of Wisconsin Press, 1994.

Goldzieher, Joseph W., and Nesaam M. Zamah. "Oral Contraceptive Side Effects: Where's the Beef?" *Contraception* 52 (1995): 327–335.

Golub, Sharon. *Periods: From Menarche to Menopause.* Newbury Park, CA: Sage, 1992.

Goodkind, Daniel M. "Vietnam's One-or-Two-Child Policy in Action." *Population and Development Review* 21 (1995): 85–111.

Grady, William R., Daniel H. Klepinger, and Anjanette Nelson-Wally. "Contraceptive Characteristics: The Perceptions and Priorities of Men and Women." *Family Planning Perspectives* 31 (1999): 168.

Grimes, David A., et al., eds. *Modern Contraception: Updates from The Contraception Report.* Totowa, NJ: Emron, 1997.

Guillebaud, John. *The Pill and Other Hormones for Contraception.* 5th ed. Oxford: Oxford University Press, 1997.

Gurstein, Rochelle. *The Repeal of Reticence: A History of America's Cultural and Legal Struggles over Free Speech, Obscenity, Sexual Liberation, and Modern Art*. New York: Hill and Wang/ Farrar, Straus, and Giroux, 1996.

"Guttmacher, Alan F(rank)." *Current Biography: 1965*. New York: H. W. Wilson, 1965.

"Gynecology." In *Encyclopedia of Medical History,* edited by Roderick E. McGrew. New York: McGraw-Hill, 1985.

Gynétics, Inc. "PREVEN Emergency Contraceptive Kit: The First and Only Emergency Contraceptive Product: Approved by The FDA." Press Release, 2 September 1998. Online: http://www.gynetics.com/gynetics/news/releases/pr199809021.html, 9 June 1999.

Hall, Ruth. *Passionate Crusader: The Life of Marie Stopes.* New York: Harcourt Brace Jovanovich, 1977.

Hankoff, Leon D., and Philip D. Darney. "Contraceptive Choices for Behaviorally Disordered Women." *American Journal of Obstetrics and Gynecology* 168.6, part 2. (1993): 1986–1989.

Harper, Michael J. K. *Birth Control Technologies: Prospects by the Year 2000.* Austin: University of Texas Press, 1983.

Harrison, Polly F., and Allan Rosenfield, eds. *Contraceptive Research and Development: Looking to the Future.* Washington, DC: National Academy Press, 1996.

———. *Contraceptive Research, Introduction, and Use: Lessons from Norplant.* Washington, DC: National Academy Press, 1998.

Haslett, Diane C. "Hull House and the Birth Control Movement: An Untold Story." *Affilia: Journal of Women and Social Work* 12 (1997): 261–277.

Hatcher, Robert A., and John Guillebaud. "The Pill: Combined Oral Contraceptives." In *Contraceptive Technology,* 17th rev ed., edited by Robert Hatcher, James Trussel, Felicia Stewart, and others, 405–466. New York: Ardent Media, 1998.

Hatcher, Robert, James Trussell, Felicia Stewart, and others. *Contraceptive Technology*. 17th rev. ed. New York: Ardent Media, 1998.

———. *Contraceptive Technology*. 16th rev. ed. New York: Irvington, 1994.

Hausfater, Glenn, and Sarah Blaffer Hrdy, eds. *Infanticide: Comparative and Evolutionary Perspectives*. New York: Aldine, 1984.

Hearts, Jack. "How to Get Fixed." *Men's Health,* July-August 1993, 58–60.

Henshaw, Stanley K. "Unintended Pregnancy in the United States." *Family Planning Perspectives* 30 (1998): 24–29.

Henshaw, Stanley K., Susheela Singh, and Taylor Haas. "The Incidence of Abortion Worldwide." *International Family Planning Perspectives* 25 (1999): S30–S38.

Herz, Barbara, and Anthony R. Measham. *The Safe Motherhood Initiative: Proposals for Action*. World Bank Discussion Papers 9. Washington, DC: World Bank, 1987.

Hicks, D. A. "What Risk of Infection with IUD Use?" *The Lancet*, 25 April 1998, 1222–1223.

Hines, Alice M., and Karen L. Graves. "AIDS Protection and Contraception among African American, Hispanic, and White Women." *Health and Social Work* 23 (1998): 186–194.

Hogue, Carol J. Rowland. "Missing the Boat on Pregnancy Prevention: Teenage Pregnancy Grabs the Headlines, But Most Unintended and Unwanted Pregnancies Occur among Adults." *Issues in Science and Technology* 13.4 (1997): 41–45.

Hole, John W. *Human Anatomy and Physiology.* 6th ed. Dubuque, IA: Wm. C. Brown, 1993.

Horner, Louse L. ed. *Black Americans: A Statistical Sourcebook*. 1998 Edition. Palo Alto, CA: Information Publications, 1998.

Houppert, Karen. "The Politics of Birth Control: How Prolife Forces Strangle Research." *Village Voice,* October 1996, 23–30.

Huezo, C. M. "Current Reversible Contraceptive Methods: A Global Perspective." *International Journal of Gynecology and Obstetrics* 62, Supplement 1 (1998): S3–S15.

Humanae Vitae: Encyclical of Pope Paul VI on the Regulation of Birth. The Vatican, 1968. Online: http://www.vatican.va/holy_father/paul_vi/encyclicals/documents/hf_p-vi_enc_25071968_humanae-vitae_en.html, 14 November 1999.

Hume, Maggie. *Contraception in Catholic Doctrine: The Evolution of an Earthly Code*. Washington, DC: Catholics for a Free Choice, 1991.

Huston, Perdita. *Motherhood by Choice: Pioneers in Women's Health and Family Planning*. New York: The Feminist Press at the City University of New York, 1992.

Imber, Jonathan B. *Abortion and the Private Practice.* New Haven, CT: Yale University Press, 1986.

"Indonesia 1994: Results from the Demographic and Health Survey." *Studies in Family Planning* 27 (1996): 119–123.

"Insertion and Removal of Levonorgestrel Subdermal Implants." *The Contraception Report,* November 1994, 4–12.

"International Medical Advisory Panel Statement on Steroidal Oral Contraception." *International Planned Parenthood Federation Medical Bulletin* 32.6 (1998): 1–6.

"International Planned Parenthood Federation Charter on Sexual and Reproductive Rights." *Women's International Network News* 24.4 (1998): 21–22.

Jacobs, Aletta. *Memories: My Life as an International Leader in Health, Suffrage, and Peace*. Trans. Annie Wright. New York: The Feminist Press at the City University of New York, 1996.

Jaffe, Frederick S. "Alan F. Guttmacher: 1898–1974." *Family Planning Perspectives* 6 (1974): 1–2.

Jejeebhoy, Shireen. *Women's Education, Autonomy, and Reproductive Behavior: Experience from Developing Countries*. Oxford: Clarendon Press, 1995.

Jiggins, Janice. *Changing the Boundaries: Women-Centered Perspectives on Population and the Environment*. Washington, DC: Island Press, 1994.

Johansson, Annika, et al. "Population Policies and Reproductive Patterns in Vietnam." *The Lancet,* 1 June 1996, 1529–1532.

"Johnson & Johnson Patch." *Wall Street Journal,* 21 July 1999, B4.

Johnson, R. Christian. "Feminism, Philanthropy, and Science in the Development of the Oral Contraceptive Pill. *Pharmacy in History* 19 (1977): 63–78.

Jones, Gavin W. "Population and the Family in Southeast Asia." *Journal of Southeast Asian Studies* 26 (1995): 184–195.

———. *Urbanization in Large Developing Countries: China, Indonesia, Brazil, and India*. New York: Oxford, 1998.

Jones, Richard, E. *Human Reproductive Biology.* San Diego, CA: Academic Press–Harcourt Brace Jovanovich: 1991.

Kahn, James G., Claire D. Brindis, and Dana A. Glei. "Pregnancies Averted among U.S. Teenagers by the Use of Contraceptives." *Family Planning Perspectives* 31 (1999): 29–34.

Kane, Penny. "Population Policy." In *The China Handbook,* edited by Christopher Hudson. Chicago: Fitzroy Dearborn, 1997.

Kaufman, K. *The Abortion Resource Handbook.* New York: Fireside–Simon and Schuster, 1997.

Kaunitz, Andrew M., and Howard Ory. "Estrogen Component of OCs." *Dialogues in Contraception* 5 (1997): 1–6.

Kennedy, David M. *Birth Control in America: The Career of Margaret Sanger*. New Haven, CT: Yale University Press, 1970.

Kessel, Elton. "Quinacrine Sterilization Revisited." Commentary. *The Lancet,* 10 September 1994, 698–700.

Kimble-Haas, Sheila L. "The Intrauterine Device: Dispelling the Myths." *The Nurse Practitioner* 23 (1998): 58.

Kingkade, Ward. *International Brief: Population Trends: Russia*. Washington, DC: U.S. Department of Commerce, Economics and Statistics Administration, Bureau of the Census, 1997.

Kirk, Dudley, and Bernard Pillet. "Fertility Levels, Trends, and Differentials in Sub-Saharan Africa in the 1980s and 1990s." *Studies in Family Planning* 29 (1998): 1–22.

Kirsh, Jonathan D. "Informed Consent for Family Planning for Poor Women in Chiapas, Mexico." *The Lancet,* 31 July 1999, 419.

Knight, James W., and Joan C. Callahan. *Preventing Birth: Contemporary Methods and Related Moral Controversies.* Ethics in a Changing World 3. Salt Lake City: University of Utah Press, 1989.

Knowles, Jon, and Marcia Ringel. *All About Birth Control: A Personal Guide.* New York: Three Rivers–Crown, 1998.

Kogan, Barry S. ed. *A Time to be Born and a Time to Die: The Ethics of Choice*. New York: Aldine de Gruyter, 1991.

Kowal, Deborah. "Abstinence and the Range of Sexual Expression." In *Contraceptive Technology,* 17th rev ed., edited by Robert Hatcher, James Trussel, Felicia Stewart, and others. New York: Ardent Media, 1998.

Kulczycki, Andrzej, Malcolm Potts, and Allan Rosenfield. "Abortion and Fertility Regulation." *Public Health* 347 (1996): 1663–1886.

Kuo, Lena. "The Lea's Shield is denied FDA approval." *The Network News,* January–February 1997, 5.

Ladd, Everett Carll, and Karlyn H. Bowman. *Public Opinion About Abortion: Twenty-five Years after* Roe v. Wade. Washington, DC: AEI Press (American Enterprise Institute), 1997.

LaMay, Craig L. "America's Censor: Anthony Comstock and Free Speech." *Communications and the Law* 19.3 (1997): 1–59.

Lande, R. E. "New Era for Injectables." *Population Reports.* Series K, no. 5. Baltimore: Johns Hopkins School of Public Health, Population Information Program, August 1995. Online: http://www.jhuccp.org/pr/k5edsum.stm, March 2000.

Larkin, Marilynn. "Easing the Way to Safer Sex." *The Lancet,* 28 March 1998, 964.

———. "Male Reproductive Health: A Hotbed of Research." *The Lancet,* 15 August 1988, 552.

"Law to Reform Food, Medical Product Regulation: President Clinton Signs FDA Modernization Act into Law." *FDA Consumer* 32.2 (1998): 3.

Leavesley, Gwen, and John Porter. "Sexuality, Fertility and Contraception in Disability." *Contraception* (Australia) 26 (1982): 417–441.

Lednicer, Daniel, ed. *Contraception: The Chemical Control of Fertility*. New York: Marcel Dekker, 1969.

Levy, Sharon Joseph. "Judaism, Population, and the Environment." *Population, Consumption, and the Environment: Religious and Secular Responses*. Albany: State University of New York Press, 1995.

Lieberman, E. James, and Karen Lieberman Troccoli. *Like It Is: A Teen Sex Guide.* Mefferson, NC: McFarland, 1998.

Lisheron, Mark. "Embracing the Complexities." *American Journalism Review,* June 1999, 40.

Lobo, Rogerio A. "The Perimenopause." *Clinical Obstetrics and Gynecology* 41.4 (1998): 895–897.

Mahler, K. "Rates of Modern Method Use Are High Among Urban Russian Women, Who Typically Want Small Families." *Family Planning Perspectives* 30.6 (1998): 293.

Martine, George. "Brazil's Fertility Decline, 1965–1995: A Fresh Look at Key Factors." *Population and Development Review* 22 (1996): 47–75.

Mastroianni, Luigi. "Future Contraceptive Methods." *The Contraceptive Report* 5 (1994): 4–12.

Matteson, Peggy. *Advocating for Self: Women's Decisions Concerning Contraception*. New York: Harrington Park Press (An Imprint of the Haworth Press), 1995.

McBride, Wayne Z. "Spontaneous Abortion." *American Family Physician* 43 (1991): 175–182.

McClamroch, Kristi. "Total Fertility Rate, Women's Education, and Women's Work: What Are the Relationships?" *Population and Environment: A Journal of Interdisciplinary Studies* 18 (1996): 175–186.

McDevitt, Thomas M. *World Population Profile: 1998*. Washington, DC: U.S. Department of Commerce, Bureau of the Census, 1999.

McDevitt, Thomas M., Arjun Adlakha, Timothy B. Fowler, and Vera Harris-Bourne. *Trends in Adolescent Fertility and Contraceptive Use in the Developing World*. Washington, DC: U.S. Department of Commerce, Bureau of the Census, 1996.

McKerns, Kenneth W., ed. *Reproductive Processes and Contraception*. New York: Plenum, 1981.

McLaren, Angus, and Arlene Tigar McLaren. *The Bedroom and the State: The Changing Practices and Politics of Contraception and Abortion in Canada, 1880–1997*. 2nd ed. Toronto: Oxford University Press, 1997.

McLaughlin, Loretta. *The Pill, John Rock, and the Church: The Biography of A Revolution*. Boston: Little, Brown, 1982.

McLucas, Bruce. "Pregnancy After Endometrial Ablation: A Case Report." *Journal of Reproductive Medicine* 40 (1995): 237–239.

The Merck Manual of Medical Information. Whitehorse Station, NJ: Merck Research Laboratories, 1997.

Merrill, Richard A. "Regulation of Drugs and Devices: An Evolution." *Health Affairs* 13.3 (1994): 47–69.

Mexico: Health Statistics Report. Washington, DC: Center of International Health Information, 1996.

Michaels, Stuart, and Alain Giami. "Sexual Acts and Sexual Relationships: Asking About Sex in Surveys." *Public Opinion Quarterly* 63 (1999): 401–420.

Mintz, Morton. *At Any Cost: Corporate Greed, Women, and the Dalkon Shield.* New York: Pantheon, 1985.

Mishell, Daniel R. "Evolution of Oral Contraception: 1960–1985." *Dialogues in Contraception* (1985): 1–6.

Mishell, Daniel R., and Patricia J. Sulak. "The IUD: Dispelling the Myths and Assessing the Potential." *Dialogues in Contraception* 2nd series, 2 (1997): 1–4.

Mitchell, Marc D., Joan Littlefield, and Suzanne Gutter. "Costing of Reproductive Health Services." *International Family Planning Perspectives* 29 (1999): S17–S29.

Moore, M. "Most U.S. Couples Who Seek Surgical Sterilization Do So for Contraception; Fewer Than 25 Percent Desire Reversal." *Family Planning Perspectives* 31 (1999): 102.

"The Morning After: Contraception." *The Economist*, 27 July 1996, 68–69.

Mosher, William D., and Christine A Bachrach. "Understanding U.S. Fertility: Continuity and Change in the National Survey of Family Growth, 1988–1995." *Family Planning Perspectives* 28 (1996): 4–12.

Mudur, Ganapati. "Indian Women's Groups Question Contraceptive Vaccine Research." *British Medical Journal,* 14 November 1998, 1340–1341.

Mukerjee, Madhusree. "Gursaran Prasad Talwar: Pushing the Envelope for Vaccines." *Scientific American,* July 1996, 38–39. Online: http://www.sciam.com/0796issue/0796profile.html, 7 March 2000.

Murray, Velma McBride, and James J. Ponzetti Jr. "American Indian Female Adolescents' Sexual Behavior: A Test of the Life-Course Experience Theory." *Family and Consumer Sciences Research Journal* 26 (1997): 75–95.

Musallam, B.F. *Sex and Society in Islam: Birth Control Before the Nineteenth Century*. Cambridge, England: Cambridge University Press, 1983.

Nadler, Richard. "Birds, Bees, and ABCs." *National Review*, 13 September 1999, 8+.

Nafis, Sadik. "Itself Far from Public Eye, UNFPA Looks Towards the Future." *UN Chronicle* 35.4 (1998): 36–37.

Nakajima, Steven T. "The New Progestins." *The Western Journal of Medicine* 161 (1994): 163.

National Institute of Child Health and Human Development, National Institutes of Health. *Facts about Vasectomy Safety.* Washington, DC: National Institutes of Health, 1996.

Nevid, Jeffrey S., and Fern Gotfried. *Choices: Sex in the Age of STDs.* Boston: Allyn and Bacon, 1995.

Newman, Lucile F., ed. *Women's Medicine: A Cross-Cultural Study of Indigenous Fertility Regulation.* New Brunswick, NJ: Rutgers University Press, 1985.

Ngom, Pierre. "Men's Unmet Need for Family Planning." *Studies in Family Planning* 28 (1997): 192–202.

Nordenberg, Tamar. "Condoms: Barriers to Bad News." *FDA Consumer* 32 (1998): 22–25.

———. *Protecting Against Unintended Pregnancy.* Rockville, MD: Department of Health and Human Services, 1997.

Nuechterlein, James. "Catholics, Protestants, and Contraception." *First Things: A Monthly Journal of Religion and Public Life,* April 1999, 10.

Obermeyer, Carla Makhlouf. "Religious Doctrine, State Ideology, and Reproductive Options in Islam." In *Power and Decision: The Social Control of Reproduction,* edited by Gita Sen and Rachel C. Snow. Boston: Harvard University Press, 1994.

O'Grada, Cormac, and Brendan Walsh. "Fertility and Population in Ireland, North and South." *Population Studies* 49 (1995): 259–279.

O'Higgins, Kathleen. "Family Planning Services in Ireland with Particular Reference to Minors." In *The Adolescent Dilemma: International Perspectives on the Family Planning Rights of Minors,* edited by Hyman Rodman and Jan Trost. New York: Praeger, 1986.

Okun, Barbara S. "Family Planning in the Jewish Population of Israel: Correlates of Withdrawal Use." *Studies in Family Planning* 28 (1997): 215–227.

Omran, Abdel Rahim. *Family Planning in the Legacy of Islam*. London: Routledge, 1992.

Oudshoorn, Nelly. *Beyond the Natural Body: An Archeology of Sex Hormones*. London: Routledge, 1994.

Packer, Corinne A. A. *The Right to Reproductive Choice*. Abo, Finland: Abo Akademi University/Institute for Human Rights, 1996.

Pasquale, Samuel A., and Jennifer Cadoff. *The Birth Control Book: A Complete Guide to Your Contraceptive Options*. New York: Ballantine, 1996.

Patton, Cindy. *Fatal Advice: How Safe-Sex Education Went Wrong*. Durham, NC: Duke University Press, 1996.

Peng, Xizhe. *Demographic Transition in China: Fertility Trends Since the 1950s*. Oxford: Clarendon Press, 1991.

Perry, Susan, and Jim Dawson. *Nightmare: Women and the Dalkon Shield.* New York: Macmillan, 1985.

Piccinino, Linda J., and William D. Mosher. "Trends in Contraceptive Use in the United States: 1982–1995." *Family Planning Perspectives* 30 (1998): 4–12.

"The Pill, Finally." *Maclean's,* 14 June 1999, 53.

Pincus, Gregory. *The Control of Fertility*. New York: Academic Press, 1965.

"The Polyurethane Vaginal Pouch: New Barrier Contraceptive May Give Women More Control over STD Prevention." *The Contraception Report* 3 (1992): 12–14.

Population Action International. *Contraceptive Choice: Worldwide Access to Family Planning*. Washington, DC: Population Action International, 1997. Online: http://www.populationaction.org/programs/rc97.htm, 11 October 1999.

———. *Fact Sheet No. 9: How are Nations Responding to the Call for Increased Funding for Reproductive Health?* Washington, DC: Population Action International, 1999.

———. *Fact Sheet No. 3: Why The United States Should Restore Funding for UNFPA*. Washington, DC: Population Action International, 1999.

———. *Why Population Matters*. Washington, DC: Population Action International, 1996.

Population Council. *Annual Report: 1998*. Online: http://www.popcouncil.org/about/ar/default.html, 6 March 2000.

———. "Contraceptives and Other Reproductive Health Products under Development by the Population Council." Online: http://www.popcouncil.org/faqs/contra97.html, 15 June 1999.

Pramik, Mary Jean. "Emergency Contraception: Is It Our Best Kept Secret?" *Drug Topics,* 4 November 1996: 35–36.

Rakel, Robert E., ed. *Saunders Manual of Medical Practice.* Philadelphia, PA: W. B. Saunders, 1996.

Ramos, Rebecca, Kathy I. Kennedy, and Cynthia M. Visness. "Effectiveness of Lactational Amenorrhea in Prevention of Pregnancy in Manila, The Philippines: Non-comparative Prospective Trial." *British Medical Journal* 313 (1996): 909–912.

Rathschmidt, Jack. "Cafeteria Catholics Don't Need to Get in Line." *U.S. Catholic* 63.1 (1998): 36–38.

Ravenholt, R. T. "Taking Contraceptives to the World's Poor." *Free Inquiry* 14.2 (1994): 1–6.

Rebar, Robert W., and Leon Speroff. "The New Progestins: Pharmacologic and Clinical Perspectives." *Dialogues in Contraception* 4.1 (1993): 1–10.

Remennick, Larissa I., Delila Amir, Yuval Elimelech, and Yliya Novikov. "Family Planning Practices and Attitudes among Former Soviet New Immigrant Women in Israel." *Social Science and Medicine* 41 (1995): 569–577.

Reynolds, Moira Davison. "Katharine McCormick." In *Women Advocates of Reproductive Rights: Eleven Who Led the Struggle in the United States and Great Britain*. Jefferson, NC: McFarland, 1994.

Richards, Arlene Kramer, and Irene Willis. *What to Do If You or Someone You Know Is Under 18 and Pregnant*. New York: Lorthrop, Lee & Shepard–William Morrow, 1983.

Richter, Judith. "'Vaccination' Against Pregnancy: The Politics of Contraceptive Research." *The Ecologist* 26.2 (1996): 53–60.

Riddle, John M. *Eve's Herbs: A History of Contraception and Abortion in the West*. Cambridge, MA: Harvard University Press, 1997.

"The Rights of Man: Contraception." *The Economist,* 16 August 1997, 63.

Roan, Shari. "A Shot in the Arm for Birth Control—Maybe." *Los Angeles Times,* 24 May 1999, home edition.

Robbins, Anthony. "Brundtland's World Health Organization: A Test Case for United Nations Reform." *Public Health Reports* 114 (1999): 30–39.

Roberts, Dorothy. *Killing the Black Body: Race, Reproduction, and the Meaning of Liberty*. New York: Pantheon, 1997.

Robertson, William H. *An Illustrated History of Contraception: A Concise Account of the Quest for Fertility Control*. Park Ridge, NJ: Parthenon, 1990.

Rock, John. *The Time Has Come: A Doctor's Proposal to End the Battle for Birth Control*. New York: Knopf, 1963.

Rose, June. *Marie Stopes and the Sexual Revolution*. London: Faber and Faber, 1992.

Rose, Lionel. *The Massacre of the Innocents: Infanticide in Britain 1800–1939*. London: Routledge and Kegan Paul, 1986.

Rosen, James E., and Shanti R. Conly. *Africa's Population Challenge: Accelerating Progress in Reproductive Health*. Country Study Series 4. Washington, DC: Population Action International, 1998.

Rosenberg, Michael, and Michael S. Waugh. "Causes and Consequences of Oral Contraceptive Noncompliance." *American Journal of Obstetrics and Gynecology* 180.2, Part 2 (1999): S276–S279.

Rosenthal, M. Sara. *The Gynecological Sourcebook*. 3rd ed. Los Angeles: Lowell House, 1999.

Rostow, W.W. *The Great Population Spike and After: Reflections on the 21st Century*. New York: Oxford University Press, 1998.

Rothman, Barbara Katz, ed. *Encyclopedia of Childbearing: Critical Perspectives.* Phoenix, AZ: Oryx Press, 1993.

Rowan, Jean P. "'Estrophasic' Dosing: A New Concept in Oral Contraceptive Therapy." *American Journal of Obstetrics and Gynecology* 180, Part 2 (1999): S302–S306.

Russell, Keith. "Does the U.S. Back Sterilization? Alleged Involvement in Involuntary Sterilization Program in Peru." *Insight on the News,* 23 March 1998, 18–19.

Sadovsky, Robert. "Oral Contraceptive Use and Risk of Cardiovascular Disease." *American Family Physician*, 58 (1998): 561–562.

Sanger, Margaret Higgins. *Margaret Sanger: An Autobiography*. 1938. Elmsford, NY: Maxwell Reprints, 1970.

Santow, Gigi. "Coitus Interruptus in the Twentieth Century." *Population and Development Review* 19 (1993): 767–792.

Santow, Gigi, and Michael Bracher. "Explaining Trends in Teenage Childbearing in Sweden." *Studies in Family Planning* 33 (1999): 169–182.

Sapolsky, Robert. "Growing Up in a Hurry." *Discover* 13 (1992): 40–45.

Schuler, Sidney Ruth, and Zakir Hossain. "Family Planning Clinics through Women's Eyes and Voices: A Case Study from Rural Bangladesh." *International Family Planning Perspectives* 24 (1998): 170–175.

Schwarts, Benjamin, et al. "Nonmenstrual Toxic Shock Syndrome Associated with Barrier Contraceptives: Report of a Case-Control Study." *Reviews of Infectious Diseases* 11, Supplement 1 (1989): S43–S49.

Sears, James T. *Sexuality and the Curriculum: The Politics and Practices of Sexuality Education*. New York: Teachers College Press, 1992.

Seeley, Rod R., Trent D. Stephens, and Philip Tate. *Anatomy and Physiology*. 5th ed. Boston: McGraw Hill, 2000.

Segal, Marian. *Cervical Cap: Newest Birth Control Choice.* Rockville, MD: Department of Health and Human Services, 1988.

———. *Norplant: Birth Control at Arm's Reach.* Rockville, MD: Department of Health and Human Services, 1991.

Sen, Gita, and Rachel C. Snow, eds. *Power and Decision: The Social Control of Reproduction.* Boston: Harvard University Press, 1994.

Shane, Barbara. *Family Planning Saves Lives*. 3rd ed. Washington, DC: Population Reference Bureau, 1996.

Singh, Susheela, Deirdre Wulf, and Heidi Jones. "Health Professionals' Perceptions about Induced Abortion in South Central and Southeast Asia." *International Family Planning Perspectives* 23 (1997): 50–67.

Skegg, David C. G., et al. "Depot Medroxyprogesterone Acetate and Breast Cancer: A Pooled Analysis of the World Health Organization and New Zealand Studies." *Journal of the American Medical Association* 273 (1995): 799–804.

Smith, Andrea. "Malthusian Orthodoxy and the Myth of Zero Population Growth." In *Defending Mother Earth: Native American Perspectives on Environmental Justice,* edited by Jace Weaver. Maryknoll, NY: Orbis Books, 1996: 122–143.

Smith, Bardwell. "Buddhism and Abortion in Contemporary Japan: Mizuko Kuyo and the Confrontation with Death." In *Buddhism, Sexuality, and Gender,* edited by Jose Ignacio Cabezon. Albany, NY: State University of New York Press, 1992.

Speroff, Leon, and Philip Darney. *A Clinical Guide for Contraception.* Baltimore: Williams and Wilkins, 1992.

Speroff, Leon, and Patricia J. Sulak. "Contraception in the Late Reproductive Years: A Valid Aspect of Preventive Health Care." *Dialogues in Contraception* 4 (1995): 1–4.

Speroff, Leon, and Carolyn L. Westhoff. "Breast Disease and Hormonal Contraception: Resolution of a Lasting Controversy." *Dialogues in Contraception* 5.3 (1997): 1–4.

Spitzer, Walter O., and Carlyle L. Saylor. *Birth Control and the Christian: A Protestant Symposium on the Control of Human Reproduction*. Wheaton, IL: Tyndale House, 1969.

Stanback, John, Andy Thompson, Karen Hardee, and Barbara Janowitz. "Menstruation Requirements: A Significant Barrier to Contraceptive Access in Developing Countries." *Studies in Family Planning* 28 (1997): 245–250.

Stanford, Joseph B., Janis C. Lemaire, and Poppy B. Thurman. "Women's Interest in Natural Family Planning." *Journal of Family Practice* 46 (1998): 652–671.

Starrs, Ann. *Preventing the Tragedy of Maternal Deaths: A Report on the International Safe Motherhood Conference, Nairobi, Kenya, February 1987*. New York: World Bank, World Health Organization, United Nations Fund for Population Activities, 1987.

Stehlin, Dori. *Depo-Provera: The Quarterly Contraceptive*. Rockville, MD: U.S. Department of Health and Human Services, 1993.

Steinbock, Bonnie. *Life Before Birth: The Moral and Legal Status of Embryos and Fetuses*. New York: Oxford University Press, 1992.

Steinem, Gloria. "Margaret Sanger: Her Crusade to Legalize Birth Control Spurred the Movement for Women's Liberation." Time 100: Leaders and Revolutionaries of the 20th Century. *Time,* 13 April 1988, 93–94.

Stephenson, Joan. "Report Offers Vision for Microbicide Development." *Journal of the American Medical Association* 281 (1999): 405.

Sternberg, Steve. "Reproductive Equality: A Male Pill?" *Science News,* 22 June 1996, 388.

Strossen, Nadine. "The Right to be Let Alone: Constitutional Privacy in *Griswold, Roe,* and *Bowers*." In *Benchmarks: Great Constitutional Controversies in the Supreme Court,* edited by Terry Eastland. Grand Rapids, MI: William B. Eerdmans, 1995.

Stryker, Jeff. "Abstinence or Else! The Just-Say-No Approach in Sex Ed Lacks One Detail: Evidence that it Works." *The Nation,* 16 June 1997, 19–21.

Studies in Family Planning 29.2 (1998). Entire issue focuses on adolescents.

Suris, Joan-Carles, Michael D. Resnick, Nadav Cassuto, and Robert W. Blum." Sexual Behavior of Adolescents with Chronic Disease and Disability." *Journal of Adolescent Health* 19 (1996): 124–131.

Taylor, Robert Joseph, James S. Jackson, and Linda M. Chatters, eds. *Family Life in Black America*. Thousand Oaks, CA: Sage, 1997.

Thorneycroft, Ian H. "Update on Androgenicity." *American Journal of Obstetrics and Gynecology* 180, part 2 (1999): S288–S294.

Tell, David. "'Responsible Adults' and Abortion." *The Human Life Review* 24.4 (1998): 99–101.

Thibodeau, Gary A., and Kevin T. Patton. *Anatomy and Physiology*. 4th ed. St. Louis, MO: Mosby, 1999.

Toulemon, Laurent, and Henri Leridon. "Contraceptive Practices and Trends in France." *Family Planning Perspectives* 30 (1998): 114–120.

Trad, Paul V. "Assessing the Patterns that Prevent Teenage Pregnancy." *Adolescence* 34 (1999): 221–240.

"Trends in Oral Contraceptive Development and Utilization: Looking to the Future." *The Contraception Report* 7.5 (1997): 4–14.

Trost, Jan E. "The Family Planning Rights of Minors in Sweden." In *The Adolescent Dilemma: International Perspectives on the Family Planning Rights of Minors,* edited by Hyman Rodman and Jan Trost. New York: Praeger, 1986.

Trussell, James, Jacqueline Koenig, Felicia Stewart, and Jacqueline E. Darroch. "Medical Care Cost Savings from Adolescent Contraceptive Use." *Family Planning Perspectives* 29 (1997): 248–255.

Trussell, James, and Barbara Vaughan. "Contraceptive Failure, Method-Related Discontinuation and Resumption of Use: Results from the 1995 National Survey of Family Growth." *Family Planning Perspectives* 31 (1999): 64–72.

Trussell, James, et al. "The Economic Value of Contraception: A Comparison of Fifteen Methods." *American Journal of Public Health* 68 (1995): 494–503.

Unger, Jennifer B., and Gregory B. Molina. "Desired Family Size and Son Preference among Hispanic Women of Low Socioeconomic Status." *Family Planning Perspectives* 29 (1997): 284–287.

United Nations Population Fund (UNFPA). *The State of World Population 1999: 6 Billion: A Time for Choices*. New York: United Nations Population Fund Information and External Relations Division, 1999. Online: http://www.unfpa.org/swp/1999, 7 March 2000.

United States Senate. "The 25th Anniversary of *Roe v. Wade*: Has It Stood the Test of Time?" Hearing Before the Subcommittee on the Constitution, Federalism, and Property Rights of the Committee on the Judiciary, 21 January 1998. Washington, DC: Government Printing Office, 1998.

"USAID Office of Women in Development." *Women's International Network News* 24 (1998): 19–20.

Van Look, Paul F. A. "Lactational Amenorrhea Method for Family Planning Provides High Protection from Pregnancy for the First Six Months after Delivery." *British Medical Journal* 313 (1996): 893–894.

Van Look, Paul F. A., and Felicia Stewart. "Emergency Contraception." In *Contraceptive Technology,* 17th rev ed., edited by Robert Hatcher, James Trussel, Felicia Stewart, and others. New York: Ardent Media, 1998

Van Phai, Nguyen, John Knodel, Mai Van Cam, and Hoang Xuyen. "Fertility and Family Planning in Vietnam: Evidence from the 1994 Inter-censal Demographic Survey." *Studies in Family Planning* 27 (1996): 1–17.

Vergano, D. "The Trouble with Condoms." *Science News,* 14 September 1996, 165.

Visaria, Leela, and Pravin Visaria. "India's Population in Transition." *Population Bulletin* 50.3 (1995): 2.

Walle, Etienne van de, and Helmut V. Muhsam. "Fatal Secrets and the French Fertility Transition." *Population and Development Review* 21 (1995): 261–280.

Wawrose, Susan C. Griswold v. Connecticut: *Contraception and the Right of Privacy*. New York: Franklin Watts/Grolier, 1996.

Weisberger, Bernard A. "Chasing Smut in Every Medium." *American Heritage* 48.8 (1997): 12–13.

Weiss, Gerson. "Risk of Venous Thromboembolism with Third-Generation Oral Contraceptives: A Review." *American Journal of Obstetrics and Gynecology* 180, part 2 (1999): S295–S301.

Wells, Elisa S. "Using Pharmacies in Washington State to Expand Access to Emergency Contraception." *Family Planning Perspectives* 30 (1998): 281–282.

Welton, K. B. *Abortion Is Not a Sin: A New-Age Look at an Age-Old Problem.* Costa Mesa, CA: Pandit Press, 1987.

Weschler, Toni. *Taking Charge of Your Fertility: The Definitive Guide to Natural Birth Control and Pregnancy Achievement.* New York: HarperCollins, 1995.

"When Your Child is Close to Puberty." *American Family Physician* 60 (1999).

Winikoff, Beverly. "Acceptability and Feasibility of Early Pregnancy Termination by Mifepristone-Misaprostol: Results of a Large Multicenter Trial in the United States." *Journal of the American Medical Association* 280 (1998): 1034. (Abstract).

Winikoff, Beverly, and Suzanne Wymelenberg. *The Whole Truth about Contraception*. Washington, DC: Joseph Henry Press, 1997.

Winstein, Merryl. *Your Fertility Signals: Using Them to Achieve or Avoid Pregnancy Naturally.* St. Louis, MO: Smooth Stone Press, 1994.

Wise, Daniel. "ACLU Battles with Ex-Unit over Breakup." *The National Law Journal,* 29 June 1992, 12.

Wissow, Lawrence S. "Infanticide." *The New England Journal of Medicine* 339 (1998): 1239–1241.

World Health Organization. *The World Health Report 1998: Life in the 21st Century: A Vision for All.* Geneva: World Health Organization, 1998.

World Health Organization Task Force on Methods for the Regulation of Male Fertility. "Contraceptive Efficacy of Testosterone-Induced Azoospermia and Oligozoospermia in Normal Men." *Fertility and Sterility* 65 (1996): 821–829.

Wulfe, Deirdre. "Family Planning Improves Child Survival and Health." *Issues in Brief*. New York: Alan Guttmacher Institute. Online: http://www.agi-usa.org/pubs/ib20.html, 10 October 1999.

———. *Sharing Responsibility: Women, Society, and Abortion Worldwide*. New York: Alan Guttmacher Institute, 1999.

Xiao, B. L., and B. G. Zhao. "Current Practice of Family Planning in China." *International Journal of Gynecology and Obstetrics* 58 (1997): 59–67.

Yuzpe, A. A., H. J. Thurlow, I. Ramzy, and J. L. Leyshon. "Postcoital Contraception—A Pilot Study." *Journal of Reproductive Medicine* 13 (1974): 53–58.

Zabin, Laurie Schwab, and Sarah C. Hayward. *Adolescent Sexual Behavior and Childbearing*. Developmental Clinical Psychology and Psychiatry 26. Newbury Park, CA: Sage, 1993.

Zhang, Jun, A. George Thomas, and Etel Leybovich. "Vaginal Douching and Adverse Health Effects: A Meta-Analysis." *American Journal of Public Health* 87 (1997): 1207–1211.

INDEX

By Debbie Lindblom

Note: Page numbers appearing in bold type refer to encyclopedia entries. Page numbers appearing in italic type refer to charts.

Marian Rengel is currently a researcher and journalist in St. Cloud, Minnesota. In the past, she has been a university instructor and a news editor. She has earned degrees in both mass communications and English.